Mind Maps in
Medical Pharmacology

A Study Resource and Review for PA, NP, and Medical Students and Clinicians

Mind Maps in Medical Pharmacology

A Study Resource and Review for PA, NP, and Medical Students and Clinicians

Jennifer Hofmann, DMSc, MS, PA-C

Clinical Professor
Director of Didactic Education
Pace University–Lenox Hill Hospital Physician
Assistant Program New York City
College of Health Professions
New York, New York
United States

CONTRIBUTOR (ANIMATIONS)

Jacob Richard Ribowsky

New York Institute of Technology
New York, New York
United States

ELSEVIER

Elsevier
1600 John F. Kennedy Blvd.
Ste 1800
Philadelphia, PA 19103-2899

MIND MAPS IN MEDICAL PHARMACOLOGY ISBN: 978-0-323-93463-3

Notice

Practitioners and researchers must always rely on their own experience and knowledge in evaluating and using any information, methods, compounds or experiments described herein. Because of rapid advances in the medical sciences, in particular, independent verification of diagnoses and drug dosages should be made. To the fullest extent of the law, no responsibility is assumed by Elsevier, authors, editors or contributors for any injury and/or damage to persons or property as a matter of products liability, negligence or otherwise, or from any use or operation of any methods, products, instructions, or ideas contained in the material herein.

International Standard Book Number: 9780323934633

Content Strategist: James T. Merritt
Content Development Manager: Ranjana Sharma
Publishing Services Manager: Shereen Jameel
Project Manager: Shereen Jameel
Design Direction: Margaret M. Reid

Printed in India

Last digit is the print number: 9 8 7 6 5 4 3 2 1

To my beautiful and brilliant sons Jake and Matthew, who inspire and teach me every day; I am eternally grateful.
In memory of my beloved sister Tara, whose life gave meaning, laughter, and joy to all fortunate enough to know her.
And to Scott, from whom love and good things come.

Preface

Mind Maps in Medical Pharmacology aims to make waves in a vast sea of medical pharmacology study guides and review books. Pharmacology is an area in which many PA, NP, and medical students often struggle due to information overload. Mind maps are multi sensory tools that can help students organize, integrate, and retain information. They help students visualize and condense extensive volumes of information and form relationships to see the "big picture." The mind maps in each chapter provide an overview of volumes of information in a visually appealing, concise "cliff notes." version of standard textbooks and slide presentations. The mind maps in each chapter highlight the following major points: central node (drug class) and sibling nodes with drug names, indications, mechanism of action, major adverse effects, warnings, and contraindications. The maps in each chapter are accompanied by explanatory, concise, practical, and up-to-date text.

The birth of mind maps occurred several years ago with basic sketches on a white board. I drew basic maps for more complex lectures, e.g., autonomic nervous system pharmacology before lectures. Students congregated at the front of the classroom enthusiastically copying or taking pictures of the rudimentary map sketches. Students requested mind maps for all drugs classes. After significant research, trial, and error, I discovered a user-friendly mind mapping tool to create concise and visually appealing maps. Student feedback and performance on exams, coupled with my interest in mapping as a valuable teaching and learning tool, led me to create *Mind Maps in Medical Pharmacology*. I hope this volume will enhance your study skills, improve performance on examinations, and, most importantly, facilitate application of drug therapy to patient care.

Jennifer Hofmann

Contents

1 Introduction   1

2 Autonomic Nervous System Pharmacology   10

3 Drugs Affecting Cardiovascular Function   16

4 Pulmonary Pharmacology   44

5 Drugs Affecting Allergic Conditions, Inflammation, Immunity, and Hematopoiesis   51

6 Hormones and Endocrine Drugs   64

7 Gastrointestinal Pharmacology   80

8 Drugs Affecting Central Nervous System   93

9 Drug Therapy for Infectious Diseases   121

10 Antineoplastic Drugs   142

11 Drug Therapy for Select Eye Diseases   146

12 Dermatologic Pharmacology   150

13 Pregnancy: Pharmacology of Select Conditions During Pregnancy   159

14 Pediatric Pharmacology   162

15 Geriatric Pharmacology   165

Index   167

Video Contents

Animation 1.1: Principles of Pharmacology
Animation 2.1: Pharmacology of the Autonomic Nervous System
Animation 3.1: Antihypertensive Medications
Animation 3.2: Heart Failure Medications
Animation 3.3: Acute Coronary Syndrome Medications
Animation 3.4: Antiarrhythmic Medications
Animation 3.5: Dyslipidemia Medications
Animation 3.6: Antiplatelet Medications
Animation 3.7: Anticoagulant Medications
Animation 4.1: Asthma Medications
Animation 4.2: COPD Medications
Animation 5.1: Nonsteroid Anti-Inflammatory Drugs (NSAIDs)
Animation 5.2: Medications for Gout
Animation 5.3: Drug-Modifying Anti-rheumatic Drugs (DMARDs)
Animation 6.1: Thyroid Medications
Animation 6.2: Women's Health Medications
Animation 6.3: Men's Health and Urologic Medications
Animation 6.4: Medications for Diabetes Mellitus
Animation 7.1: Medications for Gastroesophageal Reflux Disease (GERD) and Peptic Ulcer Disease (PUD)

Animation 7.2: Medications for Constipation
Animation 7.3: Antiemetic Medications
Animation 8.1: Sedative/Hypnotic Medications
Animation 8.2: Local Anesthetic Drugs
Animation 8.3: General Anesthetic Drugs
Animation 8.4: Antiepileptic Drugs
Animation 8.5: Drugs to Treat Parkinson's Disease
Animation 8.6: Opioids/Opiates
Animation 8.7: Antidepressant Medications
Animation 8.8: Antipsychotic Medications
Animation 9.1: Antibacterial Medications Cell Wall Inhibitors
Animation 9.2: Antibacterials Part II
Animation 9.3: Antiviral Medications
Animation 9.4: Antiviral Medications for Hepatitis Viruses
Animation 9.5: Antiretroviral Medications (HIV Treatment)
Animation 9.6: Antifungal Medications
Animation 10.1: Antineoplastic Medications
Animation 11.1: Medications for Common Eye Diseases
Animation 12.1: Medications for Common Skin Conditions
Animation 12.2: Medications for skin infections and infestations

CHAPTER 1

Introduction

INTRODUCTION TO MEDICAL PHARMACOLOGY

The approach to learning and applying pharmacology to clinical practice can be complex. Mind maps and accompanying brief text explanations will provide essential tools to organize, memorize, and visualize facts and concepts to master medical pharmacology. The chapters and maps are generally organized by the therapeutic class of drugs, for example, dermatologic medications, cardiac medications, antibacterial drugs, etc. The mind maps summarize and visually describe the text in each chapter. Mind maps and text further organize information into the most important and practical aspects of pharmacology as follows:

- Name of class
- Mechanism of action (how the drug works)
- Names (generic) of medications in the class
- Indications (use of the drug for a particular disease) and drugs of choice when applicable
- Adverse effects and toxicity
- Boxed warnings: labeled warning about increased risk of serious adverse reactions or restrictions on use of the drug
- Contraindications—specific condition or situation where drug should not be used because it may be harmful
- Drug interactions (major)

There may be additional pharmacologic information about certain drugs if it is clinically relevant, for example, long half-lives, tolerance, allergies, and harmful use during pregnancy.

Let's get started!

Definitions

Pharmacology is the study of how drugs interact with body constituents to produce therapeutic effects. Essentially, it is the effect of drugs on living systems. Pharmacology is a complex science that requires knowledge of biochemistry, physiology, organic chemistry, and molecular biology.

Clinical pharmacology is the effects of drugs on humans, which is the primary focus of clinicians. A drug is any agent that affects living systems; anything that can be used to treat, diagnose, or prevent disease. Drugs can be described by:

1. chemical name N-acetyl-p-aminophenol
2. generic or trivial name, e.g., acetaminophen

3. abbreviation, e.g., APAP
4. brand name (created by manufacturer so you will not forget it) Tylenol.

Pharmacodynamics describes the biochemical and physiologic effects of drugs and mechanisms of action. Basically, pharmacodynamics is what a drug/drugs does/do to the human body.

Pharmacokinetics is defined as the time course of drug absorption, distribution, metabolism, and excretion and describes what the body does to the drug over time.

Pharmacotherapeutics is the clinical application of drugs for prevention and treatment of disease. Pharmacotherapeutics requires careful consideration of a drug's risk, e.g., safety and tolerability to benefit (e.g., efficacy) ratio. An adverse drug reaction (or adverse drug effect) is generally defined as a negative, unwanted, and sometime dangerous effect of a drug. Toxic effects or drug toxicity most commonly relates to the negative effects of a drug in higher doses.

Toxicology is the study of poisons including recognition, treatment, and prevention of poisoning.

Teratology is the study of birth defects and how exposures during pregnancy can affect the fetus morphologically. A **teratogen** is any factor that can affect intrauterine growth, development, function, anatomic formation, and postnatal development. Maternal drug exposure to teratogenic drugs, particularly during embryogenesis and organogenesis, can cause serious birth defects.

Pharmacogenomics and **pharmacogenetics** are the study of how genetic variations affect a person's response to drugs. Although the terms are often used interchangeably, pharmacogenetics is smaller scale, e.g., how a single gene influences the response to a single drug. Pharmacogenomics is a broader study of how variations in multiple genes across the genome can influence responses to drugs. Genetic variation (polymorphisms) can affect pharmacokinetic and pharmacodynamic elements of drugs, which affect drug efficacy, tolerability, and safety. Examples of pharmacogenomic effects on drug pharmacokinetics include genetic differences in drug metabolizing enzymes and drug transporters.

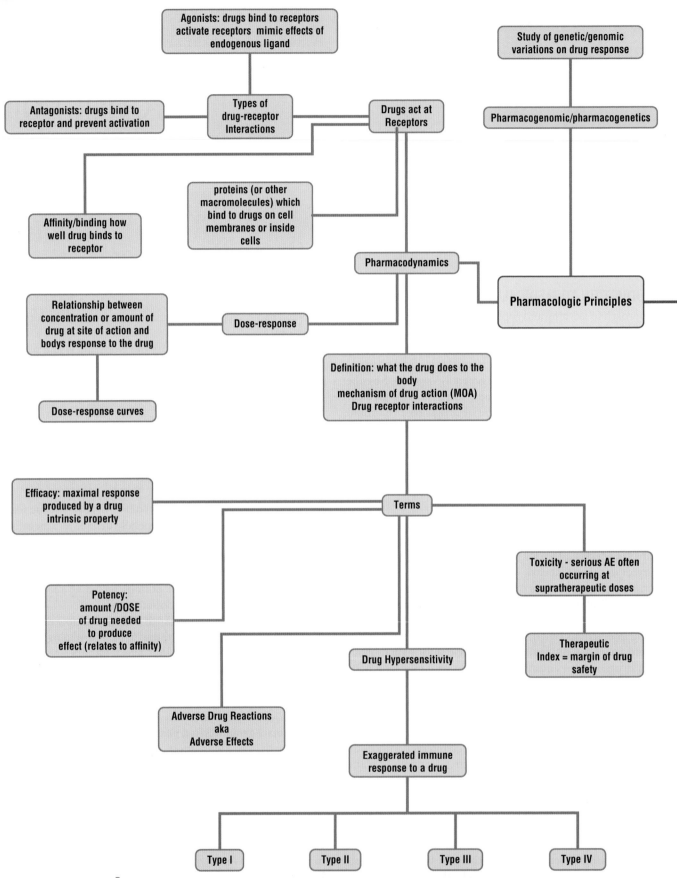

MIND MAP 1.1 Illustrates and relates basic principles of clinical pharmacology.

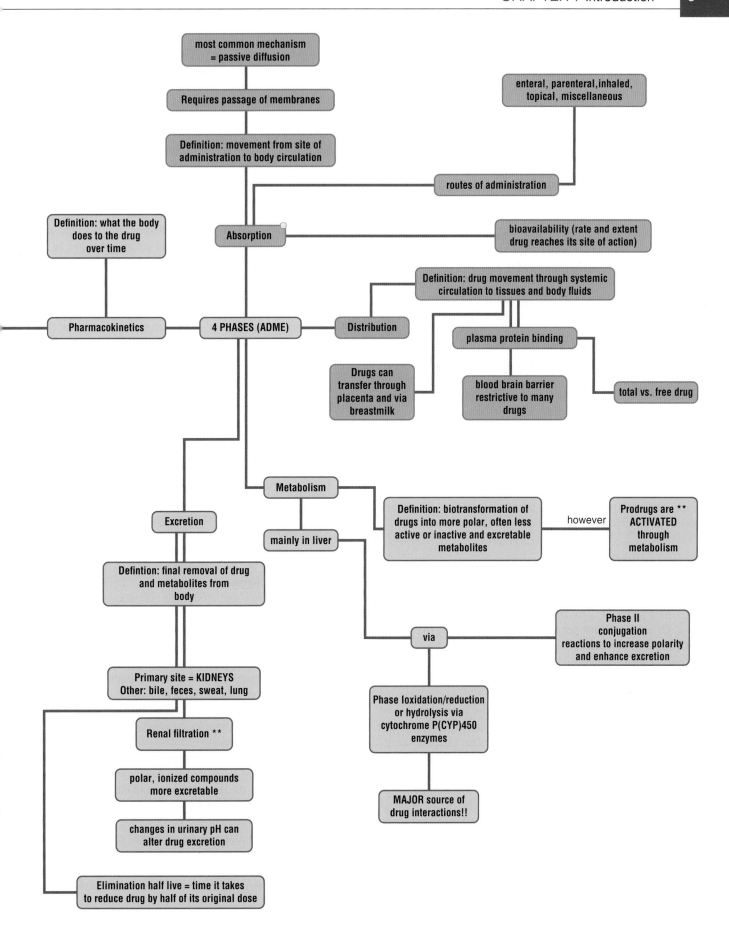

US FOOD AND DRUG ADMINISTRATION DRUG DEVELOPMENT

The drug development process includes preclinical and clinical phases. In the preclinical phase, a candidate drug compound is developed and tested on multiple animal species to assess toxicity, safety, and basic efficacy. The sponsoring company submits an Investigational New Drug (IND) application to the US Food and Drug Administration (FDA) detailing the compound and its results in animal studies and the plan for human trials. When the IND application is approved, the drug can enter the clinical phase of testing. There are three clinical phases of drug development: Phase I trials assess the safety and pharmacokinetic properties of the drug on a small number of healthy volunteers. Phase II trials assess efficacy of the drug in a larger number of patients with a certain disease, often compared to a placebo group. Phase II also evaluates dosing, drug safety, and adverse effects of the drug. Phase III evaluates the drug's effect in larger and more heterogenous population of patients. Phase III clinical trials often involve thousands of patients from multiple sites and compare the drug to placebo and other drugs used for the same condition. It further clarifies dose-response, efficacy, and additional safety information. A new drug application is submitted to the FDA by the drug sponsor to review all preclinical and clinical trial data, drug labeling, and related patient and health provider information. The FDA review team inspects the drug manufacturing facilities and approves the drug or responds to the drug sponsor's application. Phase IV is postmarketing surveillance, which occurs after the drug is marketed. Phase IV trials may be larger, longer, and affect special populations and reflect real-world use of drugs. Long-term and/or unexpected adverse drug effects may be reported in phase IV trials.[1]

PHARMACODYNAMICS

Pharmacodynamics is the study of how drugs produce their effects on the body. For drugs to produce pharmacologic effects, they must arrive at their site of action in effective concentrations. Drugs usually produce their effects by binding to biologic macromolecules called *receptors.* Receptors may be a membrane or a membrane protein, or a cytoplasmic or extracellular enzyme. The drug-binding sites on receptors have a three-dimensional structure or configuration.

The drug must bind with the receptor, and the receptor must be able to recognize the drug (specificity). There are five major types of drug-receptor interactions: G-protein coupled receptors with second messengers, ligand gated ion channels, which alter intracellular ion concentrations; membrane-bound enzymes receptors with a cytoplasmic enzyme domain, e.g., tyrosine kinase; membrane-bound receptors linked to an intracellular protein kinase; and intracellular receptors for lipid-soluble drugs and endogenous compounds, which affect gene transcription. This drug-receptor complex will produce a response, e.g., stimulate the release of a neurotransmitter or hormone, change electrical potentials to initiate a cascade-type response, change the permeability of a membrane, etc.

There are important types of drug receptors interactions and classifications of drug actions at receptors. An **agonist** is a drug or endogenous ligand that binds to and activates receptors to signal and produce a response. A **partial agonist** has high **affinity** or strong attraction for receptors but fails to produce maximal effects. **Affinity** is how avidly a drug binds to its receptor. **Inverse agonists** bind to the same receptor as an agonist but produce the opposite effect of the agonist by decreasing the activity of a receptor. An **antagonist** binds but does not activate receptor and blocks or diminishes the response of the endogenous agent. **Competitive antagonists** compete for same receptor site for the endogenous agonist, and when the antagonist is present, it occupies and blocks the agonist from binding and exerting its effects. **Non competitive antagonists** bind at different sites than the agonist but on the same receptor. This causes changes in the conformation of the receptor so the agonist cannot bind to its site on the receptor.

There is a relationship between the dose or plasma concentration of a drug and the magnitude of its effects. This relationship between drug dose or plasma concentration and effect or response can be demonstrated by a **dose response curve** (Fig. 1.1).[2] For example, let us assume there are 100 receptors at a site. Fifty receptors must be occupied for there to be an observable pharmacologic response. Assume that one molecule of drug interacts with one receptor molecule.

1. If only 25 drug molecules are present to combine with receptors, there is no observable response but there is some cellular activity.
2. As more drug molecules are introduced, there eventually will be an observable but subtherapeutic response (50–60).
3. As still more drug is added, we will see a pharmacologic response (61–75) (therapeutic range).
4. Ceiling effect: increasing the amount of the drug will not change response because there are a finite number of receptors, which can become saturated; however, toxic effects can occur at **supratherapeutic** doses.

The terms *potency* and *efficacy* are often used interchangeably although they have different meanings. **Potency** is the amount (dosage or concentration) of a drug required to produce a pharmacologic effect. Potency relates to the **affinity** of a drug for its receptor; the greater the affinity for receptors, the less of the drug is needed to produce a response. For example, drug A is more potent than drug B if the dose of drug A is less than the dose of drug B to achieve the same response. Efficacy is the magnitude of the maximum effect a drug can produce, which is an intrinsic property of a drug. Drug A is more efficacious than drug B if drug A can reduce heart rate by 10 beats per minute and drug B can reduce heart rate by 5 beats per minute regardless of the dose. Potency and efficacy are ways to compare drug doses and effects.

The **therapeutic index** of a drug (T.I.) is a margin of safety, which relates the amount of drug needed to produce therapeutic effects to the amount of the drug, which produces toxic effects. In animals, T.I. is median lethal dose (LD50)/median effective dose (ED50). In humans, T.I. is the ratio of the median toxic dose (TD50) to the ED50. Drugs with a low T.I. are not as safe to use and require closer monitoring and more precise dosing. Blood, serum, or plasma levels of the drug are used to

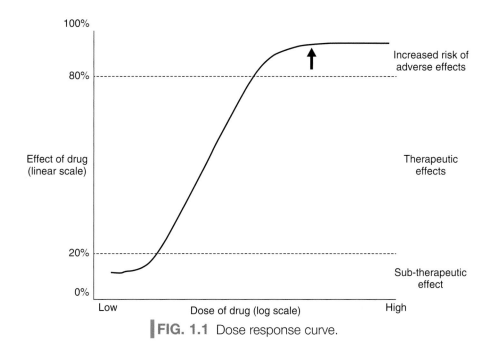

FIG. 1.1 Dose response curve.

monitor drug efficacy and toxicity. In most cases, there is a ratio between blood drug levels and tissue drug levels.

Other important terms in pharmacodynamics include:

Tolerance, which is defined as a reduced response to the same dose, or an increased dose needed for same response. Tolerance can occur due to:

1. change in receptor sensitivity to the drug.
2. change in pharmacokinetics of drug (e.g., increased metabolism or excretion).

Drug classes, which are associated with tolerance are opioids, and beta-2 agonists.

Tachyphylaxis is a type of tolerance that develops quickly and suddenly, often after one or two doses. Phenylephrine intranasal decongestants and nitroglycerin can be associated with tachyphylaxis.[3]

Dependence occurs when the person needs a drug to prevent withdrawal symptoms and signs. **Withdrawal** occurs when the drug is abruptly discontinued, and it can manifest with abnormal physical and/or psychologic effects.

A **placebo** (Latin, "I shall please") is an inactive look-alike substance response designed to have no known therapeutic effect. The placebo response is the observed response to a placebo. For example, if a patient is given inert material and told it is a potent analgesic, as many as 35% of the population will respond. In controlled clinical trials, the effects of an active drug are compared to a placebo. The placebo effect is the difference between the response to the placebo compared to no treatment.[4]

Hypersensitivity is adverse and exaggerated immune reactions that results from a previous exposure to a particular chemical or one that is structurally similar. It is divided into four categories:

The four types of hypersensitivity reactions are:

- **Type I** reactions are mediated by immunoglobulin (Ig)E antibodies. Type I reactions tend to occur quickly after challenge with sensitized allergen and are called an *immediate hypersensitivity reaction.*

  Symptoms include: urticaria, rash, vasodilation, hypotension, edema, inflammation, rhinitis, asthma, tachycardia, etc. They are the result of the release of histamine, prostaglandins, and leukotrienes (e.g., anaphylaxis to penicillin).
- **Type II** reactions are cytotoxic reactions mediated by IgG or IgM antibodies, which bind to cells and activate complement causing cell lysis. They include hemolytic anemia, thrombocytopenia, granulocytopenia, and systemic lupus erythematosus. These autoimmune reactions to drugs usually subside within several months after drug discontinuation (e.g., penicillin and hemolytic anemia).
- **Type III** reactions mediated by immune complexes. IgG immune complexes are deposited in the vascular endothelium, where a destructive inflammatory response called *serum sickness* occurs. Symptoms include erythema multiforme, arthritis, nephritis, central nervous system (CNS) abnormalities, and myocarditis (e.g., sulfonamide antibiotics).
- **Type IV** delayed reactions are mediated by T-lymphocytes and macrophages. When sensitized cells encounter the antigen, lymphokines from T-cells cause an inflammatory reaction (e.g., poison ivy).

Idiosyncrasy is defined as an unusual and unpredictable response to a drug, usually caused by genetic differences in metabolism or immunologic mechanisms.

There is significant interpatient variability with drug dose and response. A **hyperreactive** response occurs when the intensity of the effects of a given dose of a drug is greater than anticipated. A **hyporeactive** response occurs when the intensity of a given dose of a drug is less than anticipated.

PHARMACOKINETICS

There are four phases of pharmacokinetics: Absorption, Distribution, Metabolism, and Excretion.

A drug must be present in appropriate concentrations at its site of action. Drugs must cross biologic membranes to access their sites of action. The body is a series of compartments separated by membranes.

1. What's a membrane? It is a lipid bilayer made up of phospholipids and cholesterol.

   The hydrophobic ends are in the middle and the hydrophilic ends are on the outside. Chemicals that are lipophilic (fat soluble) are attracted to the membrane but not released. Large hydrophilic (water-soluble) chemicals are repelled by the lipid segment of the membrane. Most drugs have some degree of lipid and water solubility, so that they can be dissolved in an aqueous environment and be transported across the membrane. Drugs with a low molecular weight and higher lipid solubility (lipophilic) cross the membrane better than those with low lipid solubility.

   Most drugs are weakly acidic or weakly basic, so that in some pH ranges they will be charged and in others uncharged. Weak acids are hydrogen ion donors, and when they donate hydrogen ions, they become charged. Weak bases are hydrogen ion acceptors, and when they accept hydrogen ions, they become charged. In general, weak acids are more ionized (charged) in a basic environment and weak bases are more ionized (charged) in an acidic environment.

   The uncharged, unionized form of a drug is lipid soluble and therefore crosses membranes more effectively.

2. How do drugs cross membranes?

   The most common way drugs cross membranes are via passive diffusion where drugs move from high concentration to low concentration. For nonelectrolytes it is proportional to lipid solubility (partition coefficient), and for electrolytes it is related to pH. Small (<200) water-soluble molecules move with water. Since most drugs are weak acids or weak bases, they exist as both ionized and nonionized forms simultaneously.

Other forms of drug transport include facilitated diffusion, active transport, and pinocytosis. **Facilitated diffusion** is passive movement of molecules or ions across a specific via transmembrane integral proteins down their concentration gradient. **Active transport** is the transport of molecules against their concentration gradient, which requires energy (adenosine triphosphate [ATP] or electrochemical energy created by pumping ions in/out across cell membrane). **Pinocytosis** is the formation and movement of vesicles (packages) across membranes and requires energy.

Membrane drug transporter proteins transport drugs into and out of cells mainly in the liver, intestine, kidney, and blood brain barrier. There are two main superfamilies of membrane drug transporter proteins: (1) **ATP-binding cassettes** (ABC, efflux) use energy to move compounds from inside cells to outside of cells; (2) **solute carriers (SLC)** are influx transporters that move compounds from outside cells into cells. These transporter proteins are involved in movement of drugs, and competition between drugs for a drug transporter can cause drug interactions.

There are four phases of pharmacokinetics: absorption of drugs from their site of administration, distribution of drugs to body compartments and site of drug action, metabolism of drugs primarily by the liver, and excretion of drugs mainly by the kidneys.

Absorption is defined as the rate at which a drug leaves its site of administration and the extent to which it occurs.

Bioavailability is the fractional extent of the drug dosage that finally reaches the therapeutic site of action or a biological fluid that has access to that site. For example, if 1000 mg of acetaminophen is administered orally and 900 mg gets to its site of action, the oral bioavailability of acetaminophen is 90%. This may be due to the way an oral dosage form is formulated (i.e., very hard tablets do not dissolve well). Drugs that are well absorbed from the gastrointestinal tract (GI) and are extensively metabolized in the liver may have decreased bioavailability because of the first-pass effect.

First-Pass Effect is defined as the process in which a drug is metabolized at a specific location in the body, usually the liver, which reduces its concentration before it reaches systemic circulation and its site (s) of action.[5]

Important factors that also modify absorption include:
1. drug solubility (solutions>suspensions>capsules>tablets).
2. drug concentration.
3. circulation at site of absorption.
4. absorbing surface area.

ROUTES OF ADMINISTRATION
Enteral

Oral (per os or po). In general, enteral routes are convenient, less expensive, and safer than parenteral routes of drug administration. Oral absorption of drugs occurs primarily in the first third of the small intestine. Some drugs cannot be administered orally because they are too irritating. Some drugs are destroyed by stomach acids or digestive enzymes, and some are significantly altered by food or other drugs such as antacids or vitamins. The first-pass effect can limit the oral bioavailability of medications.

Sublingual (SL)

Sublingual medications are administered at the mucous membranes under the tongue and enter blood vessels without entering the GI tract. Sublingual drugs must be highly lipid soluble drugs that are very potent (i.e., nitroglycerin).

Rectal (PR)

The rectal route of administration may be useful when the oral route is not possible, for example, when the patient is unconscious, neurologically compromised, or has nausea or vomiting. Most drugs are irritating to the rectal mucosa and their absorption is unpredictable and variable. Drugs administered in the lower region of the rectum do not undergo first pass.

Parenteral

The **parenteral** route of administration occurs outside of the intestine and is often used to describe medications given by injection.

- Intravenous (IV) — no absorption phase, accurate, immediate, irreversible, must be aqueous, possible to titrate dose.

- Intramuscular (IM) — onset is slower and duration is longer than IV, absorption is delayed and is related to vascularity. Highly irritating drugs will cause tissue necrosis.
- Subcutaneous (SQ, SC) onset is slower, and duration is longer than IM because fat is less vascular than muscle.

Miscellaneous Routes of Administration

- Topical — drug is applied to the site for a local effect, e.g., creams, ointments, eye drops, ear drops, nasal sprays.
- Transdermal — unique delivery of certain molecules applied to cross the skin and enter circulation for a systemic effect (e.g., nicotine patches, estrogen, testosterone creams/solutions, clonidine patches, fentanyl patches).
- Aerosol — drug is inhaled causing very rapid onset due to extremely large surface area for absorption and good blood supply. Used mostly for a local effect on the lungs (e.g., metered dose inhalers, dry powder inhalers, nebulizers).

Drugs are distributed by movement of drug through body compartments. Each time a drug enters a new compartment, it must cross membranes. The drug then partitions between the old compartment, the membrane, and the new compartment until a dynamic equilibrium is met. The partition between the two compartments does not necessarily have to be 1:1. As a drug passes from one compartment to the next, it will also bind to other nonreceptor proteins in the plasma, fat, or muscle. Fat is also a reservoir for the drug, and highly lipophilic drugs may accumulate in fat. These nonreceptor protein-binding sites are sometimes referred to as *reservoirs*. The binding of drug to protein may significantly affect its bioavailability. DRUGS THAT ARE BOUND TO ANYTHING (other than a receptor) ARE INACTIVE. Drugs must be free or unbound to bind to receptors and produce effects. The most common nonreceptor plasma protein is albumin, which has multiple binding sites for multiple drugs. Competition for drug binding to plasma proteins is a source of drug interactions. For example, drug A and drug B can compete for binding to the same site on albumin, and drug A, which has greater affinity for the binding site, can displace drug B; this can increase the free amount of drug B. Hypoalbuminemia can affect drug distribution by increasing the amount of unbound or free drug.

There are two especially important barriers to drug distribution:
1. Blood-Brain Barrier (BBB) — The membranes separating the blood from the cerebrospinal fluid and brain are considerably more restrictive than any other membrane, and the brain is highly lipophilic. As a result, some drugs will concentrate in the brain (CNS depressants) and others may be completely excluded (many antibiotics).
2. Placental Barrier — the membranes separating the blood from the placenta are less restrictive than most other membranes. As a result, drugs pass quite easily to the developing fetus. Assume all drugs will cross.

The **volume of distribution (Vd)** is a calculated value, which describes the extent of drug distribution in body constituents, e.g., plasma, interstitial fluid, and intracellular fluid. The Vd compares the total amount of drug in the body to the plasma concentration of the drug at a given time (Volume of Distribution (L) = Amount of drug in the body (mg) / Plasma concentration of drug (mg/L)). Drugs with a large volume of distribution are widely distributed to extravascular compartments, while drugs with a low volume of distribution are less widely distributed and remain in the plasma. Some important clinical conditions that affect volume of distribution include fluid retention, e.g., kidney, heart, or liver failure or volume depletion.[6]

BIOTRANSFORMATION OR METABOLISM

In general, the body tries to convert any chemical or drug into metabolites, which are polar or charged and water soluble, so that they can be excreted often by the kidneys. Not all drugs are transformed, and some are excreted unchanged if they are sufficiently water soluble. Most drug metabolites are less active than the parent drug, but there are some active metabolites. Some drugs are administered in an inactive form called a *prodrug* and converted into the active drug by enzymes. Most, but not all, biotransformation reactions occur in the **liver.** Other organs of metabolism are the GI tract, lungs, kidneys, and brain. In general, lipophilic molecules are metabolized into more polar and less active molecules in the hepatocytes in two phases of enzymatic reactions.

Phase I reactions are oxidation-reduction reactions, which are carried out by the cytochrome P450 mixed function oxidases (abbreviated as P450 or CYP). There are numerous forms of CYP450 labeled as CYP1A2, CYP2A6, CYP2B6, CYP2C9, CYP2D6, CYP2E1, and CYP3A4; CYP3A4 is responsible for liver metabolism of most drugs. Phase I CYP450 metabolism is a **major source of drug-drug interactions**, as certain drugs inhibit CYP450 enzymes and others induce P450 enzymes.

Phase II metabolic reactions are conjugation reactions that add polar groups to parent drugs or drug metabolites from Phase I. Phase II conjugation reactions yield more water-soluble, less active, and easily excreted conjugate metabolites. Examples of phase II conjugation reactions include glucuronidation, acetylation, glycine conjugation, sulfation, and methylation. Drugs can also compete for phase II enzymes.

EXCRETION

Drugs are eliminated from the body either unchanged or as metabolites (the products of transformation reactions). The most important routes of drug excretion are: **(1) kidney, (2) feces**—either unabsorbed drug in the intestine or via **hepatobiliary excretion, and (3) breast milk**. The primary organ of excretion is the kidney, mainly by glomerular filtration, though drugs can be actively secreted. Once a drug has been transformed into a water-soluble metabolite, the control of excretion via the kidney is pH related. Water-soluble drugs are filtered into the glomerulus are not reabsorbed, and they remain in the filtrate for urinary excretion. A more alkaline urine will facilitate the excretion of ionized weak acids drugs, and acidic urine increases excretion of charged weak base drugs.

Other important terms in pharmacology include:
- **Clearance (CL)** is rate at which drug is eliminated from the body and is related to the rate of metabolism and excretion.

Clearance relates the rate of elimination (renal excretion, metabolic clearance, and all other drug clearance in body) to the drug concentration (C):

$$CL = \frac{Rate\ of\ elimination}{C}$$

- **Half-life: ($T_{1/2}$),** which is the time required for the concentration of drug to be reduced by 50% of its initial amount.
  - Plasma half-life: The time required for a drug's plasma concentration to reach half of its initial value.
- **Steady state:** with repeated dosing of a drug, a steady state is reached when the rate of drug administration is equal to the rate of drug elimination, e.g., amount of drug that goes in equals the amount that is eliminated. With repeated dosing at a regular interval, a drug accumulates and reaches a steady state at four to five half-lives.[7]
  - For example, if you administer 100 mg of a drug with a 6 hour half-life, 6 hours later you have 50 mg. You then administer the second 100 mg dose, and now the amount of drug is 150 mg. Six hours later (2 half-lives) you have 75 mg and administer the third 100 mg dose increasing the amount to 175 mg, and 6 hours later (3 half-lives) you have 87.5 mg and administer the fourth 100 mg dose, which increases amount to 187.5 mg, and 6 hours later (4 half-lives) you have 93.75 mg; after 5 half-lives, you have 96.875 mg.
- A drug with a long half-life can be administered as a larger **loading dose** to get blood plasma equivalent to steady-state condition. Loading doses are based on the desired drug concentration, drug volume of distribution, and drug bioavailability.
- **Maintenance doses** are given at regular intervals to ensure that the drug levels stay within the steady state.
  - For example, the antiplatelet drug clopidogrel is administered as a 600-mg loading dose on day 1, followed by 150 mg daily for 6 days and 75 mg daily maintenance doses thereafter.
- Drug elimination rate is also described as either **zero or first-order kinetics**. Drugs, that undergo zero-order kinetics undergo a constant elimination rate regardless of changes in drug concentration in the plasma.
  - For example, zero-order kinetics is like having a bank account that generates the same interest rate regardless of how much you add to the account.
- Most drugs undergo **first-order kinetics,** and as the plasma drug concentration increases, the rate of drug elimination increases until the system becomes saturated.
  - For example, with first-order kinetics, as you deposit more money into your account, the interest rate increases, so the more money you deposit, the higher the interest generated.[8]

Several patient-specific factors affect drug dose and effects. Age-related factors are described in Chapters 14 and 15. Pharmacogenomics/genetics relates genetic polymorphisms to variations in drug effects. Drug-disease interactions occur when drugs can have harmful effects because of an underlying disease such as chronic kidney disease, chronic liver disease, and peptic ulcer disease. Patients taking multiple medications have an increased risk of adverse drug reactions and drug-drug interactions. Drug interactions can occur by pharmacokinetic, commonly via competition for phase I cytochrome P450 enzyme metabolism and pharmacodynamic (drug-drug mode of action and adverse effects) mechanisms. Drugs that are commonly associated with drug interactions include warfarin with many drugs, nitrates, phosphodiesterase-5 inhibitors (e.g., sildenafil), statins, azole antifungals, multivalent cation antacids and tetracycline drugs, fluoroquinolone antibiotics, and thyroid drugs. An example of a pharmacodynamic drug interaction is combining CNS agents such as sedative/hypnotic drugs with alcohol. Medications that prolong the QT interval when administered concurrently can increase the risk for torsades de pointes, which is a life-threatening ventricular arrhythmia.[9,10]

Certain nutrients can interact with drugs, e.g., warfarin and vitamin K in green leafy vegetables, statin drugs and grapefruit, certain antibiotics and dairy, and alcohol with insulin or hypoglycemic medications.

SOME MECHANISMS OF DRUG INTERACTIONS

Additivity is a drug-drug interaction where the effect of two drugs combined equals the sum of their individual effects when given alone. Example: 2 + 2 = 4

Synergism is a drug-drug interaction where the total combined effect of the drugs is greater than the sum of each drug individually. Example: 2 + 2 = 10

Potentiation is a drug interaction when a drug in inactive on its own but increases the effect of another drug. For example: 0 + 3 = 5

Inhibition is a common drug-drug interaction often due to competition between drugs for Phase I CYP450 metabolism. Inhibition occurs when one drug inhibits or decreases the drug-metabolizing enzyme activity of another substrate drug. This often increases the activity of the substrate drug because its metabolism is reduced.

Common cytochrome P450 inhibitors include azole antifungal drugs, clarithromycin, erythromycin, grapefruit juice, and many selective serotonin reuptake inhibitors.

Induction is a drug-drug interaction that occurs when one drug increases or accelerates the drug-metabolizing enzyme activity of another drug, which is a substate for the enzyme. This often decreases the activity of the substate drug because its metabolism is accelerated.

Common cytochrome P450 enzyme inducers include rifampin, carbamazepine, phenobarbital, phenytoin, and St. John's wort.[11]

REFERENCES

1. US Food and Drug Administration. *The Drug Development Process.* Available at: https://www.fda.gov/patients/learn-about-drug-and-device-approvals/drug-development-process.
2. Currie GM. Pharmacology, part 2: introduction to pharmacokinetics. *Nucl Med Technol.* 2018;46:81-86.
3. Schöneberg T. Tolerance and desensitization. In: *Encyclopedia of Molecular Pharmacology.* 1203-1207. doi:10.1007/978-3-540-38918-7_140.

4. Chaplin S. The placebo response: an important part of treatment. *Prescriber*. 2006;17(5):16-22.

5. Herman TF, Santos C. First Pass Effect. [Updated 2021 Jul 28]. In: *StatPearls [Internet]*. Treasure Island, FL: StatPearls Publishing; 2022. Available at: https://www.ncbi.nlm.nih.gov/books/NBK551679/.

6. Oie S. Drug distribution and binding. *J Clin Pharmacol*. 1986;26(8):583-586.

7. Ito S. Pharmacokinetics 101. *Paediatr Child Health*. 2011;16(9):535-536. doi:10.1093/pch/16.9.535.

8. Borowy CS, Ashurst JV. Physiology, zero and first order kinetics. [Updated 2021 Sep 20]. In: *StatPearls [Internet]*. Treasure Island, FL: StatPearls Publishing; 2022. Available at: https://www.ncbi.nlm.nih.gov/books/NBK499866/.

9. Yap YG, Camm AJ. Drug induced QT prolongation and torsades de pointes. *Heart*. 2003;89(11):1363-1372.

10. Andersen L, Poulsen B, Poulsen M, Krogh M. Major drug interactions. In: *The ESC Handbook on Cardiovascular Pharmacotherapy*. Oxford, UK: Oxford University Press. Available at: https://oxfordmedicine.com/view/10.1093/med/9780198759935.001.0001/med-9780198759935-chapter-23.

11. Andersen L, Poulsen B, Poulsen M, Krogh M. Major drug interactions. In: *The ESC Handbook on Cardiovascular Pharmacotherapy*. Oxford, UK: Oxford University Press. Available at: https://oxfordmedicine.com/view/10.1093/med/9780198759935.001.0001/med-9780198759935-chapter-23. Retrieved April 13, 2022.

CHAPTER 2

Autonomic Nervous System Pharmacology

REVIEW OF AUTONOMIC PHYSIOLOGY

The autonomic nervous system (ANS) is divided into two sections; the parasympathetic and sympathetic arms. The effects of the ANS are mediated by neurotransmitters, e.g., acetylcholine, norepinephrine, and epinephrine binding to autonomic receptors on tissues and organs. Many of the drugs introduced in this section will be discussed in later sections as they relate to disease-specific therapy. The parasympathetic nervous system controls most functions of the body at rest, including digestion and elimination. The parasympathetic division is anatomically referred to craniosacral because preganglionic fibers leave the central nervous system (CNS) through the cranial nerves and sacral nerves. The primary neurotransmitter synthesized and released from parasympathetic autonomic cholinergic nerve fibers is acetylcholine, hence the terminology **cholinergic**. Acetylcholine binds to and activates nicotinic (N) receptors, which are primarily in autonomic ganglia of exiting postganglionic cholinergic fibers, and it binds and activates muscarinic (M) receptors on tissues and organs. Acetylcholine is metabolized into choline and acetate by the enzyme acetylcholinesterase in the synaptic cleft, which terminates its activity. Most clinically important medications affect M receptors. Medications can affect the parasympathetic nervous system functions by acting as direct or indirect parasympathomimetic agents. Medications that block the effects of acetylcholine are anticholinergic or antimuscarinic agents.

Some of the organ functions of the parasympathetic nervous system include:

- Eye: pupillary constriction or miosis, contraction of ciliary muscle for near accommodation.
- Pulmonary: contraction of bronchial smooth muscle (bronchoconstriction) and increased glandular secretions.
- Heart: reduction in heart rate via sinoatrial node referred to as a *negative chronotropic effect.*
- Blood vessels: relaxation of vascular smooth muscle via release of endothelium-derived relaxing factor or nitric oxide, from the endothelial cells.
- Gastrointestinal tract: activation; increase smooth muscle contraction, increased peristalsis and increased secretory

activity of gastrointestinal (GI) tract and glands including salivary glands.
- Genitourinary system: contracts bladder detrusor muscle and relaxes trigone and sphincter muscles, increases urination.
- Skin: thermoregulatory eccrine type sweat, lacrimal, and nasopharyngeal glands are activated.

The **sympathetic nervous system** predominates during extreme stress often referred to as "*fight or flight*" conditions. It is anatomically referred to as *thoracolumbar* because sympathetic preganglionic fibers leave the CNS through the thoracic, lumbar spinal nerves. Drugs that mimic sympathetic effects are referred to as *sympathomimetic drugs*, and drugs that inhibit sympathetic effects may be referred to as *sympatholytic drugs*. The primary neurotransmitters of the sympathetic nervous system are **norepinephrine (NE)** and **epinephrine**. NE and epinephrine are **catecholamine** neurotransmitters formed from the amino acid tyrosine. NE and epinephrine are metabolized by the enzymes catechol-O-methyltransferase and monoamine oxidase, which are discussed in the pharmacotherapy of Parkinson's disease and depression sections. NE and epinephrine activate the adrenergic receptors or adrenoceptors of the sympathetic nervous system; these adrenergic receptors are classed as beta receptors and alpha receptors.

There are three types of **beta receptors** with the following primary locations and functions:

- **Beta-1:** Beta-1 receptors are located on the heart and the juxtaglomerular cells in the kidneys. Functions of beta-1 activation include increasing heart rate; increasing conduction in sinoatrial, atrioventricular, and ventricular cells; increasing myocardial contractility; and increasing renin release by the juxtaglomerular cells in the kidneys.
- **Beta-2:** Beta-2 receptors are primarily located on smooth muscle in the bronchi, uterus, certain blood vessels, liver, and skeletal muscles. Activation of beta-2 receptors causes bronchodilation, relaxation of uterine smooth muscle, and vasodilation of certain blood vessels that supply large skeletal muscles. Stimulation of beta-2 receptors also increases glycogenolysis, blood glucose, and uptake of potassium by skeletal muscle.

- **Beta-3**: Beta-3 receptor activation causes relaxation of the detrusor muscle in the urinary bladder.

There are 2 types of **alpha receptors** with the following primary locations and functions:

- **Alpha-1**: Alpha-1 receptors are in vascular smooth muscle, smooth muscle of the prostate and bladder sphincter, pupillary dilator muscle, and smooth muscle of piloerector muscle. Stimulation of alpha-1 receptors causes vasoconstriction, increased blood pressure, dilation of pupils (mydriasis), contraction of bladder sphincter muscle causing retention of urine, and piloerection (goose bumps).
- **Alpha-2**: Alpha-2 receptors are inhibitory receptors primarily located in the brainstem and adrenergic and cholinergic nerve terminals. Alpha-2 receptors are a shut-off switch, and activation of alpha-2 receptors inhibits the release of norepinephrine.

Drugs that affect sympathetic nervous function are classified as adrenergic drugs, sympathomimetics or sympatholytic drugs, or antiadrenergic drugs, which are generally adrenergic receptor antagonists.

Some of the organ functions of the sympathetic nervous system include:

- Eye: pupillary dilation called mydriasis.
- Pulmonary: bronchodilation.
- Heart: increase heart rate called positive *chronotropic effect*, increase myocardial contractility called *positive inotropic effect*, increases conduction velocity or *positive dromotropic effect*.
- Blood vessels: mainly vasoconstriction, increase peripheral arterial resistance.
- Gastrointestinal tract.
- Metabolic functions: increase blood glucose via glycogenolysis in the liver, promote the uptake of potassium into cells.
- Genitourinary system: contraction of smooth muscle at bladder base, urethral sphincter, and prostate causing urinary continence.
- Skin: piloerection and increased activation of sweat glands.

An important distinction is that sweat glands are activated by the sympathetic nervous system via sympathetic postganglionic **cholinergic** fibers.

There are also **autonomic ganglia** in each arm of the ANS. Autonomic fibers that arise from cell bodies in the brainstem and spinal cord are called *preganglionic fibers*. All preganglionic fibers are cholinergic, and they synapse on autonomic ganglia, which have **nicotinic (N)** type receptors and activate postganglionic fibers. Postganglionic fibers from each arm innervate effector organs and produce either parasympathetic or sympathetic effects. Drugs that block nicotinic receptors on autonomic ganglia are referred to as *ganglionic blockers*.

PARASYMPATHOMIMETIC AND PARASYMPATHOLYTIC DRUGS

There are two categories of parasympathomimetic agents: **direct**-acting parasympathomimetic agents act as muscarinic receptor agonists, and **indirect**-acting are acetylcholinesterase inhibitors. Direct-acting agents act at muscarinic receptor agonists. Indirect-acting parasympathomimetic agents inhibit the enzyme acetylcholinesterase and decrease the metabolism of acetylcholine, which increases cholinergic activity. These agents

reversibly or irreversibly bind to and inactivate acetylcholinesterase and increase the effects of acetylcholine at nicotinic (N) and muscarinic (M) receptors. The adverse effects and toxicity of parasympathomimetic drugs reflect the extremes of normal actions of the parasympathetic systems. SLUDD (salivation, lacrimation, urination, digestion, and defecation) is an acronym used to recall the effects and adverse effects of cholinomimetic agents.

Clinically, important **muscarinic agonists** include the prototype pilocarpine, bethanechol, and cevimeline. Bethanechol is available orally for neurogenic bladder and acute postoperative and postpartum nonobstructive (functional) urinary retention. Cevimeline is available orally for xerostomia (associated with Sjögren syndrome). These agents increase in secretion of exocrine glands (such as salivary and sweat glands) and stimulate smooth muscle in the urinary and gastrointestinal tracts. Adverse effects are related to cholinergic effects and include diaphoresis; diarrhea, abdominal cramps, nausea/vomiting, urinary urgency and frequency, difficulty in visual accommodation, bradycardia, and hypotension.

Indirect-acting **acetylcholinesterase inhibitors** have some therapeutic and toxicologic considerations. Clinically, important acetylcholinesterase inhibitors include short-acting edrophonium for the diagnosis of myasthenia gravis, and neostigmine and pyridostigmine for its treatment. Myasthenia gravis is an autoimmune disease caused by destruction of the nicotinic acetylcholine postsynaptic receptors, which leads to progressive muscle weakness especially in the ocular, bulbar, facial, and neck muscles. Neostigmine is used for postoperative paralytic ileus and bladder atony. Physostigmine is a parental agent, which may be used to reverse overdose with anticholinergic agents. There are three cholinesterase inhibitors that are used for symptomatic treatment of Alzheimer disease: donepezil, rivastigmine, and galantamine are available for daily use to slow cognitive and behavioral decline in patients with Alzheimer disease.

The toxicology of acetylcholinesterase inhibitors is beyond the scope of this book. Organophosphate pesticides such as malathion and parathion are a common cause of toxicity, especially through occupational exposure. The "nerve gases"— tabun, sarin, soman, and VX are irreversible inhibitors of acetylcholinesterase and among the most toxic synthetic compounds. Clinical effects of poisoning with organophosphates include nausea and vomiting, abdominal cramps, diarrhea, localized sweating, involuntary urination, salivation, excessive lacrimation, penile erection, bradycardia, and hypotension. Muscle twitching followed by muscle weakness and paralysis, including of respiratory muscles, is most serious consequence.

Antidotes for organophosphate exposure include parenteral atropine and **pralidoxime.** Pralidoxime chloride is a parenteral (IV or subcutaneous) acetylcholinsterase reactivator, which should be administered immediately in poisoning.

Parasympatholytic drugs are muscarinic receptor antagonists that block the effects of acetylcholine at muscarinic receptors. These drugs are also referred to as *anticholinergic* or *antimuscarinic drugs*.

The adverse effects of the anticholinergic/antimuscarinic drugs include dry mouth, dry eyes, and sedation.

A classic and easy-to-recall description of anticholinergic toxicity is as follows:

- "Red as a beet"—Flushed skin due to cutaneous vasodilation to reduce heat and offset decreased sweating.
- "Dry as a bone" (anhidrosis; peripheral)—Dry skin due to decreased activity of sweat glands caused by blocked muscarinic receptors; also, dry eyes and mouth (lacrimal and salivary glands).
- "Hot as a hare"—Elevated body temperature due to decreased sweating.
- "Blind as a bat" (mydriasis)—Blurry vision caused by blockade of muscarinic input to pupillary constrictor muscles and ciliary muscle; this causes pupillary dilation and lack of accommodation, which causes blurry vision.
- "Mad as a hatter" (delirium, hallucinations; central)—Blockade of muscarinic receptors in the CNS accounts for these findings. These CNS signs and symptoms (i.e., central anticholinergic toxicity) are the most worrisome, and if they are present, the patient can be considered to have "severe" anticholinergic toxicity.

The antimuscarinic agents have variable pharmacologic properties and clinical indications. Atropine, the prototypal naturally occurring antimuscarinic agent, is derived from belladonna (Solanaceae) plants. Atropine is used to treat organophosphate or carbamate insecticide or nerve agent poisoning and, occasionally, for symptomatic bradycardia. Scopolamine, a natural antimuscarinic, is used transdermally for prevention of motion sickness. Antimuscarinic drugs such as ipratropium, tiotropium, aclidinium, and umeclidinium are inhaled agents commonly used in the treatment of chronic obstructive pulmonary disease (COPD; see Chapter 4). Oxybutynin, tolterodine, trospium chloride, darifenacin, solifenacin, and fesoterodine are muscarinic antagonists indicated for urge incontinence, also referred to as *overactive bladder*. Hyoscyamine sulfate and dicyclomine are used to treat cramping and diarrhea associated with irritable bowel syndrome. Homatropine hydrobromide, cyclopentolate hydrochloride, and tropicamide are topical ophthalmic medication used to cause mydriasis and cycloplegia in ophthalmological practice. Benztropine mesylate and trihexyphenidyl hydrochloride are adjunctive treatment for Parkinson disease and drug-induced extrapyramidal symptoms caused by antipsychotic medications.

Antimuscarinic medications have specific adverse effects and contraindications. Common adverse effects include dry mouth, constipation, blurred vision, sedation, and cognitive impairment. Contraindications to antimuscarinic agents include urinary tract obstruction, severe benign prostatic hyperplasia, GI obstruction, and angle-closure glaucoma. Toxicity of the antimuscarinic agents from accidental or intentional overdose include tachycardia, dry mouth, hot, dry, flushed skin, restlessness, dilated pupils, and blurred vision. Severe toxicity also manifests as hallucinations and delirium and coma.

SYMPATHOMIMETICS AND ADRENERGIC BLOCKERS

Drugs affecting the sympathetic nervous system are illustrated in the mind map (Mind Map 2.1).

Beta agonists are medications that act like NE or epinephrine at beta receptors. There are nonselective beta agonists that act at beta-1 and beta-2 receptors. An example of a nonselective beta-1/beta-2 agonists is isoproterenol; it was used in advanced cardiac life support for heart blocks, severe bradyarrhythmias, and cardiac arrest but has since been replaced by other drugs and procedures. Isoproterenol has cardiac stimulating properties and bronchodilating and vasodilating effects. Dobutamine is a beta agonist with some alpha-1 agonist effects, which has increased myocardial contractility and cardiac output. It can be used for severe, medically refractory heart failure and cardiogenic shock.

Beta-2 agonists are clinically important as bronchodilators specifically for bronchospastic diseases like asthma and COPD, which are discussed in detail in Chapter 4. Beta-2 agonists act at beta-2 receptors and relax smooth muscle in the airways, causing bronchodilation. Commonly used beta-2 agonists include albuterol, levalbuterol, salmeterol, formoterol indacaterol, olodaterol, and vilanterol. Most beta-2 agonists are administered via inhalation with inhalers or nebulizers. Adverse effects are mild with inhaled beta-2 agonists and include hand tremors, nervousness, palpitations, and increased heart rate.

Beta antagonists, also known as beta-blockers, act as antagonists to NE and epinephrine at beta receptors and have sympatholytic effects. Nonselective beta antagonists block beta-1 and beta-2 receptors and have more adverse effects. The primary nonselective beta antagonist is propranolol. Beta-1 selective antagonists selectively block beta-1 receptors and are commonly used for cardiac conditions such as angina, hypertension, certain cardiac arrhythmias, and stable heart failure. Beta-1 selective beta blockers include metoprolol, atenolol, nebivolol, and bisoprolol. Beta blockers reduce heart rate, decrease contractility, and reduce atrioventricular (AV) nodal conduction. They also reduce renin release from the kidney, which lowers blood pressure. **Labetalol** and **carvedilol** have both alpha-1–selective (vasodilating effects) and beta-antagonistic effects and these medications are discussed in Chapter 3.

Adverse effects of beta antagonists are divided into cardiac and noncardiac effects. Cardiac effects include bradycardia, worsening of heart blocks due to slowing of AV node conduction, and worsening of heart failure in patients with decompensated heart failure. Abrupt cessation of beta blockers can worsen ischemic heart disease, and beta blockers should be tapered to avoid this effect. Noncardiac effects include worsening of bronchospastic disease, which is more common with nonselective beta blockers due to beta-2 blocking effects. Nonselective beta blockers may mask the effects of hypoglycemia in patients with diabetes mellitus who use insulin. Nonselective beta blockers can decrease high-density lipoprotein cholesterol, increase low-density lipoprotein cholesterol, and increase triglycerides. Other nonspecific effects include fatigue, nightmares, depressed mood, and sexual dysfunction in men.

Alpha receptor agonists drugs selectively activate alpha-1 or alpha-2 receptors; there are few clinically relevant nonselective alpha agonists. The main alpha-1 agonist drug is phenylephrine, which is used orally and topically as a nasal decongestant, and topically as a mydriatic agent to dilate pupils.

Alpha-2 agonists are mostly used include clonidine, methyldopa, guanfacine, and guanabenz. These medications activate alpha-2 receptors, which reduces NE output, causing sympatholytic effects and decreasing blood pressure. Clonidine is an alpha-2 agonist used orally or transdermal patch for treatment of hypertension. Methyldopa is also available but uncommonly used for hypertension and may be associated with liver problems and autoimmune hemolytic anemia. Guanfacine is used for attention-deficit/hyperactivity disorder. Alpha-2 agonists are generally sedating; details of these medications are discussed in Chapter 3.

Alpha antagonist medications are mainly alpha-1 selective and include doxazocin, terazosin, prazosin, tamsulosin, alfuzosin, and silodosin. Alpha-1 antagonists block the effects of NE and epinephrine on alpha-1 receptors on smooth muscle, causing relaxation in the vascular smooth muscle, prostate and urethral sphincters, and iris dilator muscle. Doxazocin, terazosin, and prazosin are antihypertensive medications that reduce blood pressure by causing vasodilation. All alpha-1 blockers can be used to treat the lower urinary tract symptoms caused by benign prostatic hyperplasia (BPH). Tamsulosin, alfuzosin, and silodosin are commonly used for BPH because they are more selective for alpha-1a receptors, which are found on smooth muscle near the prostate, base of the bladder, and proximal urethra.

Adverse effects of the alpha-1 antagonists are generally attributed to their mode of action. First-dose syncope can occur, with marked postural hypotension and syncope after the initial dosage of prazosin and doxazocin. This first-dose effect can be avoided by using a low initial dosage at bedtime to minimize postural hypotension.

Other alpha antagonists include **phenoxybenzamine**, which has some alpha-1 selective effects, and **phentolamine**, which is a nonselective alpha-1 and alpha-2 receptor antagonist. Phenoxybenzamine forms a covalent bond with alpha receptors causing an irreversible blockade and long-lasting effects. Phentolamine is a nonselective alpha-1 and alpha-2 receptors competitive antagonist. Both medications are used to treat pheochromocytoma, which is a catecholamine-secreting tumor usually from chromaffin cells of the adrenal medulla and the sympathetic ganglia.

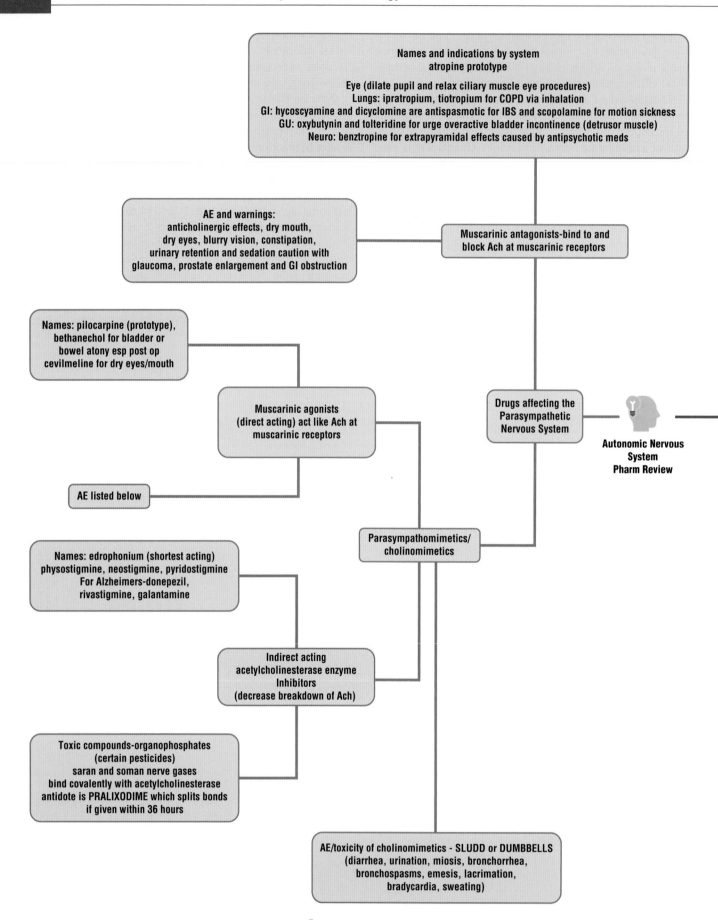

Names and indications by system
atropine prototype

Eye (dilate pupil and relax ciliary muscle eye procedures)
Lungs: ipratropium, tiotropium for COPD via inhalation
GI: hyoscyamine and dicyclomine are antispasmotic for IBS and scopolamine for motion sickness
GU: oxybutynin and tolteridine for urge overactive bladder incontinence (detrusor muscle)
Neuro: benztropine for extrapyramidal effects caused by antipsychotic meds

AE and warnings:
anticholinergic effects, dry mouth,
dry eyes, blurry vision, constipation,
urinary retention and sedation caution with
glaucoma, prostate enlargement and GI obstruction

Muscarinic antagonists-bind to and
block Ach at muscarinic receptors

Names: pilocarpine (prototype),
bethanechol for bladder or
bowel atony esp post op
cevilmeline for dry eyes/mouth

Muscarinic agonists
(direct acting) act like Ach at
muscarinic receptors

Drugs affecting the
Parasympathetic
Nervous System

Autonomic Nervous
System
Pharm Review

AE listed below

Parasympathomimetics/
cholinomimetics

Names: edrophonium (shortest acting)
physostigmine, neostigmine, pyridostigmine
For Alzheimers-donepezil,
rivastigmine, galantamine

Indirect acting
acetylcholinesterase enzyme
Inhibitors
(decrease breakdown of Ach)

Toxic compounds-organophosphates
(certain pesticides)
saran and soman nerve gases
bind covalently with acetylcholinesterase
antidote is PRALIXODIME which splits bonds
if given within 36 hours

AE/toxicity of cholinomimetics - SLUDD or DUMBBELLS
(diarrhea, urination, miosis, bronchorrhea,
bronchospasms, emesis, lacrimation,
bradycardia, sweating)

MIND MAP 2.1

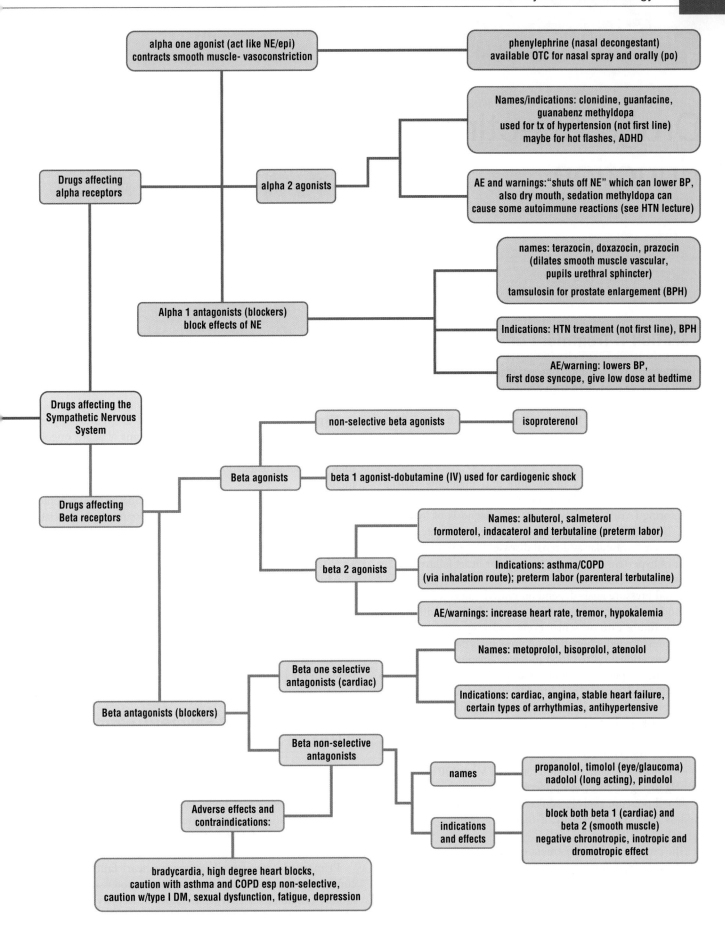

CHAPTER 3

Drugs Affecting Cardiovascular Function

SECTION 1: Treatment of Hypertension

Hypertension is a common chronic disease defined as elevated blood pressure measured with appropriate technique and classified as follows:

- Stage 1 – Systolic 130 to 139 mmHg or diastolic 80 to 89 mmHg.
- Stage 2 – Systolic at least 140 mmHg or diastolic at least 90 mmHg.

Consistent elevations in daytime and nighttime (asleep) blood pressures using home or ambulatory blood pressure monitoring (ABPM) also supports the diagnosis of hypertension. Untreated or poorly treated hypertension increases the risk for cardiovascular and renal disease. Pharmacologic treatment of hypertension reduces the risk for heart failure, stroke, and myocardial infarction.

Blood pressure goals depend on underlying risk factors and method of blood pressure measurements. Patients with higher risk for future cardiovascular events warrant more aggressive blood pressure reduction: If blood pressure is measured by routine/conventional office blood pressure (manual measurement with stethoscope or oscillometer device),[1] the goal is 125 to 130/<80 mmHg, and if measured by daytime ABPM, or home blood pressure, the goal is 120 to 125/<80 mmHg.

Low-risk patient goal blood pressure is 125 to 135/<90 mmHg (using the nonroutine [preferred] measurement methods including standardized office-based measurement, automated office BPM, home blood pressure, and ABPM) or 130 to 139/<90 mmHg (using routine [non-preferred] office measurements).

Blood pressure goals in adults aged 65 years and older may be less aggressive especially, if there is a reduced life expectancy.[1]

The preferred initial treatment options include:

- Thiazide-type diuretics.
- Angiotensin-converting enzyme (ACE) inhibitors/angiotensin II receptor blockers (ARBs).
- Calcium channel blockers (CCBs) of the dihydropyridine class.

Many patients with blood pressure greater than 20/10 mmHg above the goal require two drug combinations as initial therapy. A common combination for initial therapy is a long-acting dihydropyridine calcium channel blocker plus a long-acting ACE inhibitor/ARB.[2]

Hypertensive emergencies are defined as significantly elevated blood pressure with signs or symptoms of acute, ongoing target-organ damage, e.g., neurologic, cardiac, vascular, or renal injury. General medications used for hypertensive emergencies include:[3]

- Sodium nitroprusside, which is a vasodilator used parenterally as an infusion to lower blood pressure. It is associated with potential cyanide toxicity and causes a rapid and drastic drop in blood pressure.
- Nitroglycerin intravenously (IV), which is a vasodilator, which also dilates veins; the primary adverse effects are flushing and headache.
- Calcium channel blockers, e.g., nicardipine IV, are vasodilators.
- Labetalol IV is a beta-adrenergic and alpha-adrenergic blocker.

The major classes of antihypertensive medications are illustrated in the Mind Map 3.1 and detailed in the Table 3.1.

SECTION 2: Heart Failure: Treatment of Heart Failure

Heart failure is defined as a syndrome or pathophysiologic state in which the heart is unable to pump blood at a rate sufficient to meet the body's metabolic demands. It is caused by several diseases including coronary artery disease, diabetes mellitus, and chronic hypertension. Heart failure is staged in several ways.

Primary classes of medications for heart failure include a combination of loop diuretics, a renin-angiotensin system inhibitor (angiotensin II receptor blocker; neprilysin Inhibitor [ARNI], or ACE inhibitor, or single agent ARB), and a cardioselective beta blocker. Loop diuretics are used to alleviate symptoms and signs of fluid overload such as dyspnea and peripheral edema. The loop diuretics used in heart failure are furosemide (most common), torsemide, bumetanide. Oral loop diuretics may be continued indefinitely, and the dose can be adjusted according to daily weight. Adverse effects of loop diuretics are listed in the Table 3.2. IV loop diuretics are used for unstable or severe disease. Monitoring of loop diuretics includes renal function, blood pressure, fluid status, serum electrolytes.

One of the renin-angiotensin system inhibitors (ARNI, or ACE inhibitor, or single agent ARB) medications are a mainstay of treatment for patients with heart failure. The choice depends on tolerability and cost; the angiotensin II receptor blocker and neprilysin inhibitor, sacubitril/valsartan, is expensive and has the highest risk of hypotension. ACE inhibitors for heart failure include captopril (dosed TID), enalapril, lisinopril, and ramipril. ARBs include candesartan, valsartan, and losartan. All these drugs are detailed in Mind Map 3.2 and in Table 3.2. Adverse effects include hypotension, increased serum potassium, worsening renal function with increased blood urea nitrogen (BUN) and creatinine, cough, and risk for angioedema. Monitoring in patients taking the renin-angiotensin system inhibitors includes blood pressure, BUN, serum creatinine, and serum potassium. ARBs, e.g., valsartan or candesartan, are alternatives to ACE inhibitors with less cough and angioedema.

Beta-antagonists are indicated for many patients with stable heart failure. The beta-blockers used for heart include one of the following: carvedilol (immediate release or extended release), extended-release metoprolol succinate, or bisoprolol. Beta-blockers are initiated at very low doses after patients are started on angiotensin system blocker (ACE inhibitor, ARNI, or ARB). The antihypertensive chart and map and heart failure chart describes the pharmacology of beta-blockers.

Secondary pharmacotherapy options for heart failure include mineralocorticoid receptor antagonist, sodium-glucose cotransporter 2 inhibitor (described in diabetes mellitus Mind Map Chapter 6), ivabradine, hydralazine plus nitrate, and digoxin. Mineralocorticoid receptor antagonist (MRA), e.g., spironolactone, can be added to usual therapy for patients with low ejection fraction heart failure who are symptomatic on initial therapy. Indications for other secondary pharmacologic therapies are detailed in the heart failure chart.[5]

Treatment of acute decompensated heart failure, which is new or a worsening of heart failure symptoms, may require hospitalization. General pharmacotherapeutic medications include IV loop diuretics, vasodilators, e.g., nitroprusside, and potentially positive inotropic agents such as dobutamine or milrinone.[6]

SECTION 3: Treatment of Angina Pectoris

Angina pectoris, or angina, is chest pain or discomfort associated with myocardial ischemia when myocardial oxygen demand exceeds supply. Angina is usually caused by coronary artery disease, which in itself has several risk factors. Angina medications are used intermittently to treat acute symptoms and daily to prevent attacks of angina.

There are three primary classes of medications used to treat angina caused by coronary artery disease: nitrates, beta-blockers, and CCBs. Table 3.2 details the classes of medications for angina. Beta-1 selective-blockers are the preferred prophylactic medications for angina. Other prophylactic medications for angina include CCBs, long-acting nitrates, and ranolazine.

Nitrates are available in sublingual, buccal, oral, spray, ointment, and transdermal preparations. The nitrates are vasodilators, which relax vascular smooth muscle in veins and arteries, including coronary arteries. The nitrates reduce myocardial oxygen demand and may increase coronary artery blood flow. The commonly used nitrates include nitroglycerin, which is most used as a sublingual tablet for acute attacks of angina. Nitroglycerin is also available as a sublingual metered dose spray. Nitroglycerin sublingual tablets and spray are rapid acting with onset of action of 2 to 5 minutes and the duration of action of 15 to 30 minutes. The most used long-acting nitrate is extended-release isosorbide mononitrate, which is administered orally once daily for angina prophylaxis. The most common adverse effects of the nitrates are flushing and headache; lightheadedness can occur due to hypotension. Nitrate **tolerance** is a common problem with the use of nitrates as chronic antianginal therapy. Nitrate tolerance can be mitigated by using intermittent therapy and providing a nitrate-free interval of 8 to 10 hours per day.

Prophylactic therapy for chronic stable angina is detailed in Table 3.3. Cardio-selective beta blockers, e.g., metoprolol or atenolol, are first-line daily therapy for prevention of anginal symptoms. Beta-blockers reduce heart rate and contractility and reduce angina episodes and improve exercise tolerance. Alternative therapies include CCBs, e.g., diltiazem or amlodipine, or isosorbide mononitrate. CCBs reduce angina episodes and improve exercise tolerance; they reduce blood pressure and afterload. Verapamil and diltiazem reduce heart rate and contractility. Isosorbide mononitrate is a long-acting nitrate, which improves exercise tolerance and time to onset of angina. Combination therapy is appropriate for patients who are symptomatic on monotherapy. Ranolazine can be added as a third medication for symptomatic patients with chronic stable angina. Ranolazine inhibits late inward sodium channels in diseased myocardial cells, which may affect calcium entry and decrease diastolic tension.[8]

SECTION 4: Treatment of Acute Coronary Syndrome

Acute coronary syndrome (ACS) refers to three clinical conditions that cause acute myocardial ischemia or infarction. Non-ST-elevation myocardial infarction (NSTEMI), ST-elevation MI (STEMI), and unstable angina are the primary types of **ACS**, although unstable angina is often diagnosed as NSTEMI due to increased high-sensitivity troponin testing. STEMI and NSTEMI have elevated troponins, and the distinguishing feature are electrocardiogram (ECG) findings of ST-elevation or new left bundle branch block in patients with STEMI. ACS often presents with chest discomfort and/or dyspnea often associated with exercise or increased activity, which can radiate to

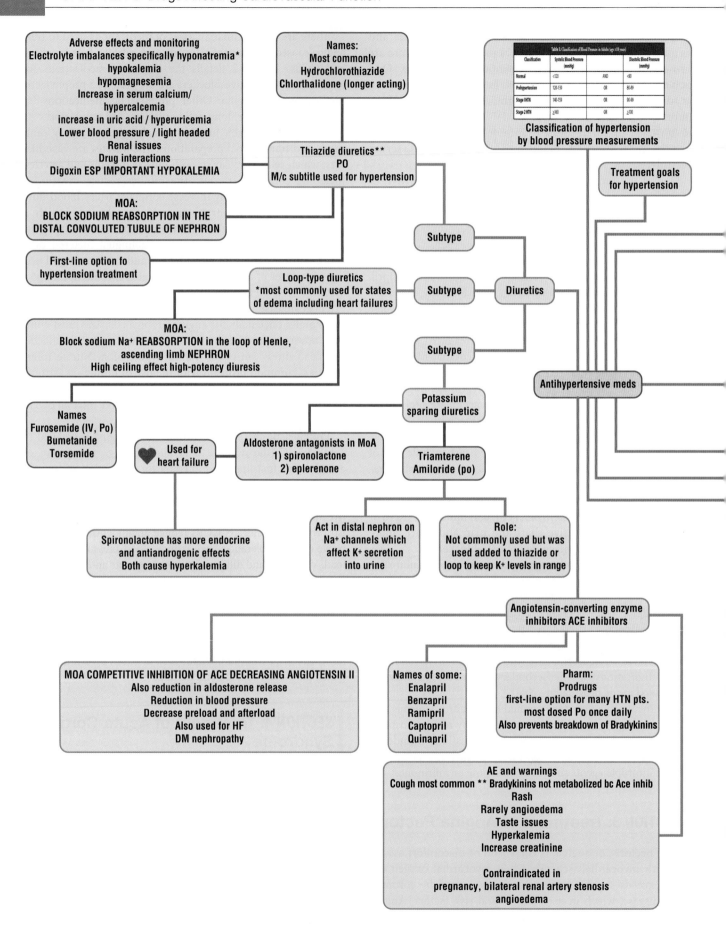

Adverse effects and monitoring
Electrolyte imbalances specifically hyponatremia*
hypokalemia
hypomagnesemia
Increase in serum calcium/
hypercalcemia
increase in uric acid / hyperuricemia
Lower blood pressure / light headed
Renal issues
Drug interactions
Digoxin ESP IMPORTANT HYPOKALEMIA

Names:
Most commonly
Hydrochlorothiazide
Chlorthalidone (longer acting)

Classification of hypertension
by blood pressure measurements

Thiazide diuretics**
PO
M/c subtitle used for hypertension

Treatment goals
for hypertension

MOA:
BLOCK SODIUM REABSORPTION IN THE
DISTAL CONVOLUTED TUBULE OF NEPHRON

Subtype

First-line option fo
hypertension treatment

Loop-type diuretics
*most commonly used for states
of edema including heart failures

Subtype

Diuretics

MOA:
Block sodium Na+ REABSORPTION in the loop of Henle,
ascending limb NEPHRON
High ceiling effect high-potency diuresis

Subtype

Antihypertensive meds

Names
Furosemide (IV, Po)
Bumetanide
Torsemide

Potassium
sparing diuretics

Used for
heart failure

Aldosterone antagonists in MoA
1) spironolactone
2) eplerenone

Triamterene
Amiloride (po)

Spironolactone has more endocrine
and antiandrogenic effects
Both cause hyperkalemia

Act in distal nephron on
Na+ channels which
affect K+ secretion
into urine

Role:
Not commonly used but was
used added to thiazide or
loop to keep K+ levels in range

Angiotensin-converting enzyme
inhibitors ACE inhibitors

MOA COMPETITIVE INHIBITION OF ACE DECREASING ANGIOTENSIN II
Also reduction in aldosterone release
Reduction in blood pressure
Decrease preload and afterload
Also used for HF
DM nephropathy

Names of some:
Enalapril
Benzapril
Ramipril
Captopril
Quinapril

Pharm:
Prodrugs
first-line option for many HTN pts.
most dosed Po once daily
Also prevents breakdown of Bradykinins

AE and warnings
Cough most common ** Bradykinins not metabolized bc Ace inhib
Rash
Rarely angioedema
Taste issues
Hyperkalemia
Increase creatinine

Contraindicated in
pregnancy, bilateral renal artery stenosis
angioedema

MIND MAP 3.1

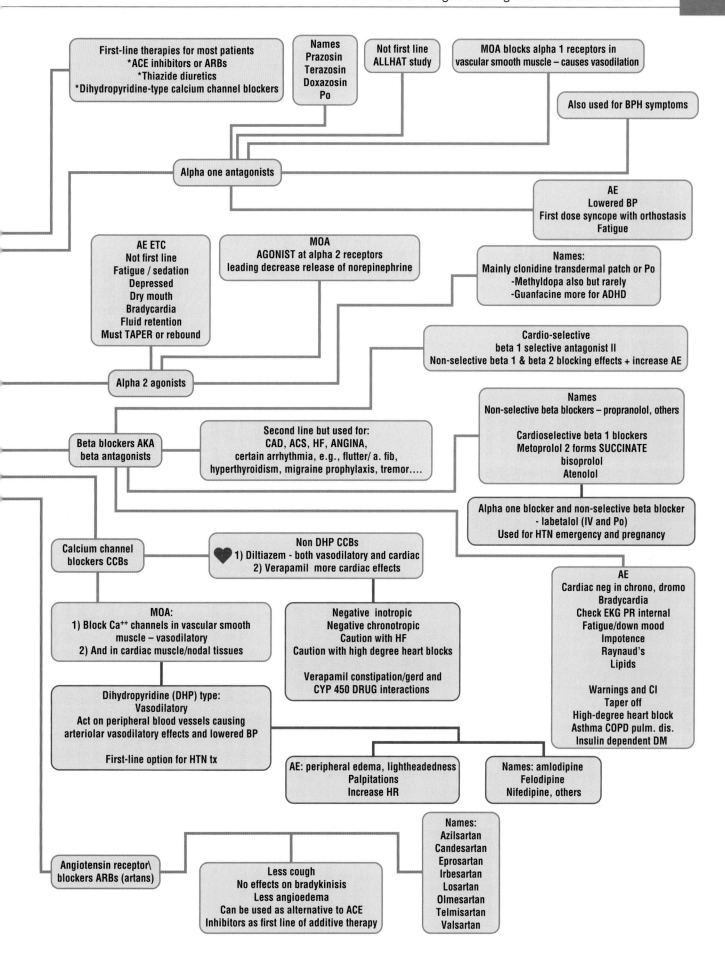

TABLE 3.1   Chart of Hypertension Medications

Class of Drugs	Names, Dosing and Administration	Mechanism of Action / Indications	Adverse Effects/ Toxicity	Warnings and Contraindications
Thiazide Type Diuretics	Chlorthalidone 12.5–25 mg/day Hydrochlorothiazide 12.5–25 mg/day Indapamide: 1.25 mg/day of indapamide	Inhibit sodium transport in the distal convoluted tubule cells of nephrons and decrease Na+ reabsorption, may have some vasodilating effects	Hypokalemia, hyponatremia, hyperuricemia, hyperglycemia, hyperlipidemia, hypomagnesemia occasionally, hypercalcemia sexual dysfunction in men	Potentially sulfonamide allergies Anuria
Loop Diuretics (used for heart failure and edema NOT first line for HTN) These are included in this chart and in the heart failure chart	Furosemide: oral dosage IV 20–40 mg once then titrate as needed max daily dose 600 mg/day Bumetanide (IV, po forms): initially Initial: 0.5–1 mg once daily and titrate (weight, fluid status) Torsemide initial: 10–20 mg once daily; may increase gradually by doubling dose max is 200 mg/day Ethacrynic acid: oral dose: 50–200 mg/day in 1–2 divided doses, IV 50 mg or 0.5–1 mg/kg/dose	Inhibit Na-K-2 Cl carrier in ascending limb of loop of Henle, significantly reducing Na+ reabsorption	Profound diuresis with water and electrolyte depletion	Anuria Warning but not contraindication Sulfonamide ("sulfa") allergy unclear if cross-reactivity with nonantibiotic and antibiotic sulfonamides
Potassium sparing diuretics • Aldosterone antagonists • Amiloride and triamterene directly block sodium channels in principal cells of collecting ducts	Aldosterone antagonists Not first line for initial management • Eplerenone: Initial: 50 mg once daily can increase to 50 mg BID • Spironolactone: Initial: 25 mg once daily; titrate as needed based on response and tolerability up to 100 mg once daily Amiloride 5–10 mg in 1–2 divided doses (better tolerated than triamterene) Triamterene 100 mg po twice daily	Eplerenone Spironolactone inhibit the mineralocorticoid receptors in collecting ducts, which reduce urinary excretion of K+ and increases Na and water reabsorption Amiloride and triamterene directly block sodium channels in principal cells of collecting ducts, which reduces K+ excretion into urine	All can cause hyperkalemia Spironolactone: gynecomastia, menstrual abnormalities, impotence, and decreased libido Triamterene can cause nephrotoxicity and increase kidney stone formation	Hyperkalemia Anuria Severe liver or kidney disease Caution with other drugs, which increase potassium including potassium supplements Caution with eplerenone and Addison disease
Calcium Channel Blockers: dihydropyridine type ('PINEs')	Nifedipine Nicardipine 20 mg orally 3 times daily; usual dosage: 20–40 mg 3 times daily Long acting: Isradipine 5–10 mg/day in 2 divided doses felodipine, 2.5–10 mg once daily Nisoldipine: 17–34 mg once daily Amlodipine: Initial: 2.5–5 mg once daily up to 10 mg /day levamlodipine: 1.25–2.5 mg once daily	Inhibit calcium influx into arterial smooth muscle cells causing vasodilation	Most common peripheral edema (not fluid retention) with ankle and leg swelling Less common: flushing, headache, dizziness	Caution with: Aortic stenosis Hypotension Hypertrophic cardiomyopathy

Drug class	Description	Adverse effects	Contraindications
Calcium channel blockers: non-dihydropyridine type (verapamil and diltiazem) (not first line for HTN)	Verapamil (dose varies if immediate release or extended release) Diltiazem (dose varies if immediate release or extended release) There are IV formulations of these drugs These drugs are not first line for essential hypertension They are used for rate control in patients with atrial fibrillation and certain SVTS and option for chronic therapy in chronic stable angina	Non-dihydropyridines (verapamil and diltiazem) are dose-dependent constipation	Verapamil: Diltiazem: sick sinus syndrome second- or third-degree AV block (except in patients with a functioning artificial pacemaker); hypotension (systolic <90 mm Hg acute MI and pulmonary congestion Atrial fibrillation or flutter associated with accessory bypass tract (e.g., Wolff-Parkinson-White syndrome, short PR syndrome) Ventricular tachycardia (with wide-complex tachycardia [QRS ≥0.12 seconds][4]
Beta-antagonists	Cardio selective beta- antagonists: atenolol metoprolol bisoprolol: 5–10 mg po once daily max: 20 mg/day nebivolol: 5 mg po daily may increase to maximum of 40 mg/day Nonselective beta blockers: Propranolol Beta blockers with alpha-1 antagonist activity: Carvedilol Labetalol	Beta-1 receptors, which are found primarily in heart muscle. Blocking beta-1 receptors decreases in heart rate (negative chronotropic), decreases contractility (negative inotropic), decreases AV conduction (negative dromotropic) Also reduce renin release from kidney Nonselective beta antagonists have more AE because they affect beta-2 receptors	Cardiac AE: Bradycardia Worsen heart failure if decompensated Worsen AV heart blocks Abrupt withdrawal can worsen underlying heart conditions Noncardiac: Can worsen bronchospasm-caution with asthma and COPD Fatigue Depression Sexual dysfunction Increase HDL and triglycerides Caution with insulin dependent DM caused by masking of hypoglycemic symptoms May worsen severe peripheral vascular disease	Severe bradycardia Second- and third-degree heart blocks Cardiogenic shock Decompensated heart failure Sick sinus syndrome Caution with asthma and COPD

Continued

TABLE 3.1 Chart of Hypertension Medications—cont'd

Class of Drugs	Names, Dosing and Administration	Mechanism of Action / Indications	Adverse Effects/ Toxicity	Warnings and Contraindications
ACE inhibitors (First line for HTN)	Benazepril Captopril Enalapril Enalaprilat (IV) Fosinopril Lisinopril Moexipril Quinapril Ramipril Trandolapril	Inhibits ACE, which prevents the formation of angiotensin II, thereby decreasing the amount of angiotensin and its negative effects	Dry cough hypotension, acute kidney injury, hyperkalemia, and problems during pregnancy Rarely angioedema	Pregnancy Angioedema Hyperkalemia Bilateral renal artery stenosis
Angiotensin Receptor Blockers (First-line option for HTN)	Azilsartan Candesartan Eprosartan Irbesartan Losartan Olmesartan Telmisartan Valsartan	Blocks angiotensin II (AT2) receptors prevents Ang II effects, e.g., vasoconstriction, aldosterone release, vasopressin, hypertrophic effects on myocardium	Lower rates of cough and angioedema than ACE inhibitors otherwise similar effects	Pregnancy Caution with hypotension Caution with renal artery stenosis
Alpha-1 antagonists	Doxazosin Terazosin Prazosin (all oral)	Block alpha-1 receptors on vascular smooth muscles causing vasodilation Not indicated first-line therapy but may benefit men with BPH and low cardiovascular risk	First-dose syncope with postural hypotension (start with low dose and dose at bedtime)	Hypersensitivity to doxazosin
Alpha-2 agonists	Clonidine po twice daily or once weekly transdermal patch NOT first line for HTN	Stimulates alpha-2 receptors in the brain stem resulting in reduced sympathetic outflow from the CNS and reduced blood pressure	Patch: contact dermatitis xerostomia, drowsiness, dizziness	Hypersensitivity to clonidine

ACE, Angiotensin converting enzyme; AE, adverse effect; AV, atrioventricular; BID, twice per day; BPH, benign prostatic hyperplasia; COPD, chronic obstructive pulmonary disease; CNS, central nervous system; DM, diabetes mellitus; HDL, high-density lipoprotein; HTN, hypertension; IV, intravenous; MI, myocardial infarction; po, orally; SVTs, supraventricular tachycardias.

TABLE 3.2   Chart of Heart Failure Medications

Class of Drugs	Names	Mechanism of Action /Indications	Adverse Effects/Toxicity	Contraindications
Loop Diuretics	(see Table 3.1)	(see Table 3.1)	(see Table 3.1) Monitor for: hypokalemia, metabolic alkalosis, and hyperuricemia Monitor for hypotension and hypovolemia Monitor BUN and creatinine Furosemide, bumetanide, and torsemide are sulfonamides, so potential for hypersensitivity reactions Ototoxicity w deafness can occur with high-dose intravenous therapy	Anuria Caution with uncorrected electrolyte depletion, hypovolemia, hypotension;
ARNI	Sacubitril/valsartan po	Sacubitril: inhibits neprilysin (neutral endopeptidase), which increases natriuretic peptides; induces vasodilation and natriuresis Valsartan: blocks angiotensin II (AT2) receptors and prevents Ang II effects e.g., vasoconstriction, aldosterone release, vasopressin, hypertrophic effects on myocardium		Pregnancy Do not administer within 36 hours of switching to or from an ACE inhibitor
ACE inhibitors	Captopril Lisinopril Enalapril Ramipril	Inhibit formation of angiotensin II, thereby decreasing the amount of angiotensin and its negative effects	See antihypertensive chart With heart failure assess renal function and hypokalemia after initiation	Pregnancy Bilateral renal artery stenosis Angioedema Avoid combining with sacubitril/ valsartan
Angiotensin II receptor blockers (ARBs)	Candesartan Valsartan Losartan	Blocks AT2 receptors prevents Ang II effects e.g., vasoconstriction, aldosterone release, vasopressin, hypertrophic effects on myocardium	See antihypertensive chart With heart failure assess renal function and hypokalemia after initiation	Pregnancy Angioedema
Beta Blockers	Metoprolol succinate Bisoprolol Carvedilol (nonselective beta blocker/alpha₁ antagonist	Reduce effects of catecholamines, reduce heart rate, reduce myocardial oxygen demand, decrease ventricular remodeling[7]	See antihypertensive chart	Active bronchospasm Heart block greater than first degree (unless the patient has a permanent pacemaker), those with first-degree heart block and a PR interval >0.30 seconds Severe bradycardia

Continued

TABLE 3.2 Chart of Heart Failure Medications—cont'd

Class of Drugs	Names	Mechanism of Action /Indications	Adverse Effects/Toxicity	Contraindications
Mineralocorticoid receptor antagonists (MRA)	Spironolactone (po) Eplerenone (po)	Blocks negative effects of aldosterone in diseased heart. Indications: Added to initial therapy for persistent symptoms and post MI with LVEF ≤35%	Hyperkalemia Endocrine effects with spironolactone	Hyperkalemia; Addison disease
Digoxin	Digoxin (po) once daily	Positive inotropic effects by Increases vagal tone decreasing heart rate and AV nodal conduction. Indications: Persistent NYHA functional class III and IV symptoms despite optimal initial therapy plus all other indicated secondary pharmacologic therapies indications	Arrhythmias, conduction disturbances GI: nausea, vomiting visual disturbances, e.g., blurred or yellow vision Requires serum drug monitoring and serum electrolytes especially potassium and magnesium	Significant sinus or AV block (unless the block has been addressed with a permanent pacemaker Cautions: Narrow therapeutic index Caution: increased toxicity with hypokalemia
Ivabradine	Ivabradine orally twice daily	Inhibits (HCN) channels (f-channels) within the sinoatrial (SA) node, slows SA node and reduces heart rate. Indications: LVEF ≤35% in sinus rhythm with a resting heart rate ≥70 beats per minute despite a maximum tolerated dose of beta blocker or with contraindications to beta blockers	Bradycardia May increase risk atrial fibrillation Visual Phosphenes	Third-degree heart blocks Sick sinus syndrome Symptomatic bradycardia Decompensated heart failure
Hydralazine/isosorbide dinitrate	Orally three times per day	Vasodilating effects. Indications: alternative to angiotensin system blocker if neither ACE inhibitor, ARNI, nor single agent ARB is tolerated	Flushing, hypotension, tachycardia palpitations	Contraindications: Use of nitrates with phosphodiesterase-5 inhibitors Contraindicated in patients with mitral valve rheumatic heart disease Caution with coronary artery disease
Sodium-glucose cotransporter 2 (SGLT2) inhibitors	dapagliflozin, empagliflozin canagliflozin	patients with HFrEF with type 2 DM	Vulvovaginal candidiasis and urinary tract infections Increase the risk of DKA Acute kidney injury	Type 1 DM Type 2 with history of DKA Volume depletion end-stage kidney disease

ACE, Angiotensin converting enzyme; *ARNI*, angiotensin II receptor blocker; neprilysin inhibitor; *AV*, atrioventricular; *BUN*, blood urea nitrogen; *DM*, diabetes mellitus; *DKA*, diabetic ketoacidosis; *GI*, gastrointestinal; *HCN*, hyperpolarization-activated cyclic nucleotide-gated; *HDL*, high-density lipoprotein; *HFrEF*, heart failure with reduced ejection fraction; *LVEF*, left ventricular ejection fraction; *MI*, myocardial infarction; *NYHA*, New York Heart Association; *po*, orally.

TABLE 3.3 Drugs Used to Treat Angina

Class of Drugs	Names, Dosing and Administration	Indications	Adverse Effects	Contraindications
Short-acting Nitrates	Sublingual nitroglycerin Nitroglycerin spray IV nitroglycerin (used for ACS)	Acute attacks of angina	Flushing and headache	Hypertrophic cardiomyopathy Suspected right ventricular infarction Use of phosphodiesterase Type 5 inhibitors
Long-acting Nitrates	Extended-release isosorbide mononitrate once daily 120 mg	Prevention of angina pectoris caused by coronary artery disease	Flushing and Headache Tolerance	Hypertrophic cardiomyopathy Suspected right ventricular infarction Use of phospho-diesterase Type 5 inhibitors
Beta-blockers	Atenolol Metoprolol Various dosages	First-line therapy to control symptoms in patients with chronic stable angina	Decreases in heart rate, contractility, and atrio-ventricular (AV) node conduction Bronchoconstriction Fatigue Worsening of Raynaud's Nightmares Erectile dysfunction	Active bronchospasm Heart block greater than first degree (unless the patient has a permanent pacemaker), those with first-degree heart block and a PR interval >0.30 seconds Severe bradycardia
Calcium Channel Blockers (CCBs)	Verapamil 60–480 mg/day Diltiazem 240–360 mg/day Dihydropyridine (DHP) types: Amlodipine Felodipine	Daily therapy for Chronic stable angina if there are contraindications or adverse reactions to either beta blockers or nitrates[9]	Dose-dependent constipation Bradycardia Reduced cardiac output DHP-class CCBs Headache lightheadedness flushing Dose-dependent peripheral edema	Use with beta blockers Heart failure with reduced ejection fraction (HFrEF), sick sinus syndrome Second- or third-degree atrioventricular block DHP types CCBs Use extreme caution in patients with severe aortic stenosis[10]
Ranolazine	ranolazine 500 mg twice daily	Management of chronic stable angina-adjunctive therapy	Increase in the QT interval- monitor ECG dizziness	Hepatic cirrhosis

ACS, Acute coronary syndrome; *ECG,* electrocardiogram; *IV,* intravenous.

many places including arms (upper and forearm), wrist, hands, neck and throat, lower jaw and teeth, and upper abdomen. Risk factors for ACS include age, family history, male sex, diabetes, hypertension, dyslipidemia, and cigarette smoking. Older patients, women, and people with diabetes may have atypical presentations of ACS.

Treatment of ACS should be initiated immediately with several medication interventions. Mind Map 3.3 highlights the classes of medications for ACS. Unstable angina and NSTEMI have the same treatment while STEMI patients may be candidates for fibrinolytic therapy. Supplemental oxygen is administered to patients in respiratory distress and arterial saturation less than 90%. Sublingual nitroglycerin is administered for chest pain (three sublingual nitroglycerin tablets), and IV nitroglycerin may be used for continuous chest pain. Patients with hypotension, right ventricular infarction, and aortic stenosis cannot take nitrates. Nitrates cannot be administered if a patient took a phosphodiesterase inhibitor for erectile dysfunction within the previous 24 hours.

Antithrombotic therapy is a critical component of medical therapy for ACS. There are three antiplatelets classes used in the treatment of ACS. Aspirin is an antiplatelet agent, which acts as a cyclooxygenase (COX) enzyme inhibitor and blocks thromboxane production and inhibits platelet aggregation. Aspirin should be administered immediately at 325 mg of uncoated formulation followed by a maintenance dose of 75 to 81 mg/day. Other antiplatelets drugs that are added to aspirin in ACS include oral platelet P2Y12 receptor blockers, e.g., ticagrelor, prasugrel, or clopidogrel, and the choice depends on approach to treatment. Cangrelor is an IV P2Y12 inhibitor also available for ACS. The antiplatelet P2Y12 receptor blockers reduce platelet aggregation by blocking the adenosine diphosphate (ADP) P2Y12 receptors on platelets. The third class of antiplatelet drugs for ACS are the IV platelet glycoprotein (GP) IIb/IIIa inhibitors tirofiban, eptifibatide, and abciximab, which may be added in certain patients with high-risk ACS. These drugs inhibit platelet aggregation by blocking GP IIb/IIIa receptor

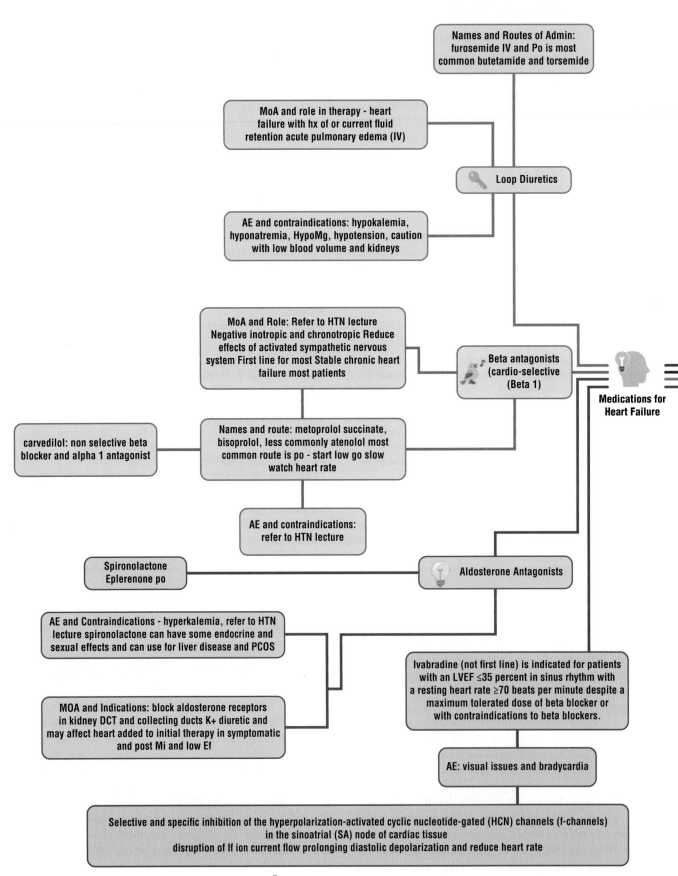

Names and Routes of Admin: furosemide IV and Po is most common butetamide and torsemide

MoA and role in therapy - heart failure with hx of or current fluid retention acute pulmonary edema (IV)

Loop Diuretics

AE and contraindications: hypokalemia, hyponatremia, HypoMg, hypotension, caution with low blood volume and kidneys

MoA and Role: Refer to HTN lecture Negative inotropic and chronotropic Reduce effects of activated sympathetic nervous system First line for most Stable chronic heart failure most patients

Beta antagonists (cardio-selective (Beta 1)

Medications for Heart Failure

carvedilol: non selective beta blocker and alpha 1 antagonist

Names and route: metoprolol succinate, bisoprolol, less commonly atenolol most common route is po - start low go slow watch heart rate

AE and contraindications: refer to HTN lecture

Spironolactone Eplerenone po

Aldosterone Antagonists

AE and Contraindications - hyperkalemia, refer to HTN lecture spironolactone can have some endocrine and sexual effects and can use for liver disease and PCOS

Ivabradine (not first line) is indicated for patients with an LVEF ≤35 percent in sinus rhythm with a resting heart rate ≥70 beats per minute despite a maximum tolerated dose of beta blocker or with contraindications to beta blockers.

MOA and Indications: block aldosterone receptors in kidney DCT and collecting ducts K+ diuretic and may affect heart added to initial therapy in symptomatic and post Mi and low Ef

AE: visual issues and bradycardia

Selective and specific inhibition of the hyperpolarization-activated cyclic nucleotide-gated (HCN) channels (f-channels) in the sinoatrial (SA) node of cardiac tissue disruption of If ion current flow prolonging diastolic depolarization and reduce heart rate

MIND MAP 3.2

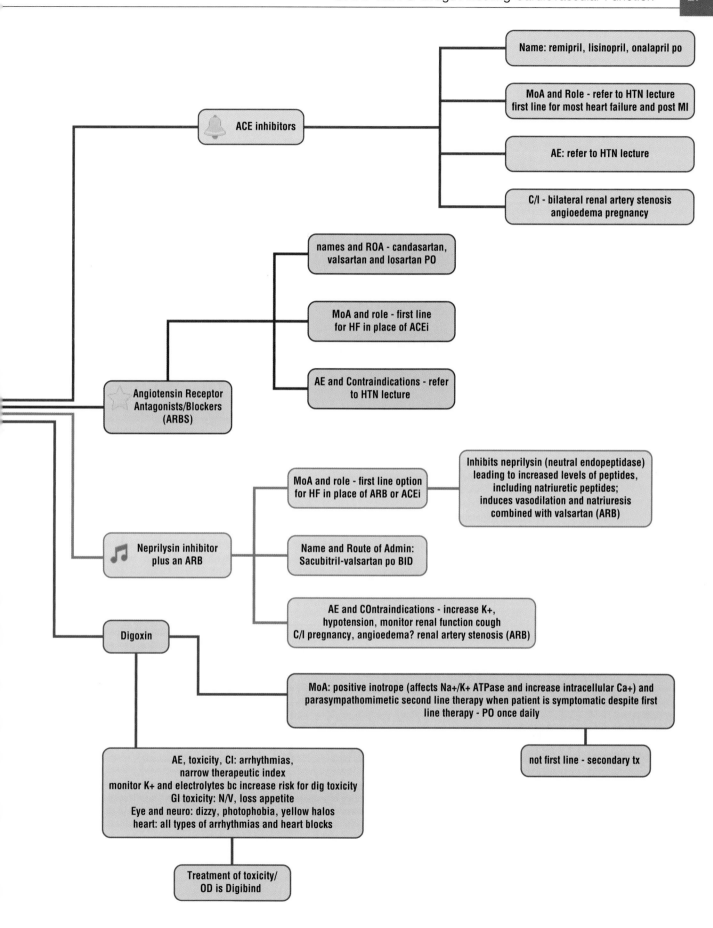

ACE inhibitors

- Name: remipril, lisinopril, onalapril po
- MoA and Role - refer to HTN lecture first line for most heart failure and post MI
- AE: refer to HTN lecture
- C/I - bilateral renal artery stenosis angioedema pregnancy

Angiotensin Receptor Antagonists/Blockers (ARBS)

- names and ROA - candasartan, valsartan and losartan PO
- MoA and role - first line for HF in place of ACEi
- AE and Contraindications - refer to HTN lecture

Neprilysin inhibitor plus an ARB

- MoA and role - first line option for HF in place of ARB or ACEi
  - Inhibits neprilysin (neutral endopeptidase) leading to increased levels of peptides, including natriuretic peptides; induces vasodilation and natriuresis combined with valsartan (ARB)
- Name and Route of Admin: Sacubitril-valsartan po BID
- AE and COntraindications - increase K+, hypotension, monitor renal function cough C/I pregnancy, angioedema? renal artery stenosis (ARB)

Digoxin

- MoA: positive inotrope (affects Na+/K+ ATPase and increase intracellular Ca+) and parasympathomimetic second line therapy when patient is symptomatic despite first line therapy - PO once daily
  - not first line - secondary tx
- AE, toxicity, CI: arrhythmias, narrow therapeutic index monitor K+ and electrolytes bc increase risk for dig toxicity GI toxicity: N/V, loss appetite Eye and neuro: dizzy, photophobia, yellow halos heart: all types of arrhythmias and heart blocks
  - Treatment of toxicity/ OD is Digibind

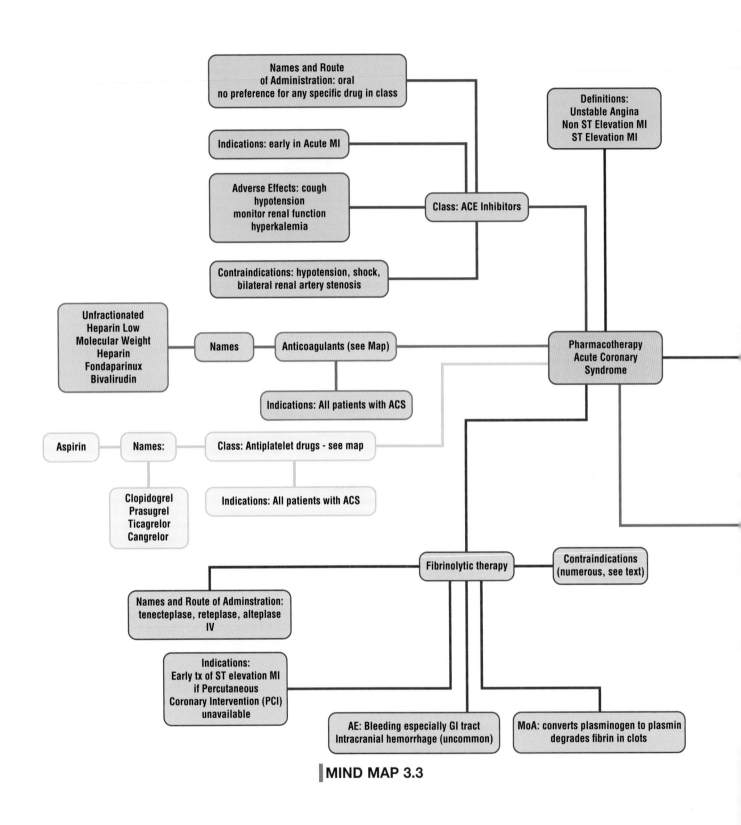

Names and Route of Administration: oral no preference for any specific drug in class

Definitions:
Unstable Angina
Non ST Elevation MI
ST Elevation MI

Indications: early in Acute MI

Adverse Effects: cough
hypotension
monitor renal function
hyperkalemia

Class: ACE Inhibitors

Contraindications: hypotension, shock, bilateral renal artery stenosis

Unfractionated Heparin Low Molecular Weight Heparin Fondaparinux Bivalirudin

Names

Anticoagulants (see Map)

Pharmacotherapy Acute Coronary Syndrome

Indications: All patients with ACS

Aspirin

Names:

Class: Antiplatelet drugs - see map

Clopidogrel
Prasugrel
Ticagrelor
Cangrelor

Indications: All patients with ACS

Fibrinolytic therapy

Contraindications (numerous, see text)

Names and Route of Adminstration: tenecteplase, reteplase, alteplase IV

Indications:
Early tx of ST elevation MI if Percutaneous Coronary Intervention (PCI) unavailable

AE: Bleeding especially GI tract Intracranial hemorrhage (uncommon)

MoA: converts plasminogen to plasmin degrades fibrin in clots

MIND MAP 3.3

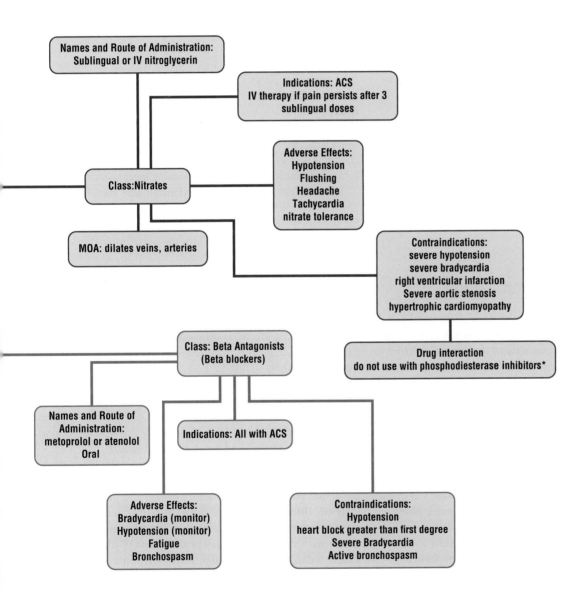

Names and Route of Administration:
Sublingual or IV nitroglycerin

Indications: ACS
IV therapy if pain persists after 3
sublingual doses

Adverse Effects:
Hypotension
Flushing
Headache
Tachycardia
nitrate tolerance

Class:Nitrates

MOA: dilates veins, arteries

Contraindications:
severe hypotension
severe bradycardia
right ventricular infarction
Severe aortic stenosis
hypertrophic cardiomyopathy

Drug interaction
do not use with phosphodiesterase inhibitors*

Class: Beta Antagonists
(Beta blockers)

Names and Route of
Administration:
metoprolol or atenolol
Oral

Indications: All with ACS

Adverse Effects:
Bradycardia (monitor)
Hypotension (monitor)
Fatigue
Bronchospasm

Contraindications:
Hypotension
heart block greater than first degree
Severe Bradycardia
Active bronchospasm

interactions. All antiplatelet drugs can increase bleeding risks. Aspirin is continued indefinitely, and antiplatelet P2Y12 receptor blocker therapy is continued for variable duration depending on management of ACS.

Three classes of anticoagulants used in the management of ACSs include heparins, such as unfractionated heparin (UFH) and low-molecular-weight heparins (LMWH); fondaparinux, which is non-heparin factor Xa inhibitor; or the direct thrombin inhibitor bivalirudin. One of the aforementioned anticoagulants is added to other medications in patients with ACS. Anticoagulants are used in the inpatient management of ACS. Bleeding is a risk associated with anticoagulants. Heparin-induced thrombocytopenia (HIT) is a risk associated with heparin, especially UFH treatment for more than 4 days.[11]

Refer to the details of the anticoagulants in Mind Map 3.7.

Fibrinolytic drugs may be indicated in certain patients with STEMI. The fibrinolytic drugs, specifically tenecteplase, reteplase, and alteplase, are administered IV as soon as possible in patients with STEMI in the absence of contraindications. There are several contraindications and adverse effects of fibrinolytic agents, which are detailed in Section 9.

Additional therapies for ACS include oral beta-blockers for most patients with ACS usually with either metoprolol or atenolol within the first 24 hours in the absence of contraindications. Details of the beta-blockers are in Section 1 of this chapter. High-intensity statin therapy to reduce low-density lipoprotein (LDL) cholesterol level is initiated during ACS in the absence of contraindications and is continued indefinitely. Statin drugs are discussed in Section 6.

SECTION 5: Antiarrhythmic Drugs

Arrhythmias are the disturbances of the normal electrical conduction of impulses in the heart. The heart beat can be too fast, too slow, or irregular and can originate in the atrium, atrioventricular (AV) junction, or ventricles. Normally, the sinoatrial node (SA) spontaneously depolarizes and sets the rate for the heart by conducting action potentials through the atria, to the AV node, to the His Purkinje fibers in the ventricles, causing contraction. Action potentials are conducted through the conducting system with the opening and closing of ions and ion channels. Action potentials in the heart are either fast or slow response and they have five phases: phase 0 is depolarization (fast Na^+ channels open, Na^+ influx into cells), phase 1 is brief repolarization (fast Na^+ channels close and K^+ open), phase 2 plateau phase (slow Ca^{2+} open), phase 3 is repolarization (K^+ channels open K^+ efflux), and phase 4 return to resting membrane potential. The atria and ventricles and specialized infranodal conduction system are fast response cells. The SA and AV nodes are slow-response tissues, and phase 0 depolarization is controlled by slower-velocity Ca^{2+} (not sodium) channels.

The different antiarrhythmic (AR) drugs are classified by their effects on cardiac action potential generation and propagation, effects on ion channels (sodium [Na^+], potassium [K^+], chloride [Cl^-], and calcium [Ca^{2+}]), and beta-adrenergic receptors. The Vaughan Williams classification system organizes AR drugs into four main classes: **Class I** drugs act by modulating or blocking the sodium channels; **Class II** drugs inhibit sympathetic activity, primarily beta-blockers; **Class III** drugs block the potassium channels, prolonging repolarization and refractory period; and **Class IV** drugs are CCBs, specifically verapamil and diltiazem. There are also miscellaneous unclassified medications such as adenosine and digoxin. Mind Map 3.4 highlights the AR drugs. Many AR drugs can have proarrhythmogenic effects and require close monitoring.

Class I AR drugs are Na^+ channel blockers and block sodium entry into cells during depolarization. They are divided into classes Ia, Ib, and Ic. Classes Ia drugs (**quinidine, procainamide, and disopyramide**) block Na^+ channels and also affect K^+ channels, have anticholinergic activity, and prolong the action potential and refractory periods. Quinidine has prominent gastrointestinal side effects and cinchonism may cause tinnitus, hearing loss, confusion, delirium, and disturbances in vision when administered) in high doses. Procainamide can cause lupus-like syndrome and has an active toxic metabolite called *NAPA*. Disopyramide has the most prominent anticholinergic effects. Class Ia drugs can cause a ventricular arrhythmia called *Torsades de Pointes*, which can also occur with some of the class III agents. Class Ib drugs (lidocaine IV and mexiletine oral [po]) block Na^+ channels in depolarized cells and are more effective for ventricular tachyarrhythmias. Lidocaine is also a local anesthetic agent.

Class Ic drugs include **propafenone** and **flecainide**; they block fast sodium channels during phase 0 and are both used for supraventricular tachycardia (SVT) and certain ventricular arrhythmias. Both drugs can have proarrhythmic effects in patients with structural heart disease. Flecainide can cause bradycardia and heart blocks, dizziness, headaches, and nausea. Propafenone has negative inotropic, chronotropic, and dromotropic effects and can cause bradycardia, heart blocks as well as nausea, taste changes, and dizziness.

Class II ARs are **beta-antagonists**, which are discussed in Chapter 2 and in the hypertension section of this chapter. Esmolol is a short-acting IV beta-blocker often used during or after surgery, propranolol is non selective, and metoprolol is beta-1 selective antagonist. Beta-blockers can be used to control rate in atrial fibrillation, treat certain SVTs, and suppress ventricular ectopic depolarizations. They are also used post-myocardial infarction and for stable heart failure.

Class III ARs are heterogeneous but generally block potassium channels during repolarization phase 3, which prolongs the action potential and refractory period and prolongs the QT interval. **Ibutilide** (IV) and **dofetilide** (po) are indicated for conversion and maintenance of atrial flutter or atrial fibrillation to normal sinus rhythm. They prolong the QT interval and can induce a dangerous ventricular tachyarrhythmia called *Torsades de pointes*. **Sotalol** is a beta-antagonist with class III potassium channel blocking effects, and it is used for atrial fibrillation and ventricular arrhythmias.

Amiodarone (IV, po) has multiple AR effects in addition to class III **potassium blocking**, beta-antagonist, Na^+ and calcium channels. It is indicated IV to terminate sustained ventricular tachycardia and ventricular fibrillation. Amiodarone has a long half-life about 40 days and a delayed onset of action, which requires loading doses. Amiodarone is used orally for suppression of SVT and ventricular arrhythmias, but it is limited by several serious adverse effects. Amiodarone can cause thyroid abnormalities, especially hypothyroidism, which requires monitoring. A potentially fatal reaction is pulmonary fibrosis, which requires monitoring with chest radiographs and pulmonary function tests. Corneal deposits are common and usually benign. Skin reactions can occur including photosensitivity and bluish-gray discoloration (blue man syndrome), especially on the face. Liver function tests should be monitored periodically to detect hepatic injury.

Class IV ARs are the **CCBs verapamil** (po, IV) and **diltiazem** (po, IV), which are described in the antihypertensive section of this chapter. They have negative dromotropic effects especially on the AV node. Verapamil and diltiazem are used to treat and suppress certain SVTs and control rate in atrial fibrillation.

Miscellaneous AR drugs include **digoxin, adenosine,** and **ivabradine**. Digoxin is described in the heart failure section of this chapter. Digoxin increases vagal tone, decreases heart rate, and slows AV node conduction velocity; it is a positive inotropic agent, which is used for rate control in atrial fibrillation and heart failure. Digoxin has multiple adverse effects including cardiac arrhythmias, neurologic, and gastrointestinal and requires serum drug monitoring. **Adenosine** is a rapid-acting (half-life of 10 seconds) IV medication used to terminate SVTs. It binds to adenosine receptors, which causes hyperpolarization and inhibits AV nodal conduction. Adverse effects are flushing, chest pressure, and shortness of breath. **Ivabradine** (po) reduces heart rate by inhibiting SA pacemaker modulating "f-current" (If). It is indicated in certain patients with reduced ejection fraction heart failure with a resting heart rate ≥ 70 beats per minute despite a maximum tolerated dose of beta-blocker or with contraindications to beta-blockers. Ivabradrine can cause bradycardia and visual disturbances of light images called *phsophenes*.[12]

SECTION 6: Treatment of Dyslipidemia

Lipids, such as cholesterol and triglyceride in the plasma are attached to carriers called *major lipoproteins*: chylomicrons; very low-density lipoprotein (VLDL); intermediate-density lipoprotein; LDL; and high-density lipoprotein (HDL). These lipoproteins transport lipids to tissues and the liver for energy utilization, steroid hormone production, and bile acid formation in the liver. A serum lipid panel detects various abnormalities in lipids (dyslipidemias) and can be used to screen, diagnose, and manage patients with dyslipidemia. Dyslipidemia is very common and elevated total, and LDL cholesterol levels are one of the risk factors for atherosclerotic cardiovascular disease (CVD). Lipid-lowering medications may be added to lifestyle modifications such as weight loss in overweight or obese patients, increased aerobic exercise, and diets lower in saturated fats, for primary prevention of CVD in high-risk patients. Ten-year cardiovascular risk assessment in addition to determination of LDL-C levels guide therapy for patients. Lipid-lowering medications are recommended for secondary

prevention in patients with existing CVD to reduce the risk of subsequent events.

Medications used to treat dyslipidemia include the following classes/drugs:
- 3-Hydroxy-3-methylglutaryl-coenzyme A (HMG-CoA) reductase inhibitors or statins.
- fibric acid derivatives (fibrates).
- nicotinic acid derivatives (niacin).
- bile acid resins.
- ezetimibe, an inhibitor of intestinal cholesterol absorption.
- inhibitors of proprotein convertase subtilisin/kexin type 9 (PCSK9).
- bempedoic acid and oral inhibitor of adenosine triphosphate (ATP) citrate lyase.
- Evinacumab is a fully human monoclonal antibody against angiopoietin-like protein 3 (ANGPTL3).
- lomitapide is an inhibitor of microsomal triglyceride transfer protein (MTP).

These medications are highlighted in Mind Map 3.5.

The **HMG coenzyme A reductase inhibitors**, aka **statins**, are the most used medications and are the generally preferred lipid-lowering medications for primary and secondary prevention of CVS. Statins include atorvastatin, simvastatin, rosuvastatin, pitavastatin, as well as fluvastatin, pravastatin, and lovastatin, which are less efficacious. The statins inhibit cholesterol synthesis in the liver by competitively inhibiting HMG coenzyme A reductase, which is the enzyme that catalyzes the rate-limiting step of cholesterol synthesis. Statins are administered orally once daily in various dosages to lower LDL-C as well as cholesterol. The dosage of statin depends on the intensity of LDL lowering required; high-intensity statin therapy ($\geq 50\%$ LDL-C reduction) is recommended for secondary prevention and very high LDL primary prevention, whereas moderate-intensity statin therapy (30–50% LDL-C reduction) is recommended for primary prevention in patients with 10-year cardiovascular risk $>10\%$. LDL-C is monitored 6 to 8 weeks after initiation of lipid-lowering therapy to assess response and annually thereafter.

The primary adverse effects of statins are hepatic dysfunction and muscle injury. Liver function tests are indicated prior to initiation of therapy and if clinically indicated. Muscle symptoms are variable with statins, but severe muscle injury with myonecrosis is rare. The presence of muscle weakness and soreness with elevated creatine kinase levels within weeks to months of initiating statin therapy may necessitate temporary discontinuation. Risk factors for statin-associated muscle symptoms include hypothyroidism, low vitamin D, chronic liver and kidney disease, and use of fibrates and concomitant medications that inhibit CYP3A4. Statins are substrates for CYP3A4 and may be associated with drug interactions; pitavastatin is less metabolized than other statins. Statins should not be used during pregnancy or breastfeeding or in patients with active liver disease.

Fibrates are generally used for moderate to severe hypertriglyceridemia despite lifestyle interventions. Fibrates are agonists for the nuclear transcription factor peroxisome proliferator-activated receptor-alpha), which inhibits VLDL synthesis, increases VLDL catabolism, and increases lipoprotein lipase,

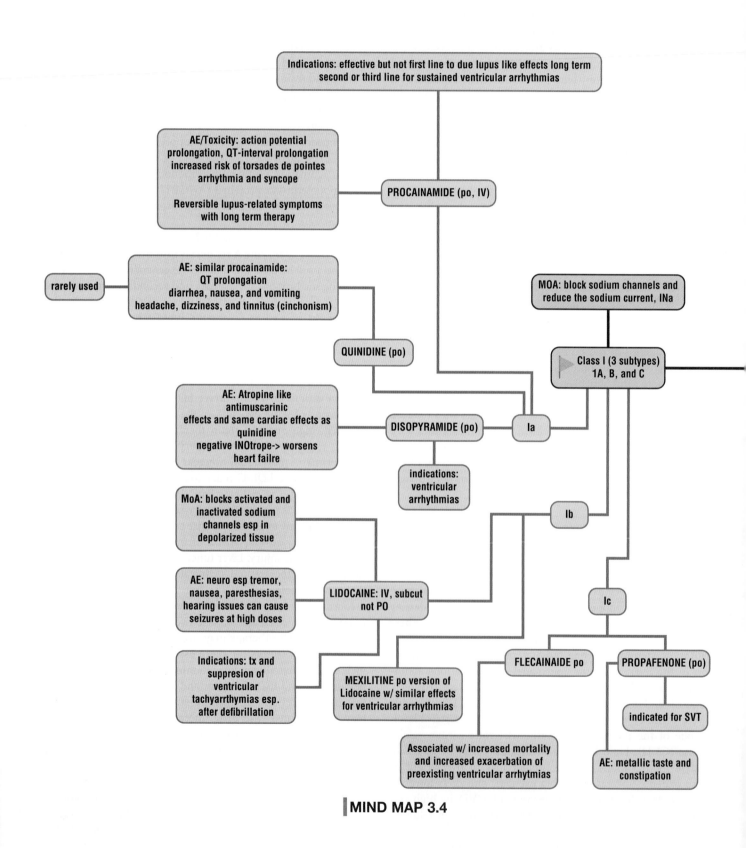

MIND MAP 3.4

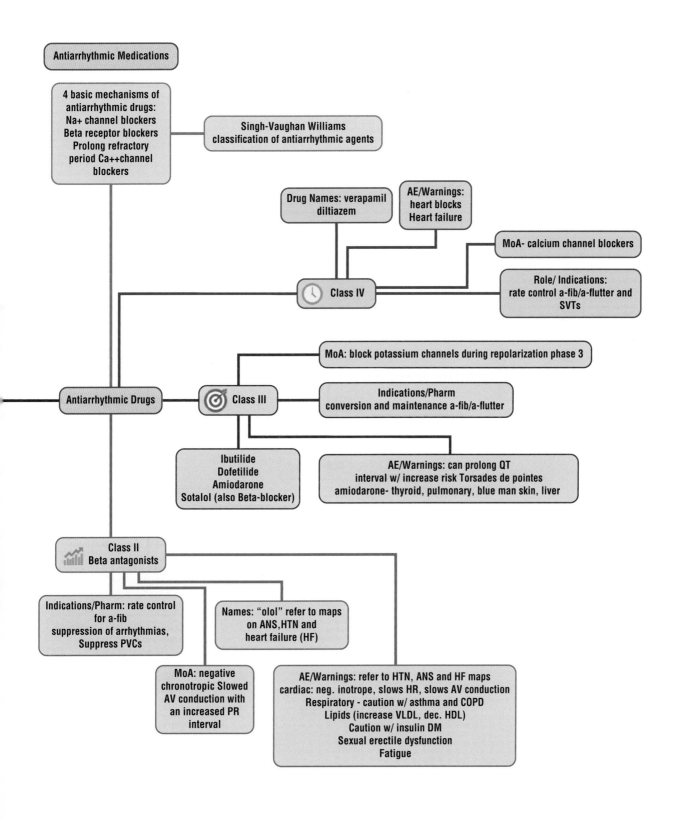

Antiarrhythmic Medications

4 basic mechanisms of antiarrhythmic drugs:
Na+ channel blockers
Beta receptor blockers
Prolong refractory period Ca++channel blockers

Singh-Vaughan Williams classification of antiarrhythmic agents

Drug Names: verapamil diltiazem

AE/Warnings: heart blocks Heart failure

MoA- calcium channel blockers

Class IV

Role/ Indications: rate control a-fib/a-flutter and SVTs

MoA: block potassium channels during repolarization phase 3

Antiarrhythmic Drugs

Class III

Indications/Pharm conversion and maintenance a-fib/a-flutter

Ibutilide
Dofetilide
Amiodarone
Sotalol (also Beta-blocker)

AE/Warnings: can prolong QT interval w/ increase risk Torsades de pointes
amiodarone- thyroid, pulmonary, blue man skin, liver

**Class II
Beta antagonists**

Indications/Pharm: rate control for a-fib
suppression of arrhythmias, Suppress PVCs

Names: "olol" refer to maps on ANS,HTN and heart failure (HF)

MoA: negative chronotropic Slowed AV conduction with an increased PR interval

AE/Warnings: refer to HTN, ANS and HF maps
cardiac: neg. inotrope, slows HR, slows AV conduction
Respiratory - caution w/ asthma and COPD
Lipids (increase VLDL, dec. HDL)
Caution w/ insulin DM
Sexual erectile dysfunction
Fatigue

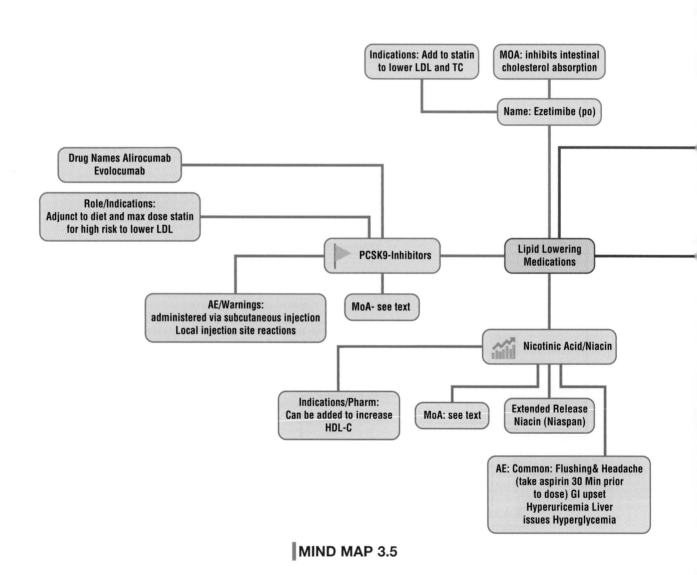

Indications: Add to statin to lower LDL and TC

MOA: inhibits intestinal cholesterol absorption

Name: Ezetimibe (po)

Drug Names Alirocumab Evolocumab

Role/Indications: Adjunct to diet and max dose statin for high risk to lower LDL

PCSK9-Inhibitors

Lipid Lowering Medications

AE/Warnings: administered via subcutaneous injection Local injection site reactions

MoA- see text

Nicotinic Acid/Niacin

Indications/Pharm: Can be added to increase HDL-C

MoA: see text

Extended Release Niacin (Niaspan)

AE: Common: Flushing& Headache (take aspirin 30 Min prior to dose) GI upset Hyperuricemia Liver issues Hyperglycemia

MIND MAP 3.5

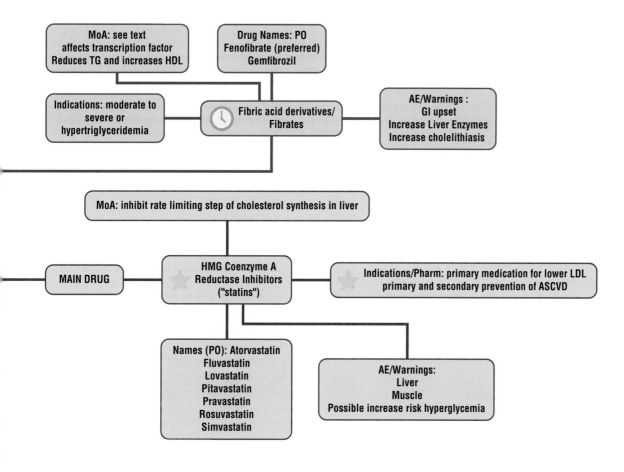

MoA: see text
affects transcription factor
Reduces TG and increases HDL

Drug Names: PO
Fenofibrate (preferred)
Gemfibrozil

Indications: moderate to
severe or
hypertriglyceridemia

Fibric acid derivatives/
Fibrates

AE/Warnings :
GI upset
Increase Liver Enzymes
Increase cholelithiasis

MoA: inhibit rate limiting step of cholesterol synthesis in liver

MAIN DRUG

HMG Coenzyme A
Reductase Inhibitors
("statins")

Indications/Pharm: primary medication for lower LDL
primary and secondary prevention of ASCVD

Names (PO): Atorvastatin
Fluvastatin
Lovastatin
Pitavastatin
Pravastatin
Rosuvastatin
Simvastatin

AE/Warnings:
Liver
Muscle
Possible increase risk hyperglycemia

causing a decrease in triglycerides. Fibrates can also increase HDL levels. Available fibrates include oral fenofibrate once daily in various preparations and gemfibrozil orally twice daily; fenofibrate is preferred because it is better tolerated and has few drug interactions. The main adverse effects of the fibrates are drug-induced liver injury and myopathy, especially when gemfibrozil is combined with statin.

Bile acid resins are uncommonly used for dyslipidemia because they are not well tolerated and less effective at lowering LDL than statins. The available bile acid resins cholestyramine, colestipol, and colesevelam bind bile acids in the intestine and reduce reabsorption of bile acids causing reduction in the intrahepatic cholesterol, which increases the liver's LDL receptors thereby increasing hepatic uptake of LDL-C. Gastrointestinal adverse effects including nausea, bloating, and constipation are very common. Bile acid resins affect absorption of other drugs, so other drugs should be administered 1 hour before or 4 hours after the bile acid resin. Colesevalam is best tolerated of the bile acid resins and can be used in pregnancy.

Nicotinic acid derivatives (niacin) can be used for increasing HDL-C and lowering triglycerides, although it is not specifically associated with a cardiovascular benefit to increase isolated low HDL-C levels.[13] Niacin may work by increasing lipoprotein lipase activity, which reduces triglycerides and decreasing the breakdown of HDL.[14] Nicotinic acid derivatives are limited by significant adverse effects including flushing, which is very common and can be accompanied by nausea, pruritus, and paresthesias. Ibuprofen or aspirin administration 1 hour prior to niacin reduces flushing and related symptoms. Niacin can increase blood glucose, increase liver enzymes with potential for hepatotoxicity, and should be avoided in patients with gout because it can cause hyperuricemia. Niacin is available by prescription as controlled-release niacin, which is a controlled-release formulation of nicotinic acid that is administered once daily. There are also several over-the-counter formulations of nicotinic acid.

Ezetimibe, an inhibitor of intestinal cholesterol absorption, can be used as monotherapy in patients who are intolerant to statins or as adjunctive therapy to diet and an HMG-CoA reductase inhibitor to lower triglycerides and LDL-C. It is administered orally once daily. The adverse effects of ezetimibe include an increased risk for liver and muscle injury with concomitant statin use, but it is otherwise well tolerated.

PCSK9 inhibitors are antibodies that interfere with PCSK9 enzymes; PCSK9 enzymes degrade LDL-C receptors on the liver, which increases LDL-C in the blood. PCSK9 inhibitors are indicated for homozygous FH to reduce LDL-C as an adjunct to diet in combination with other LDL-C-lowering therapies in adults with primary hyperlipidemia. Alirocumab and evolocumab are PCSK9 inhibitors, which are administered subcutaneously once or twice a month and are expensive. They are well tolerated with injection site reactions and occasionally hypersensitivity reactions such as rash, pruritus, and urticaria.

Bempedoic acid is an oral inhibitor of ATP citrate lyase, which is an enzyme in the cholesterol biosynthesis pathway in the liver. It is indicated to reduce LDL-C, as an adjunct to diet,

and maximally tolerated statin therapy for secondary prevention of established atherosclerotic CVD and for heterozygous FH. It can cause hyperuricemia and gout, especially in the first 4 weeks of therapy.[15]

Evinacumab is a fully human monoclonal antibody against ANGPTL3 and is US Food and Drug Administration approved for homozygous FH as an adjunct to other LDL-lowering therapies. It is administered as IV infusion every 4 weeks. Evinacumab inhibits ANGPTL3, which inhibits lipoprotein lipase and endothelial lipase, leading to reduced triglycerides and LDL-C. Adverse effects include nasopharyngitis and infusion reactions, and it should not be used in pregnant women.[16]

Lomitapide is an oral inhibitor of MTP approved for homozygous FH as an adjunct to diet and other lipid-lowering treatments. Gastrointestinal adverse effects including diarrhea, nausea, dyspepsia, and vomiting are common. It has a boxed warning of hepatotoxicity and hepatic fat accumulation, and it is contraindicated in pregnancy. Lomitapide is associated with potential drug interactions.

Combination lipid-lowering therapy may be required for secondary prevention of CVD in people who do not meet LDL goals despite maximal statin doses. Ezetimibe is usually added to statin therapy in these patients. PCSK9 inhibitors may be added if LDL levels are not at goal levels despite statins and ezetimibe.[17]

SECTION 7: Antiplatelets (Mind Map 3.6)

Platelets play an essential role in hemostasis; after injury to a blood vessel, vasospasm occurs and platelets adhere, activate, and aggregate to the site to form a platelet plug. Antiplatelet therapies include medications from four classes that target different aspects of platelet biology; (1) COX inhibitors, which decrease thromboxaneA_2 (aspirin); (2) ADP P2Y12 receptor blockers (clopidogrel, ticlopidine, prasugrel, ticagrelor, cangrelor); (3) GP IIb/IIIa antibodies and receptor antagonists (e.g., abciximab, tirofiban, eptifibatide); and (4) protease-activated receptor-1, or PAR-1, antagonists (vorapaxar). Miscellaneous antiplatelet drugs include **dipyridamole**, combined with aspirin for secondary prevention of cerebrovascular disease; and **cilostazol**, which is used for intermittent claudication in patients with peripheral arterial disease (PAD).

Dual antiplatelet therapy with aspirin and an ADP P2Y12 receptor blocker is standard treatment for most patients with ACS.

Aspirin is a nonsteroidal antiinflammatory drug (NSAID) that inhibits platelet aggregation by irreversibly inhibiting COX enzymes in platelets and decreasing thromboxaneA_2. Aspirin is administered orally for acute treatment of ACS and transient ischemic attacks (TIA), PAD, secondary prevention of MI and thromboembolic stroke, and primary prevention in certain patients with multiple cardiovascular risk factors. Adverse effects of aspirin include gastrointestinal injury, ulceration and bleeding, kidney dysfunction, and, in high doses, salicylism. Contraindications to aspirin include hypersensitivity to NSAIDs; patients with asthma, allergic rhinitis, and nasal polyps; and use in children or teenagers for viral infections.

The antiplatelet class of ADP P2Y12 receptor blockers include **clopidogrel, ticlopidine, prasugrel, ticagrelor**, and **cangrelor**. These drugs bind to P2Y12 receptors and inhibit ADP binding and platelet aggregation. Clopidogrel and prasugrel are oral prodrugs and are activated by the cytochrome P450 (CYP) system. Clopidogrel is associated with more drug interactions and potential for decreased efficacy in patients with two loss-of-function alleles of the *CYP2C19* gene. Ticagrelor (po) and cangrelor (IV) are active drugs with a rapid onset of action. ADP P2Y12 receptor blockers are used in combination with aspirin for ACS for primary and secondary prevention of MI or stroke in high-risk patients with coronary artery disease. The dosage of aspirin should be <100 mg/day when given with ticagrelor. Adverse effects are mainly bleeding, both minor and major types. Contraindications include active abnormal bleeding, and prasugrel is also contraindicated in patients with history of TIA or stroke.

GP IIb/IIIa antibodies and receptor antagonists (e.g., **abciximab, tirofiban, eptifibatide**) block the final step in platelet aggregation. They are administered IV in some patients with ACS undergoing percutaneous coronary intervention. Bleeding is the major adverse effect, and there are multiple contraindications, including active abnormal bleeding, severe uncontrolled hypertension, history of hemorrhagic stroke.

Protease-activated receptor-1, or PAR-1, antagonist (**vorapaxar**) is an oral antiplatelet drug used for prevention of thrombotic cardiovascular events in patients with history of MI or PAD. Vorapaxar binds to PAR-1 and inhibits thrombin-mediated platelet activation. The most common adverse effect is bleeding, and vorapaxar is contraindicated in patients with a history of stroke or active abnormal bleeding.

SECTION 8: Anticoagulants
(Mind Map 3.7)

Anticoagulant medications interfere with blood coagulation by affecting various components of the coagulation cascade. Fig. 3.1 illustrates the coagulation cascade. Primary indications for anticoagulant therapy include prevention and treatment of venous thromboembolism (VTE), e.g., deep vein thrombosis, and pulmonary embolism, prevention of ischemic stroke, and other embolic events in patients with atrial fibrillation, prevention of valve thrombosis, and thromboembolic events in patients with prosthetic heart valves.

There are several classes of anticoagulants:
- Antithrombin inhibitors, which include heparins (UFH), LMWH, and fondaparinux.
- Vitamin K antagonists (VKA) (e.g., warfarin).
- Direct-acting oral anticoagulants ("non-vitamin K antagonist oral anticoagulants" or NOACs), which include
  - direct thrombin inhibitors (e.g., dabigatran) and
  - direct factor Xa inhibitors (e.g., rivaroxaban, apixaban, edoxaban).

Heparins, including **UFH** and a variety of **LMW heparin** products (enoxaparin, dalteparin, tinzaparin), are administered subcutaneously or IV. Heparins inhibit the clotting factors thrombin (IIa), IXa, and Xa by binding to and potentiating the effects of endogenous anticoagulant antithrombin. The dosage form for most forms of heparin is units; enoxaparin and fondaparinux are dosed in milligrams.

Heparin requires monitoring for efficacy and toxicity. Laboratory monitoring of heparin includes primarily partial thromboplastin time (PTT) to determine efficacy and overdosage and platelet counts to assess thrombocytopenia. Adverse effects of heparin include bleeding and HIT. HIT is a drug-induced immunologic condition that causes thrombosis and thrombocytopenia. HIT is more common in surgical patients taking UFH for more than 4 days. Treatment of HIT is cessation of heparin and initiation of parenteral direct thrombin inhibitors or fondaparinux.[18] Contraindications to heparin are active bleeding, history of HIT, hemophilia, significant thrombocytopenia, and advanced liver or kidney disease. Excessive heparin and associated bleeding are treated by heparin discontinuation and IV **protamine sulfate**.

Fondaparinux is a long-acting small heparin-like molecule that binds to antithrombin and inhibits factor Xa. It is administered once daily subcutaneously. It is an option for prevention and treatment of VTE in patients with acute or remote histories of HIT. Bleeding is the primary adverse effect, including spinal hematomas in patients undergoing epidural or spinal anesthesia. Bleeding can be reversed with the antidote, **andexanet alfa**. Contraindications to fondaparinux include severe renal impairment and active major bleeding.[19]

Vitamin K antagonists (VKA) (e.g., **warfarin**) are administered orally once daily for prevention of venous thromboembolism, prevention of thrombotic complications of prosthetic valves, and prevention of stroke in patients with atrial fibrillation. Warfarin inhibits vitamin K epoxide reductase in the liver, which depletes functional vitamin K and reduces the synthesis of active clotting factors, proteins C and S. Warfarin has a delayed onset of anticoagulation, and its full therapeutic effect takes 5 to 7 days after initiation of therapy. Patients who require immediate anticoagulation generally receive a heparin product to bridge warfarin therapy. Regular monitoring of the **international normalized ratio** blood test is required in patients taking warfarin. Warfarin has multiple drug and food interactions; specifically foods high in vitamin K (e.g., leafy green vegetables) can decrease the anticoagulant effect of warfarin. Genetic variations in vitamin K epoxide reductase and *CYP2C9* gene can cause variations in warfarin dose requirements. Adverse effects of warfarin include minor and major bleeding and gastrointestinal effects. Warfarin-associated bleeding is reversed with oral or IV **vitamin K,** and in cases of serious major bleeding, IV 4-factor prothrombin complex concentrate is administered. Warfarin is contraindicated in pregnancy (teratogenic), abnormal active bleeding, malignant hypertension, and recent surgeries.[20]

Direct factor Xa inhibitors (e.g., rivaroxaban, apixaban, edoxaban) are oral anticoagulants that inactivate circulating and clot-bound factor Xa. Direct factor Xa inhibitors have similar indications as warfarin, but they are not used for mechanical heart valves, pregnancy, or antiphospholipid syndrome. Routine laboratory monitoring is not required, but baseline serum creatinine, prothrombin time (PT), PTT, and

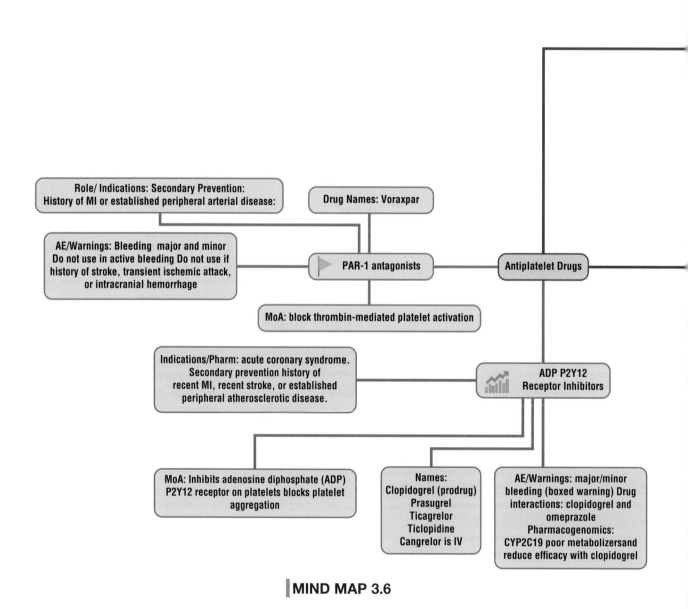

Role/ Indications: Secondary Prevention: History of MI or established peripheral arterial disease:

Drug Names: Voraxpar

AE/Warnings: Bleeding major and minor Do not use in active bleeding Do not use if history of stroke, transient ischemic attack, or intracranial hemorrhage

PAR-1 antagonists

Antiplatelet Drugs

MoA: block thrombin-mediated platelet activation

Indications/Pharm: acute coronary syndrome. Secondary prevention history of recent MI, recent stroke, or established peripheral atherosclerotic disease.

ADP P2Y12 Receptor Inhibitors

MoA: Inhibits adenosine diphosphate (ADP) P2Y12 receptor on platelets blocks platelet aggregation

Names: Clopidogrel (prodrug) Prasugrel Ticagrelor Ticlopidine Cangrelor is IV

AE/Warnings: major/minor bleeding (boxed warning) Drug interactions: clopidogrel and omeprazole Pharmacogenomics: CYP2C19 poor metabolizersand reduce efficacy with clopidogrel

MIND MAP 3.6

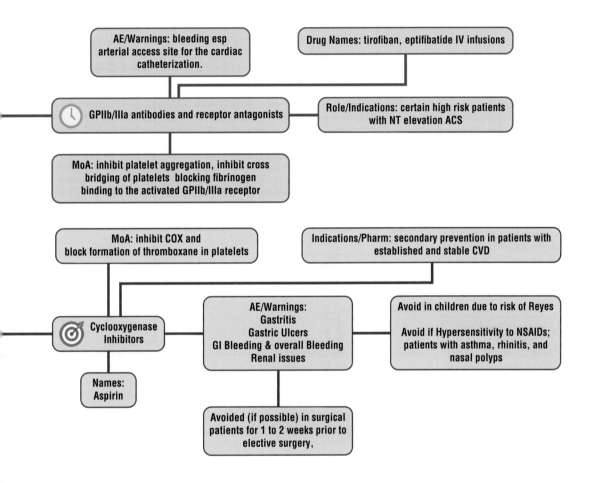

AE/Warnings: bleeding esp arterial access site for the cardiac catheterization.

Drug Names: tirofiban, eptifibatide IV infusions

GPIIb/IIIa antibodies and receptor antagonists

Role/Indications: certain high risk patients with NT elevation ACS

MoA: inhibit platelet aggregation, inhibit cross bridging of platelets blocking fibrinogen binding to the activated GPIIb/IIIa receptor

MoA: inhibit COX and block formation of thromboxane in platelets

Indications/Pharm: secondary prevention in patients with established and stable CVD

Cyclooxygenase Inhibitors

AE/Warnings:
Gastritis
Gastric Ulcers
GI Bleeding & overall Bleeding
Renal issues

Avoid in children due to risk of Reyes

Avoid if Hypersensitivity to NSAIDs; patients with asthma, rhinitis, and nasal polyps

Names:
Aspirin

Avoided (if possible) in surgical patients for 1 to 2 weeks prior to elective surgery,

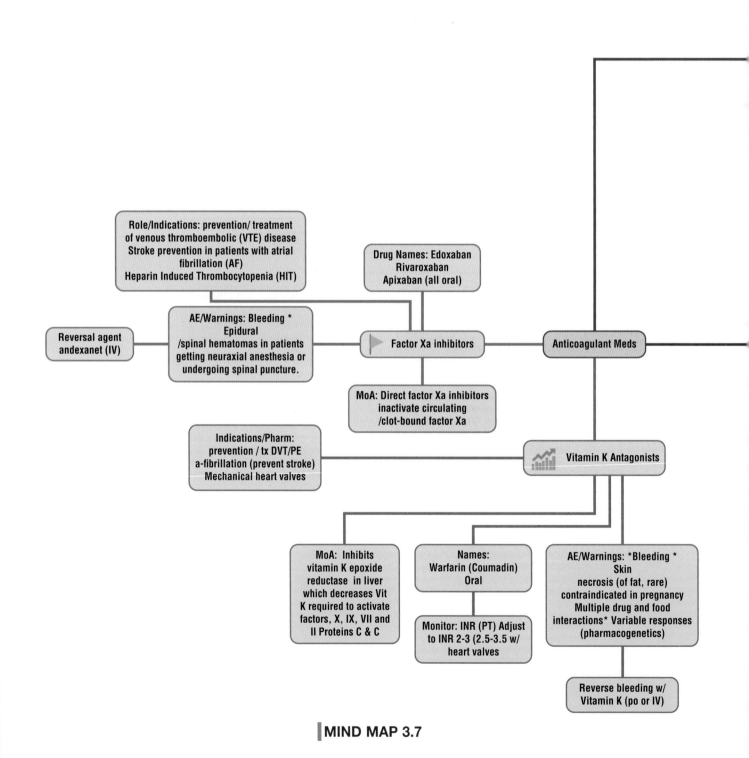

Role/Indications: prevention/ treatment of venous thromboembolic (VTE) disease Stroke prevention in patients with atrial fibrillation (AF) Heparin Induced Thrombocytopenia (HIT)

Drug Names: Edoxaban Rivaroxaban Apixaban (all oral)

Reversal agent andexanet (IV)

AE/Warnings: Bleeding * Epidural /spinal hematomas in patients getting neuraxial anesthesia or undergoing spinal puncture.

Factor Xa inhibitors

Anticoagulant Meds

MoA: Direct factor Xa inhibitors inactivate circulating /clot-bound factor Xa

Indications/Pharm: prevention / tx DVT/PE a-fibrillation (prevent stroke) Mechanical heart valves

Vitamin K Antagonists

MoA: Inhibits vitamin K epoxide reductase in liver which decreases Vit K required to activate factors, X, IX, VII and II Proteins C & C

Names: Warfarin (Coumadin) Oral

AE/Warnings: *Bleeding * Skin necrosis (of fat, rare) contraindicated in pregnancy Multiple drug and food interactions* Variable responses (pharmacogenetics)

Monitor: INR (PT) Adjust to INR 2-3 (2.5-3.5 w/ heart valves)

Reverse bleeding w/ Vitamin K (po or IV)

MIND MAP 3.7

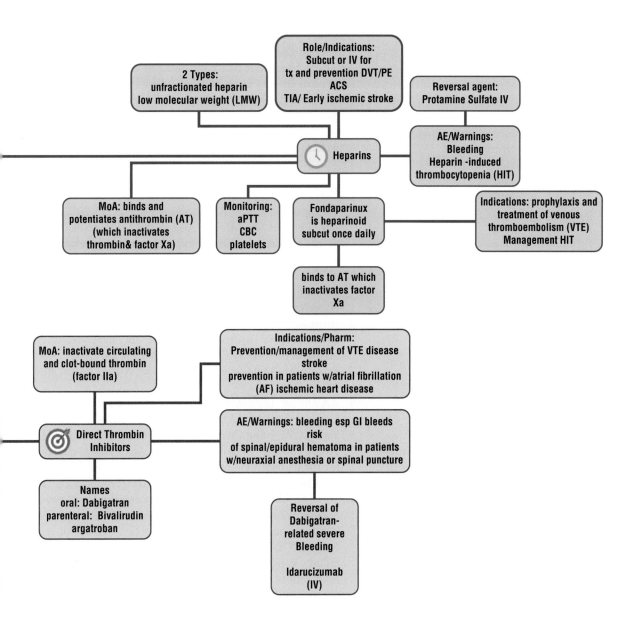

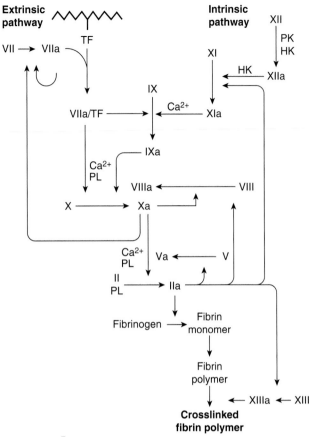

FIG. 3.1 Coagulation cascade.

platelet counts should be established. Bleeding is the primary risk associated with direct Xa inhibitors, and the emergency reversal agent is IV **andexanet**.

Direct thrombin inhibitors (e.g., dabigatran) are anticoagulants that inactivate circulating and clot-bound thrombin (factor IIa). Parenteral direct thrombin inhibitors include **bivalirudin** and **argatroban**, which are indicated for percutaneous coronary interventions and HIT. Dabigatran is an oral direct thrombin inhibitor indicated for thromboembolism prevention in atrial fibrillation and prevention and treatment of VTE. Bleeding is the main adverse effect of direct thrombin inhibitors; dabigatran can also cause dyspepsia. **Idarucizumab** is a monoclonal antibody that can emergently reverse the effects of dabigatran. Routine monitoring of the direct-acting Xa and direct thrombin inhibitors is not required, but baseline laboratories PT, PTT, platelets, and renal function should be established.[21]

SECTION 9: Fibrinolytic drugs

Fibrinolytic drugs lyse thrombi by converting plasminogen into plasmin, which degrades fibrin clots. Alteplase, reteplase, and tenecteplase are parenteral tissue plasminogen activators that activate plasminogen that is bound to fibrin. Indications for the fibrinolytic drugs include STEMI, hemodynamically unstable pulmonary embolism, severe DVT, and acute ischemic stroke

within 3 hours of symptom onset. Bleeding, internal and external, especially at vascular access sites, and intracranial hemorrhage are the most serious adverse effects.

There are several contraindications including active internal bleeding; history of recent stroke; recent (within 3 months [American College of Cardiology Heart Failure Classification/American Heart Association: within 2 months]) intracranial or intraspinal surgery or serious head trauma; presence of intracranial conditions that may increase the risk of bleeding (e.g., intracranial neoplasm, arteriovenous malformation, aneurysm); known bleeding diathesis; and severe uncontrolled hypertension.[22]

REFERENCES

1. Whelton PK, Carey RM, Aronow WS, et al. 2017 ACC/AHA/AAPA/ABC/ACPM/AGS/APhA/ASH/ASPC/NMA/PCNA Guideline for the prevention, detection, evaluation, and management of high blood pressure in adults: a report of the American College of Cardiology/American Heart Association Task Force on Clinical Practice Guidelines. *Hypertension.* 2018;71:e13.
2. Jamerson K, Weber MA, Bakris GL, et al. Benazepril plus amlodipine or hydrochlorothiazide for hypertension in high-risk patients. *N Engl J Med.* 2008;359:2417.
3. Peixoto AJ. Acute severe hypertension. *N Engl J Med.* 2019; 381:1843.
4. AA-Diltiaz (diltiazem) [product monograph]. Vaughan, Ontario, Canada: AA Pharma Inc; April 2020.
5. Yancy CW, Jessup M, Bozkurt B, et al. 2017 ACC/AHA/HFSA Focused Update of the 2013 ACCF/AHA guideline for the management of heart failure: a report of the American College of Cardiology/American Heart Association Task Force on Clinical Practice Guidelines and the Heart Failure Society of America. *Circulation.* 2017;136:e137.
6. Writing Committee Members, Yancy CW, Jessup M, et al. 2013 ACCF/AHA guideline for the management of heart failure: a report of the American College of Cardiology Foundation/American Heart Association Task Force on practice guidelines. *Circulation.* 2013;128:e240.
7. Groenning BA, Nilsson JC, Sondergaard L, et al. Anti Remodeling effects on the left ventricle during beta-blockade with metoprolol in the treatment of chronic heart failure. *J Am Coll Cardiol.* 2000;36:2072.
8. Beyder A, Strege PR, Reyes S, et al. Ranolazine decreases mechanosensitivity of the voltage-gated sodium ion channel Na(v)1.5: a novel mechanism of drug action. *Circulation.* 2012;125:2698.
9. Fihn SD, Blankenship JC, Alexander KP, et al. 2014 ACC/AHA/AATS/PCNA/SCAI/STS focused update of the guideline for the diagnosis and management of patients with stable ischemic heart disease: a report of the American College of Cardiology/American Heart Association Task Force on Practice Guidelines, and the American Association for Thoracic Surgery, Preventive Cardiovascular Nurses Association, Society for Cardiovascular Angiography and Interventions, and Society of Thoracic Surgeons. *J Am Coll Cardiol.* 2014;64:1929.

10. Norvasc (amlodipine) [prescribing information]. New York, NY: Pfizer Labs; January 2019.

11. Martel N, Lee J, Wells PS. Risk for heparin-induced thrombocytopenia with unfractionated and low-molecular-weight heparin thromboprophylaxis: a meta-analysis. *Blood.* 2005; 106:2710.

12. Corlanor (ivabradine) [prescribing information]. Thousand Oaks, CA: Amgen Inc; August 2021.

13. AIM-HIGH Investigators, Boden WE, Probstfield JL, et al. Niacin in patients with low HDL cholesterol levels receiving intensive statin therapy. *N Engl J Med.* 2011;365:2255.

14. Niaspan (niacin) extended-release tablet [prescribing information]. North Chicago, IL: AbbVie Inc; September 2020.

15. Nexletol (bempedoic acid) [prescribing information]. Ann Arbor, MI: Esperion Therapeutics Inc; September 2021.

16. Evkeeza (evinacumab) [prescribing information]. Tarrytown, NY: Regeneron Pharmaceuticals Inc; February 2021.

17. Rosenson RS, Hegele RA, Fazio S, Cannon CP. The evolving future of PCSK9 inhibitors. *J Am Coll Cardiol.* 2018; 72:314.

18. Greinacher A. Clinical practice. Heparin-induced thrombocytopenia. *N Engl J Med.* 2015;373:252.

19. Andexxa (andexanet alfa) [prescribing information]. Boston, MA: Alexion Pharmaceuticals Inc; February 2021.

20. Coumadin (warfarin) [prescribing information]. Princeton, NJ: Bristol-Meyers Squibb Company; December 2019.

21. Reilly PA, Lehr T, Haertter S, et al. The effect of dabigatran plasma concentrations and patient characteristics on the frequency of ischemic stroke and major bleeding in atrial fibrillation patients: the RE-LY Trial (Randomized Evaluation of Long-Term Anticoagulation Therapy). *J Am Coll Cardiol.* 2014;63:321.

22. Cathflo Activase (alteplase) [prescribing information]. South San Francisco, CA: Genentech Inc; February 2019.

CHAPTER 4

Pulmonary Pharmacology

DRUGS USED TO TREAT ASTHMA

Asthma is a common, often chronic condition of the airways caused by underlying inflammation and bronchial hyperreactivity. The clinical presentation is variable and is characterized by recurring respiratory symptoms such as cough, wheezing, and difficulty breathing or shortness of breath. Spirometry testing is used to evaluate and diagnose patients, stage asthma, and assess response and control of asthma with medications. Assessment of asthma is based on frequency and intensity of asthma symptoms, nocturnal symptoms, frequency of rescue/relief inhaler use, impairment of activities, and number of asthma exacerbations. Asthma severity is categorized as one of the following: mild intermittent, mild persistent, moderate persistent, severe persistent, and severe persistent that is poorly controlled. Pharmacotherapy is determined by asthma severity in a "stepwise" approach and level of asthma control. According to asthma experts, well-controlled asthma is characterized by daytime symptoms no more than twice per week and nighttime awakening due to asthma no more than twice per month.[1]

Goals of asthma treatment include relief of symptoms, improvement in ability to perform activities, and reduction or elimination of acute exacerbations. The route of administration for most asthma medications is via inhalation using inhalers and nebulizers. The types of medications are bronchodilators, antiinflammatory drugs, and biologic agents.

TYPES OF DEVICES

The primary route of administration for asthma medication is via inhalation using various types of inhaler devices. There are three main types of inhaler devices: the pressurized metered-dose inhaler (pMDI), the dry-powder inhaler (DPI), and the soft-mist inhaler (SMI). The metered-dose inhaler is a pressurized canister that contains a drug suspended with inactive propellants and other ingredients. Most MDIs propel a dose of medicine in each "puff" that is released by pressing the top of the inhaler; a breath-actuated MDI delivers a dose when patient breathes in thorough the mouthpiece. Most MDIs must be shaken before each use and primed before initial use. Priming an inhaler requires shaking and spraying two to four doses in

the air to ensure mixing of medication with propellant. Patients should be instructed to press the inhaler while breathing in and then hold breath for 5 to 10 seconds with each puff.

Other inhalers include the DPI and SMI. DPIs are breath-actuated devices that deliver micronized powdered drug particles by inhalation with single- or multi dose inhaler devices. Patients insert mouthpiece of inhaler into their mouth, close lips tightly around the mouthpiece, and breathe in quickly and forcefully, then remove the inhaler and hold breath for 5 to 10 seconds. Soft-mist inhalers (SMIs) are propellant-free inhalers used for chronic obstructive pulmonary disease (COPD), which produces a lower-velocity, sustained-release mist. Techniques for using SMIs and MDIs are similar.

Valved holding chambers (VHCs) and spacers extend the mouthpiece of the inhaler and decrease the deposition of medication in the oropharynx. A spacer is usually an open-ended tube or bag, and a VHC is a spacer with a one-way valve to direct inspiratory flow and prevent accidental exhalation into the device. Spacers and VHCs are spacers that are used with inhaled corticosteroids to decrease oropharyngeal drug deposition, thrush, and voice changes. They are helpful for young children and in patients with difficulty coordinating breathing with actuation of the MDI. Spacers can be fitted with masks for use in young children and infants.

Nebulizers are also used to deliver medications via inhalation by aerosolizing liquid medications using different technologies. There are three main types of nebulizers: jet (also known as *pneumatic*), ultrasonic, and mesh. Nebulized medications are administered intermittently or continuously using a mouthpiece or a facemask.

TYPES OF MEDICATIONS

Medications for asthma are illustrated in Mind Map 4.1.

The medications for asthma include the following:

Bronchodilators

Three main classes of bronchodilators are discussed in the following section.
- Beta-2 adrenergic agonists:
  The primary mechanism of action of beta-2 adrenergic agents is binding and activation of beta-2 receptors on

bronchial smooth muscle cells causing smooth muscle relaxation and bronchodilation. Beta-2 adrenergic agonists are delivered to the lungs via inhalation using nebulizers or inhalers. The adverse effects of the inhaled beta-2 adrenergic agonists are mild and usually include tremor, excitability, nervousness, tachycardia, and occasionally hypokalemia. Reflex bronchospasm can also occur, which worsens underlying asthma or COPD.

- Short-acting beta-adrenergic agonists inhaled (SABAs): albuterol and levalbuterol are used for quick relief of acute asthma symptoms. The onset of action is within 5 minutes and duration of action is 4 to 6 hours. SABAs should be used as needed, and increasing use of SABAs indicates poor control and need for improved maintenance therapy. Tolerance to SABAs can occur, which may reduce the duration and effectiveness of bronchodilation.
- Long-acting beta-adrenergic agonists inhaled (LABAs): salmeterol, formoterol, and vilanterol are added to inhaled glucocorticoids for daily maintenance therapy. Formoterol has rapid onset of action within 3 minutes and is long-acting (up to 12 hours of bronchodilation). Vilanterol is ultra-long acting with up to 24 hours of bronchodilation. These medications are delivered via inhalers once or twice daily. LABAs SHOULD NOT be used as monotherapy because of an increased risk for risk of serious adverse events (SAEs) and asthma-related deaths.[2]

- Theophylline is an oral medication taken daily and is infrequently used for maintenance in asthma and COPD. It is classified as a methylxanthine drug, which has caffeine-like effects. It works by inhibiting phosphodiesterase enzymes, which has bronchodilator and antiinflammatory effects. It is indicated mainly as an additive therapy to other first-line maintenance medications for poorly controlled asthma or COPD. There is an intravenous (IV) form of theophylline, which can be administered during an acute exacerbation of asthma for patients on chronic theophylline who are unable to tolerate their usual oral theophylline. There are multiple oral dosage forms of theophylline, and sustained release is generally preferred oral formulation. Theophylline clearance is affected by age (reduced clearance less than 1 and older than 60 years) and cigarette smoking status (decreased clearance with recent smoking cessation) as well as certain concomitant drugs. Theophylline is usually well tolerated at therapeutic doses. The primary adverse effects include headache, nausea, and sometimes vomiting, abdominal discomfort, and restlessness.
  - Theophylline has a narrow therapeutic index, and it requires careful titration and periodic serum drug level monitoring. Therapeutic dosages of theophylline generally provide a PEAK serum concentration of 10 to 20 mg/L (mcg/mL). Clinical features of theophylline toxicity include coarse tremor, abdominal pain, vomiting, seizures, which are difficult to control, and arrhythmias including tachycardia, supraventricular tachycardia, and fatal ventricular arrhythmias.
- Muscarinic receptor antagonists, also known as *antimuscarinic agents*, are used via inhalation primarily in COPD but may be used in asthma in certain specific situations. Antimuscarinic drugs are competitive antagonists at muscarinic

receptors in bronchial smooth muscle and other bronchial cells; they block the effects of acetylcholine, resulting in bronchodilation and reduced mucus secretion. An inhaled antimuscarinic agent that is short acting is **ipratropium** (onset of action within 15 minutes and duration 4–5 hours); it is used for immediate relief of asthma symptoms or acute exacerbations. Inhaled long-acting antimuscarinic agents (e.g., tiotropium) may be added for long-term maintenance treatment in asthma as add-on therapy to inhaled corticosteroids and LABAs. These medications are delivered via inhalers or nebulizers. The inhaled antimuscarinics are less effective as bronchodilators than beta agonists in asthma. However, in COPD, the inhaled antimuscarinic agents are effective bronchodilators and play a central role in treatment of patients with COPD.

Antiinflammatory Drugs

Glucocorticosteroids (inhaled and systemic)

Inhaled glucocorticosteroids (ICS) are the mainstay of maintenance controller therapy for asthma. ICS have broad-spectrum antiinflammatory effects, and as glucocorticosteroids, they bind to the intracellular glucocorticoid receptors and affect gene transcription to suppress genes for most inflammatory cytokines, promote antiinflammatory genes, and inhibit phospholipase and cyclooxygenase enzymes. Some of the common ICS include beclomethasone (Qvar), budesonide (Pulmicort), ciclesonide (Alvesco), and fluticasone (ArmonAir, Arnuity, Flovent). ICS are also available in combination with LABAs as budesonide and formoterol, fluticasone propionate and salmeterol, fluticasone furoate and vilanterol, mometasone and formoterol. Local adverse effects include topical candidiasis (thrush) and dysphonia (hoarseness) and, occasionally, reflex cough. Topical candidiasis can be minimized by using a spacer with an MDI and rinsing the mouth after using the inhaler.

Systemic steroids can be used briefly for 5 to 7 days during exacerbations of asthma. Names of systemic steroids include prednisone, prednisolone, and methylprednisolone. Adverse effects of short-term use are sleep disturbance, increased appetite, and moodiness. Adverse effects of long-term systemic glucocorticosteroids are detailed in Chapter 6 and include osteoporosis, cataracts, skin changes, myopathy, Cushing syndrome, hyperglycemia, insomnia, and mood changes, especially elevated mood and, sometimes, mania. Hypothalamic-pituitary-adrenal axis suppression can occur if long-term oral steroids are not tapered (reduce 10–20% every 1–2 weeks if >3 weeks).

Antileukotrienes

Leukotriene receptor antagonists include montelukast (zafirlukast) and 5′-lipoxygenase enzyme inhibitors (zileuton). These oral medications act by reducing the effect of inflammatory leukotrienes, which cause bronchoconstriction, mucous production, and recruitment of proinflammatory cells such as mast cells, eosinophils, and lymphocytes. Montelukast is an oral once-daily medication commonly used for mild-to-moderate persistent asthma maintenance therapy either as monotherapy or added to other medications such as ICS.

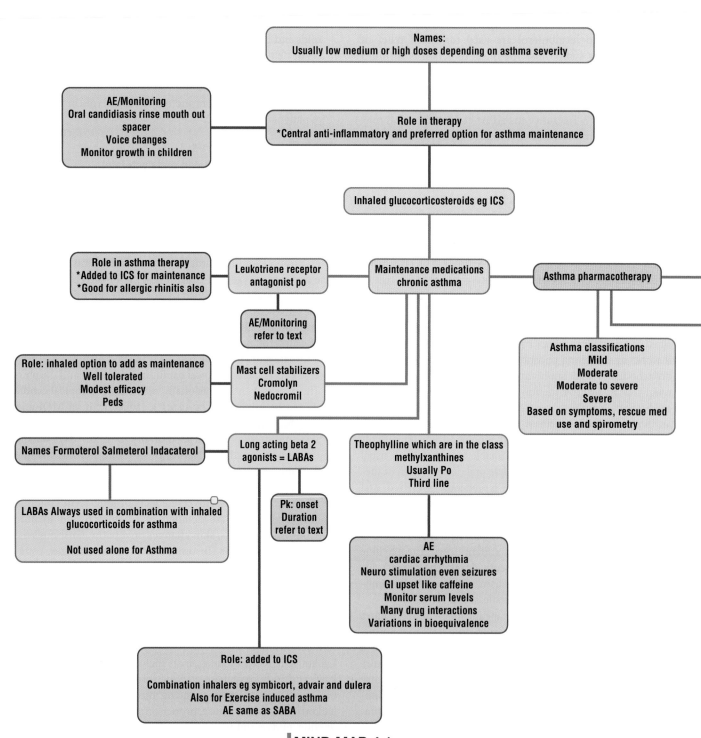

MIND MAP 4.1

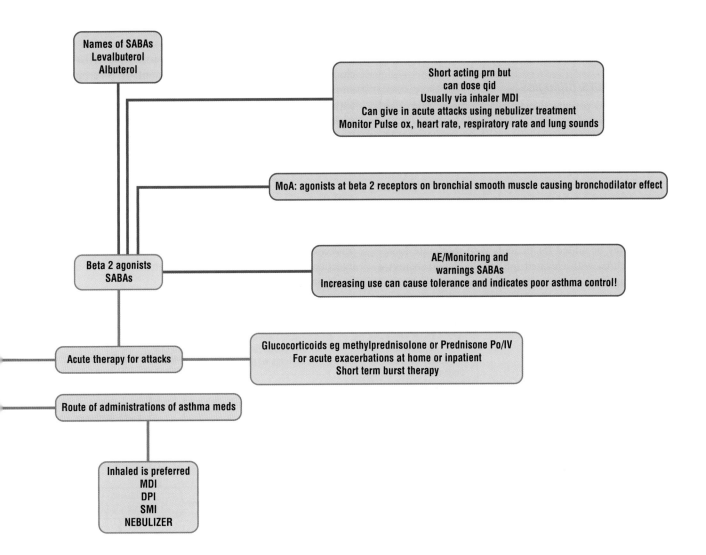

Names of SABAs
Levalbuterol
Albuterol

Short acting prn but
can dose qid
Usually via inhaler MDI
Can give in acute attacks using nebulizer treatment
Monitor Pulse ox, heart rate, respiratory rate and lung sounds

MoA: agonists at beta 2 receptors on bronchial smooth muscle causing bronchodilator effect

Beta 2 agonists
SABAs

AE/Monitoring and
warnings SABAs
Increasing use can cause tolerance and indicates poor asthma control!

Acute therapy for attacks

Glucocorticoids eg methylprednisolone or Prednisone Po/IV
For acute exacerbations at home or inpatient
Short term burst therapy

Route of administrations of asthma meds

Inhaled is preferred
MDI
DPI
SMI
NEBULIZER

Montelukast and zafirlukast are well tolerated. The US Food and Drug Administration issued a boxed warning on montelukast about potential neuropsychiatric events (e.g., agitation, depression, insomnia, suicidal thoughts and actions). Zileuton has more adverse effects including liver inflammation and increased drug interactions and is rarely used in the United States.

Immunomodulators/Biologics

These are specialized parenteral maintenance medications used for certain phenotypes of persistently uncontrolled asthma despite use of multiple maintenance medications.

Anti-IgE receptor therapy

Omalizumab is a humanized monoclonal antibody that blocks the binding of immunoglobulin (Ig)E to high-affinity IgE receptors (FcεR1) on mast cells and thus prevents their activation by allergens. This medication is administered via subcutaneous injection and may be added for patients with moderate to severe allergic asthma with elevated IgE levels. Hypersensitivity reactions ranging from injection site reactions to anaphylaxis to omalizumab can occur, and patients should be observed in office for 30 minutes after injection and bring epinephrine autoinjector(s).

Anti-IL-5 therapy

Mepolizumab and reslizumab are anti-interleukin (IL)-5 monoclonal antibodies; benralizumab is an anti-IL-5 receptor alpha antibody. Mepolizumab is a subcutaneous injection for patients with severe eosinophilic asthma. Adverse effects of mepolizumab include headache, herpes zoster, and injection site reactions. Reslizumab is an IV infusion administered every 4 weeks. Adverse effects of reslizumab include mouth and throat pain and IV infusion reactions with rare anaphylaxis.

Anti-IL-4 receptor alpha subunit antibody

Dupilumab is a fully human monoclonal antibody that binds to the alpha subunit of the IL-4 receptor. Indicated for moderate-to-severe, eosinophilic asthma and administered via subcutaneous injections. Adverse effects include elevated blood eosinophils and injection site reactions.

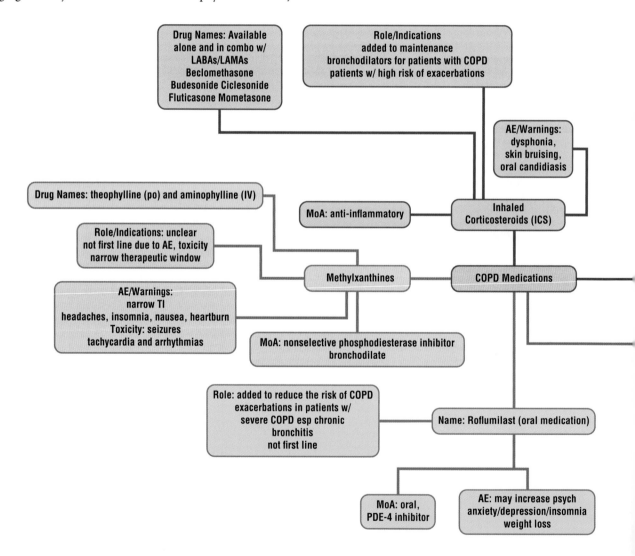

MIND MAP 4.2

Overview

Medications used for acute relief of asthma symptoms include inhaled SABAs. Preferred maintenance controller therapies for are ICS. LABAS can be added to ICS but are not used alone due to increased risk for serious adverse effects and asthma-related deaths. Other controller maintenance therapies for asthma include oral leukotriene receptor antagonist (montelukast). Theophylline is an oral medication that may be added if patients have symptoms despite other controller medications, e.g., ICS. Biologic agents are parenteral agents that may be added for persistently uncontrolled asthma with certain features.

COPD PHARMACOTHERAPY

COPD is another common chronic pulmonary disorder. It is characterized by persistent airflow limitation with abnormal airways and alveoli causing respiratory symptoms. The most common cause is cigarette smoking. The most common symptoms are exertional dyspnea, cough especially at night, and sputum production. The Global Initiative for Chronic Obstructive Lung Disease GOLD system categorizes patients with COPD into one of four groups (A, B, C, D), based on symptoms, number of, and risk of future exacerbations and hospitalizations:

- Group A: Minimally symptomatic, low risk of future exacerbations: Modified Medical Research Council (mMRC) grade 0 to 1 or COPD Assessment Test [CAT] score <10; 0 to 1 exacerbation per year and no prior hospitalization for exacerbation
- Group B: More symptomatic, low risk of future exacerbations: mMRC grade ≥2 or CAT score ≥10; 0 to 1 exacerbation per year and no prior hospitalization for exacerbation
- Group C: Minimally symptomatic, high risk of future exacerbations: mMRC grade 0 to 1 or CAT score <10; ≥2 exacerbations per year or ≥1 hospitalization for exacerbation
- Group D: More symptomatic, high risk of future exacerbations: mMRC grade ≥2 or CAT score ≥10; ≥2 exacerbations per year or ≥1 hospitalization for exacerbation.[3]

In general, the drugs used to treat COPD are like those used for asthma (see Mind Map 4.2). The inhaled bronchodilators beta-2 agonists and inhaled muscarinic antagonists are primary therapies for COPD. SABAs, e.g., albuterol and levalbuterol or

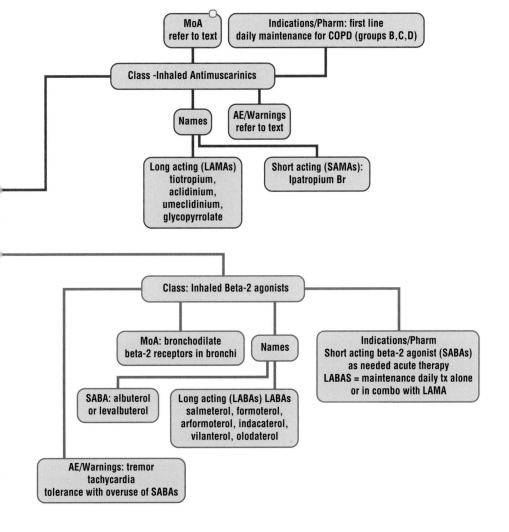

ipratropium and the short-acting muscarinic antagonist (SAMAs), are used for quick relief of intermittent respiratory symptoms. LABAs and long-acting muscarinic antagonists (LAMAs) are used for symptomatic patient for daily control of symptoms. The LABAs include salmeterol, formoterol, aformoterol, indacaterol, vilanterol, and olodaterol. The LAMAs include tiotropium, aclidinium, umeclidinium, and glycopyrrolate and revefenacin. LABAs or LAMAs are administered via DPIs, SMIs or via nebulizer once or twice daily. LABAs or LAMAs can be used for group B COPD, and LAMAs are preferred for groups C and D. The adverse effects of inhaled SAMAs and LAMAs are mild and include dry mouth, headache, and cough. Use caution in patients with benign prostatic hyperplasia due to potential risk for urinary retention, and monitor heart rate especially in patients with preexisting cardiovascular conditions.

Combination LAMA/LABA inhalers such as aclidinium 400 mcg/formoterol 12 mcg, glycopyrrolate 15.6 mcg/indacaterol 27.5 mcg, glycopyrrolate 50 mcg/indacaterol 110 mcg, glycopyrrolate 9 mcg/formoterol 4.8 mcg, tiotropium 2.5 mcg/olodaterol 2.5 mcg per actuation, or umeclidinium 62.5 mcg/vilanterol 25 mcg can be used for patients with persistent dyspnea and limitation in activities. These combination bronchodilator inhalers are more convenient and not associated with increased risks or adverse effects.[4,5]

The ICS play a different role in COPD compared to asthma. The inhaled corticosteroids may be added to inhaled bronchodilators in patients with persistent symptoms, repeated exacerbations, or severe exacerbations despite long-acting inhaled bronchodilators, e.g., LAMA/LABA. Patients with elevated blood eosinophils and COPD exacerbations may be considered for additive ICS therapy. The adverse effects of ICS are reviewed in Mind Map 4.1 and in the asthma section of this chapter.

Certain patients with COPD are symptomatic and/or have repeated exacerbations despite maximal first-line therapies. Pharmacologic option includes adding theophylline or oral roflumilast. Roflumilast is an oral, phosphodiesterase-4 inhibitor that reduces airway inflammation and may cause bronchodilation. It can be added once daily to usual maintenance therapies in patients with repeated exacerbations but with modest overall benefits. Roflumilast can cause anxiety, depression, insomnia, as well as diarrhea, nausea, and vomiting. Patients with stable chronic, severe hypoxemia at rest are candidates for long-term, continuous oxygen (O_2) therapy.

In addition to medications, cigarette smoking cessation is essential for all COPD patients who smoke. Pharmacologic interventions to assist smoking cessation include nicotine replacement therapy, bupropion, and varenicline, which are most effective in combination with counseling.[3]

REFERENCES

1. Global Initiative for Asthma. *Global Strategy for Asthma Management and Prevention.* 2022. Available at: www.ginasthma.org.
2. FDA Drug Safety Communication. *Drug Labels Now Contain Updated Recommendations on the Appropriate Use of Long-Acting Inhaled Asthma Medications Called Long-Acting Beta-Agonists (LABAs).* Available at: https://www.fda.gov/drugs/drug-safety-and-availability/fda-drug-safety-communication-fda-review-finds-no-significant-increase-risk-serious-asthma-outcomes#:~:text=Using%20LABAs%20alone%20to%20treat,risk%20of%20asthma%2Drelated%20death.
3. Global Initiative for Chronic Obstructive Lung Disease. *Global Strategy for the Diagnosis, Management and Prevention of Chronic Obstructive Pulmonary Disease: 2020 Report.* Available at: www.goldcopd.org. Accessed February 10, 2021.
4. Yu AP, Guérin A, Ponce de Leon D, et al. Therapy persistence and adherence in patients with chronic obstructive pulmonary disease: multiple versus single long-acting maintenance inhalers. *J Med Econ.* 2011;14:486.
5. Singh D, Ferguson GT, Bolitschek J, et al. Tiotropium + olodaterol shows clinically meaningful improvements in quality of life. *Respir Med.* 2015;109:1312.

CHAPTER 5

Drugs Affecting Allergic Conditions, Inflammation, Immunity, and Hematopoiesis

SECTION 1: Drugs for Allergic Diseases

ALLERGIC DISEASES

These are diverse and involve complex immunologic and inflammatory components. Several chemical medicators including histamine, serotonin, prostaglandins, and leukotrienes (LTs) play important roles in allergic and inflammatory conditions. Histamine is a biologically active amine that is synthesized and stored in mast cells and basophils, and in enterochromaffin cells in the stomach and in the brain. The effects of histamine include the cardinal signs of inflammation: redness, swelling, increased heat, and pruritus. Histamine is released locally when there is tissue injury and causes local vasodilation, increased capillary permeability, and inflammation. Mast cells and basophils are leukocytes that release histamine and other inflammatory mediators when they are sensitized by certain antigens or allergens and immunoglobulin (Ig)E antibodies attached to receptors on their cell surfaces. Histamine acts on histamine (H) receptors, which are in smooth and cardiac muscle, on vascular endothelial and nerve cells, on parietal cells in the stomach, and on inflammatory cells. Antihistamines, specifically histamine type 1 (H1) receptor antagonists, are a common class of medications used to treat a variety of allergic and inflammatory conditions including allergic rhinitis, urticaria, angioedema, and pruritus. H2 antagonists are used for gastrointestinal (GI) diseases including gastroesophageal reflux disease and peptic ulcer disease, which are discussed in Chapter 7. Other medications used to treat allergic conditions include glucocorticosteroids (see Chapter 6), LT antagonists, and mast cell stabilizers.

Antihistamines block the actions of histamines at H1 receptors, and are divided into first-generation and second-generation agents. First-generation antihistamines are more sedating because they distribute into the central nervous system, and they can affect autonomic receptors. First-generation antihistamines include diphenhydramine, dimenhydrinate, chlorpheniramine, hydroxyzine, meclizine, promethazine, and cyproheptadine. Most of the first-generation antihistamines have antimuscarinic effects; promethazine is also an alpha-1 antagonist with

antiemetic/antinausea effects, which can cause orthostasis. Meclizine and dimenhydrinate are effective agents for the prevention of motion sickness. First-generation antihistamines are shorter acting and generally administered orally a few times a day. Adverse effects of the first-generation antihistamines are sedation, which may impair motor skills, and anticholinergic effects, including dry mouth and eyes, urinary hesitancy, and confusion. Second-generation antihistamines are minimally sedating and do not affect autonomic receptors. Second-generation antihistamines include cetirizine, levocetirizine, loratadine, desloratadine, and fexofenadine. Second-generation antihistamines are administered orally once daily, and they are well tolerated.[1,2]

There are also antihistamine nasal sprays (azelastine and olopatadine) used for allergic rhinitis, and ophthalmic solutions including olopatadine, alcaftadine, bepotastine, azelastine hydrochloride, cetirizine, ketotifen fumarate, and emedastine for allergic conjunctivitis.

EICOSANOIDS (PROSTAGLANDINS, LEUKOTRIENES)

The eicosanoids are a diverse group of molecules derived from arachidonic acid and include prostaglandins, thromboxanes (TXs), and LTs. In response to various stimuli, arachidonic acid is released by phospholipase A2 from the cell membranes. Arachidonic acid is enzymatically converted into (1) prostanoids (prostaglandins [PG], prostacyclin, and TX) by cyclooxygenase (COX) enzymes and (2) LTs by the lipooxygenases. Prostaglandins and TXs have multiple effects on platelets, inflammatory cells, kidneys, the nervous system, eyes, and in the smooth muscle in the vasculature, airways, and GI and reproductive tracts. Prostaglandins, especially PGI2 and PGE2, cause vasodilation while TXA2 is a potent vasoconstrictor. In platelets, PGI2 (prostacyclin) inhibits aggregation and TXA2 increases platelet aggregation. PGE2 and PGI2 increase inflammation and fever.

Clinical use of prostaglandins is diverse and includes induction of labor and abortion, treatment of pulmonary hypertension, maintaining the patency of the neonate's ductus arteriosus in certain congenital heart diseases, topical ophthalmic treatment of glaucoma, and for certain GI indications. COX inhibitors are antiinflammatory and inhibit the formation of prostanoids and are discussed in Section 2, Nonsteroidal Antiinflammatory Drugs (NSAIDS). Synthetic prostaglandins dinoprostone and misoprostol are used for cervical ripening for labor induction; misoprostol is an abortifacient, which is administered after mifepristone for medication abortions. Oral prostacyclin receptor agonists, for example, selexipag, parenteral prostanoids epoprostenol and treprostinil, and inhaled iloprost are used for pulmonary arterial hypertension. Misoprostol has protective effects on the stomach and can be used to protect against NSAID-induced ulcers; lubiprostone is a prostaglandin E1 derivative used for constipation in inflammatory bowel syndrome. Latanoprost, bimatoprost, travoprost, and tafluprost are topical ophthalmic prostaglandin analogs used for glaucoma.

LTs are derived from arachidonic acid via lipoxygenase enzymes. LT act on receptors and cause potent bronchoconstriction and inflammation in the airways. LT receptor antagonists, specifically montelukast, are used to treat asthma and allergic rhinitis. LT antagonists, for example, montelukast, are discussed in Chapter 4.

SECTION 2: Nonsteroidal Antiinflammatory Drugs and Acetaminophen

The NSAIDs are highlighted in Mind Map 5.1. NSAIDs are inhibitors of COX enzymes that prevent the formation of prostaglandins and TXA2. NSAIDS have analgesic, antipyretic, and antiinflammatory effects. Acetaminophen inhibits COX enzymes, but it does not have antiinflammatory effects. There are two isoforms of COX enzymes; COX-2 enzymes are expressed during inflammation and form inflammatory prostaglandins and prostacyclin formation. COX-1 enzymes are constitutively expressed and form TXA2, which causes platelet aggregation and PGE2, which has gastric cytoprotection. Prostaglandins also regulate renal blood flow, sodium, and water excretion.

NSAIDs are indicated for a wide range of musculoskeletal conditions including arthritis, inflammatory pain, dysmenorrhea, and fever. Aspirin is also indicated for treatment of acute coronary syndrome, as well as primary and secondary prevention of cardiovascular disease.

NSAIDs are generally administered orally or topically, and they are grouped by chemical classification and COX selectivity. The nonselective COX inhibitor NSAIDs include aspirin, which is an irreversible COX inhibitor, other salicylates such as methyl salicylate, and diflunisal. Indomethacin is a nonselective highly potent antiinflammatory NSAID with very high incidence of adverse effects including GI distress, diarrhea, and neurologic effects, most commonly frontal headache. Diclofenac, which has topical formulations, and etodolac, which has dose-dependent COX 2 selectivity, are in the same chemical class as indomethacin. Ibuprofen, naproxen, oxaprozin, and ketoprofen are in the same chemical class; ibuprofen is shorter acting, dosed every 6 hours, naproxen is longer acting, dosed every 12 hours, and oxaprozin is long acting, and dosed once daily.

COX-2 selective inhibitors or "coxibs" include **celecoxib**, which is the only approved coxib in the United States. Meloxicam, nabumetone, etodolac, and possibly diclofenac are not coxibs, but they have COX-2 selectivity at lower doses.[3] The COX-2 selective NSAIDs have a reduced risk of gastroduodenal toxicity compared with nonselective NSAIDs; the coxibs NSAIDs do not inhibit platelet aggregation and are less likely to cause bronchospasm in patients with aspirin-induced asthma.

The major adverse effects of NSAIDS include:
- GI effects: dyspepsia, NSAID-induced peptic ulcer disease, and GI bleeding.
- Renal effects due to lack of prostaglandins, including acute renal failure, hyperkalemia, hyponatremia especially in patients with preexisting renal disease and volume depletion.
- Cardiovascular: NSAIDs can reduce the effectiveness of antihypertensive medications, elevate blood pressure, and increase the risk for myocardial infarction, stroke, and heart failure.
- Hematologic: aspirin and nonselective NSAIDs have antiplatelet effects; patients should stop aspirin for at least 1 week prior to surgery to reduce risk for bleeding.

Aspirin toxicity is associated with tinnitus, vertigo, nausea, vomiting, tachypnea, acid-base disturbances, and mental status changes. Aspirin overdoses are managed with activated charcoal, supplemental glucose, and alkalinization of the urine with sodium bicarbonate to enhance urinary excretion.

Aspirin is also contraindicated in children or teenagers who have any viral infection, with or without fever, because of possible Reye's syndrome warning, and it is contraindicated in patients allergic to NSAIDs and in patients with asthma, rhinitis, and nasal polyps.[4]

NSAIDs are contraindicated in patients with NSAID hypersensitivity or salicylate hypersensitivity, as well as in patients who have experienced an allergic reaction (urticaria, asthma, etc.) after taking NSAIDs, patients who have recently undergone coronary artery bypass graft surgery, and during the third trimester of pregnancy.

SECTION 3: Treatment of Gout

Gout (monosodium urate crystal deposition disease) is caused by precipitation of urate acid crystals, which incite tissue inflammation and damage. Hyperuricemia (typically defined as serum urate concentration >6.8 mg/dL) is caused by underexcretion of uric acid by the kidneys, excessive uric acid production, or reduced intestinal excretion. Urate production comes from the breakdown of dietary and endogenous purines into xanthine and uric acid. The clinical manifestations of gout include acute flares of inflammatory, often painful monoarticular lower extremity arthritis, chronic gouty arthritis, and tophaceous gout with accumulation of collections of solid urates that deposit around joints, soft tissues, tendons, and bursa. Renal manifestations and complications of chronic gout include uric acid nephrolithiasis and chronic urate nephropathy.

Pharmacotherapy of gout includes management of acute flares and chronic treatment to reduce recurrent gout and hyperuricemia. Treatment of acute flares includes systemic and intraarticular glucocorticoids, NSAIDs, and colchicine. Mind Map 5.2 illustrates the medications used to treat gout. Oral glucocorticoids (e.g., prednisone or prednisolone) are used in doses of 30 to 40 mg per day until the flare-up starts to resolve, and then tapered over 7 to 10 days. Intraarticular glucocorticosteroids, e.g., triamcinolone acetonide or methylprednisolone acetate, can be an alternative in patients with one or two affected joints, confirmed gout, and treated by an experienced clinician.[5] Potent NSAIDS such as naproxen 500 mg twice daily or indomethacin 50 mg three times daily are another first-line option for acute gout. NSAIDS should be initiated within 48 hours of the attack and continued until resolution usually 5 to 7 days. Adverse effects and contraindications of NSAIDS are discussed in Section 2.

Low-dose colchicine is another option for acute gout flares and prophylaxis, particularly in patients who cannot tolerate or have contraindications to NSAIDS and glucocorticosteroids. Colchicine is most effective within 24 hours of a flare, and it has variable dosing options, including an initial dose of 1.2 mg of oral colchicine, followed 1 hour later by another 0.6 mg, for a total dose on the first day of therapy of 1.8 mg. The mechanism of action of colchicine may be decreased due to neutrophil recruitment and adhesion to inflamed tissues. GI symptoms, especially diarrhea and abdominal cramping, as well as abdominal pain, nausea, and vomiting, are common with colchicine. Colchicine is also associated with some toxicities including peripheral neuropathy, myopathy, bone marrow suppression, and severe skin reactions.[6] Colchicine has a narrow therapeutic index, the dose must be reduced in hepatic and renal impairment, and it is associated with several drug interactions.

Management of recurrent gout flares and damage to joints and tissues involves lifestyle modification and pharmacotherapy to lower the serum urate level. Urate-lowering therapy includes uricosuric drugs and xanthine oxidase inhibitors (XOIs), which lower serum uric acid levels, reduce gout flares, and prevent or decrease tophi. Allopurinol and febuxostat are oral XOIs that inhibit the breakdown of purine metabolites, xanthine, and hypoxanthine into uric acid. Allopurinol is generally preferred, and it is started at a low dose and titrated to maintain serum urate <6 mg/dL (<357 micromol/L).[7] Allopurinol can precipitate a gout flare if it is initiated close to a recent flare. Adverse effects include rash, diarrhea, and leukopenia or thrombocytopenia. Patients who are human leukocyte antigen-B*5801 positive, which is more common in Thai, Chinese, Korean, and African Americans, have a higher incidence of severe cutaneous reactions and hypersensitivity and should not use allopurinol. Drug reaction with eosinophilia and systemic symptoms syndrome consists of an erythematous rash, fever, hepatitis, and eosinophilia, and acute renal failure is a rare but serious syndrome that can occur with allopurinol. Allopurinol dosing must be reduced in patients with renal impairment. Allopurinol is also associated with some drug interactions.

Feuxostat is another oral XOI. It is associated with hepatic abnormalities and cardiovascular adverse effects. There is a boxed warning about increased mortality in patients with existing cardiovascular disease and it should be reserved for use in patients who cannot tolerate allopurinol.[8]

Uricosuric agents increase renal uric acid excretion by inhibiting proximal tubule urate-anion exchangers in the kidney.[9] Probenecid is the only uricosuric in the United States and is not commonly used. Probenecid is associated with an increase in uric acid urolithiasis, and it should not be used with patients with nephrolithiasis; rash and GI intolerance are other common adverse effects.

Pegloticase is an intravenous recombinant mammalian urate oxidase (uricase) reserved for certain patients with severe, symptomatic refractory gout. Pegloticase converts uric acid to allantoin, which is soluble and excretable. Adverse effects include precipitation of gout flare, as well as infusion reactions including anaphylaxis and formation of inactivating antibodies. Premedication with antihistamines and corticosteroids is required before infusions.

SECTION 4: Immunosuppressants

Immunosuppressive drugs are used to suppress the immune response in organ/tissue transplantation and certain autoimmune diseases. The primary classes of immunosuppressants include glucocorticoids (see Chapter 6), calcineurin inhibitors, antiproliferative/antimetabolic agents, and biologics (antibodies, Section 6). Glucocorticoids (prednisone, methylprednisolone) are first-line therapy for solid organ and hematopoietic stem cell transplant recipients, but they are associated with long-term toxicities such as increased risk for infections, Cushing syndrome, adrenal suppression, obesity, hyperglycemia, hypertension, mood disturbances, and bone and muscle disorders.

Calcineurin inhibitors, cyclosporine and tacrolimus, interrupt the activation of T cells by inhibiting calcineurin, which in turn inhibits activation of a T cell–specific transcription factor and decreases gene transcription of interleukin (IL)-2, IL-3, interferon-γ. **Cyclosporine is** available intravenously and orally and is used in combination regimens for graft-versus-host disease (GVHD) and kidney, liver, heart, and other organ transplantation. Cyclosporine is associated with several drug interactions, adverse effects, and toxicities. The primary adverse effects of cyclosporine are renal dysfunction and hypertension; other adverse effects include tremor, gum hyperplasia, hirsutism, hyperlipidemia, and increased risk for infections and neoplasia. Nephrotoxicity is the major reason for discontinuation of cyclosporine.[10]

Tacrolimus is another calcineurin inhibitor, which can be administered orally or intravenously for organ rejection prophylaxis. Tacrolimus adverse effects are similar to those of cyclosporine, including **nephrotoxicity, hypertension,** neurotoxicity mainly tremor, hyperkalemia, hyperglycemia, and diabetes. It is also associated with increased risk for opportunistic infections and malignancies, especially squamous cell skin cancer and lymphomas.

Antiproliferative/antimetabolic agents include sirolimus, mycophenolate mofetil, methotrexate, and azathioprine. **Sirolimus** (rapamycin) is orally administered for prophylaxis of organ rejection in patients receiving renal transplants. It suppresses cytokine-mediated T-cell proliferation and inhibits cell

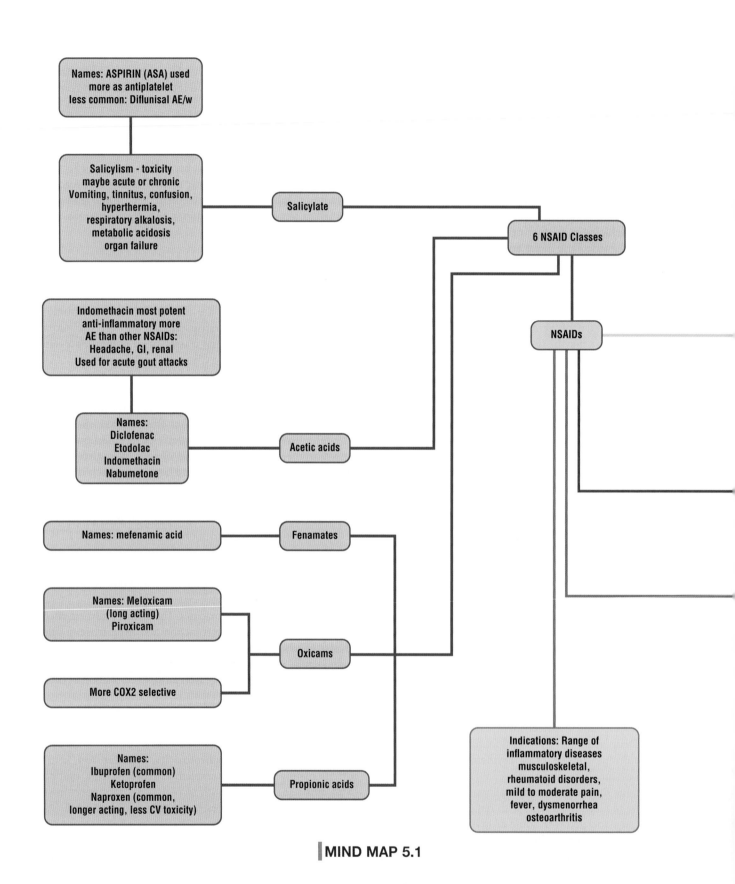

MIND MAP 5.1

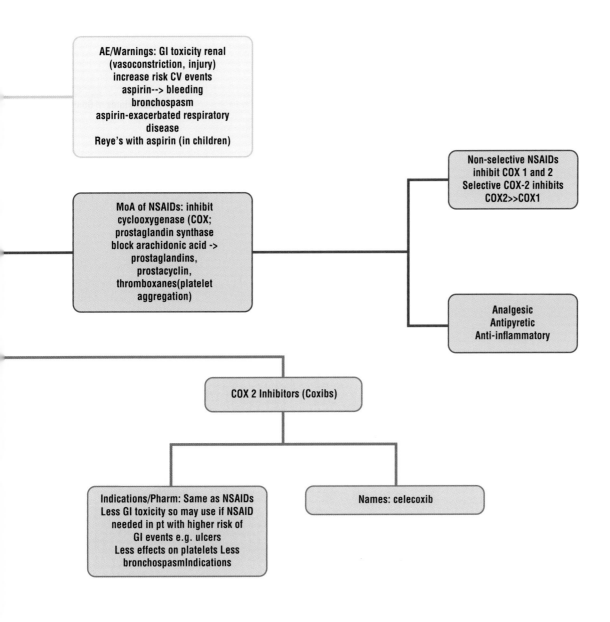

AE/Warnings: GI toxicity renal (vasoconstriction, injury) increase risk CV events aspirin--> bleeding bronchospasm aspirin-exacerbated respiratory disease Reye's with aspirin (in children)

MoA of NSAIDs: inhibit cyclooxygenase (COX; prostaglandin synthase block arachidonic acid -> prostaglandins, prostacyclin, thromboxanes(platelet aggregation)

Non-selective NSAIDs inhibit COX 1 and 2 Selective COX-2 inhibits COX2>>COX1

Analgesic Antipyretic Anti-inflammatory

COX 2 Inhibitors (Coxibs)

Indications/Pharm: Same as NSAIDs Less GI toxicity so may use if NSAID needed in pt with higher risk of GI events e.g. ulcers Less effects on platelets Less bronchospasmIndications

Names: celecoxib

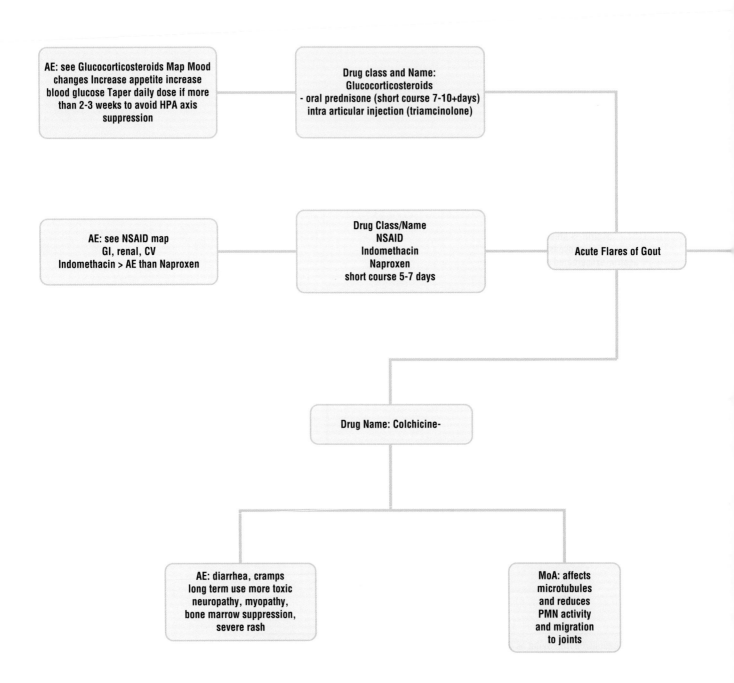

AE: see Glucocorticosteroids Map Mood changes Increase appetite increase blood glucose Taper daily dose if more than 2-3 weeks to avoid HPA axis suppression

Drug class and Name:
Glucocorticosteroids
- oral prednisone (short course 7-10+days)
intra articular injection (triamcinolone)

AE: see NSAID map
GI, renal, CV
Indomethacin > AE than Naproxen

Drug Class/Name
NSAID
Indomethacin
Naproxen
short course 5-7 days

Acute Flares of Gout

Drug Name: Colchicine-

AE: diarrhea, cramps long term use more toxic neuropathy, myopathy, bone marrow suppression, severe rash

MoA: affects microtubules and reduces PMN activity and migration to joints

MIND MAP 5.2

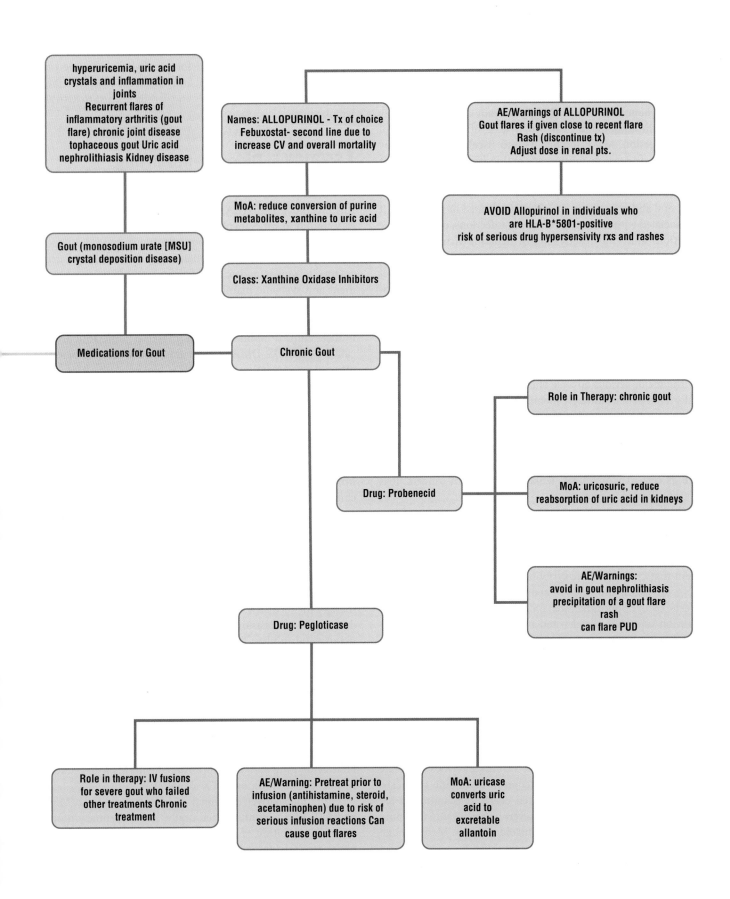

hyperuricemia, uric acid crystals and inflammation in joints
Recurrent flares of inflammatory arthritis (gout flare) chronic joint disease tophaceous gout Uric acid nephrolithiasis Kidney disease

Names: ALLOPURINOL - Tx of choice
Febuxostat- second line due to increase CV and overall mortality

AE/Warnings of ALLOPURINOL
Gout flares if given close to recent flare
Rash (discontinue tx)
Adjust dose in renal pts.

MoA: reduce conversion of purine metabolites, xanthine to uric acid

AVOID Allopurinol in individuals who are HLA-B*5801-positive
risk of serious drug hypersensitivity rxs and rashes

Gout (monosodium urate [MSU] crystal deposition disease)

Class: Xanthine Oxidase Inhibitors

Medications for Gout

Chronic Gout

Role in Therapy: chronic gout

Drug: Probenecid

MoA: uricosuric, reduce reabsorption of uric acid in kidneys

AE/Warnings:
avoid in gout nephrolithiasis
precipitation of a gout flare
rash
can flare PUD

Drug: Pegloticase

Role in therapy: IV fusions for severe gout who failed other treatments Chronic treatment

AE/Warning: Pretreat prior to infusion (antihistamine, steroid, acetaminophen) due to risk of serious infusion reactions Can cause gout flares

MoA: uricase converts uric acid to excretable allantoin

cycle progression. Sirolimus has less nephrotoxicity than calcineurin inhibitors but more GI effects, especially bowel changes including diarrhea and/or constipation, as well as liver function abnormalities. Other common adverse effects include elevated cholesterol, hypertriglyceridemia, and a **decrease in platelets and leukocytes.**

Mycophenolate mofetil (MMF) is orally and intravenously available in combination for prophylaxis of various types of organ rejection. MMF inhibits T- and B-cell proliferation by inhibiting de novo guanosine nucleotide synthesis. The major side effect of MMF is reversible myelosuppression (primarily delayed onset neutropenia) and GI nausea and vomiting, diarrhea, and abdominal pain. It is contraindicated in pregnancy. It is associated with an increased risk for infections, opportunistic infections and viral reactivation of hepatitis viruses, and the risk for lymphoma and skin malignancy is increased.[11]

Azathioprine and **mercaptopurine** are antimetabolites that interfere with purine nucleic acid metabolism and inhibit proliferation of antigenically stimulated lymphoid cells. Azathioprine is available orally and intravenously and has been used to prevent kidney transplant rejection and in several autoimmune diseases including Crohn disease, ulcerative colitis, and rheumatoid arthritis.

The major serious adverse effect is myelosuppression, especially leukopenia, although anemia and thrombocytopenia may also occur. Common adverse effects include nausea, vomiting, and diarrhea. As an immunosuppressant, azathioprine increases the risk for bacterial infections, viral infections, fungal infections, protozoal infections, and opportunistic infections as well as certain lymphomas, leukemias, and skin cancers. It is contraindicated in pregnancy.

Cyclophosphamide is another potent immunosuppressant mainly used for various malignancies but also for certain autoimmune diseases and prophylaxis of GVHD. Cyclophosphamide is available orally and intravenously; it is an alkylating agent that cross-links deoxyribonucleic acid (DNA), decreases DNA synthesis, and leads to apoptosis. Major serious adverse effects of cyclophosphamide include dose-related myelosuppression especially platelet and neutrophils, nausea/vomiting, and serious hemorrhagic cystitis, which can be prevented or treated with intravenous (IV) mesna (see Chapter 10). Cardiotoxicity and rarely pulmonary toxicities have been reported with cyclophosphamide, and it can increase the risk for secondary malignancies (see Chapter 10).[12]

Methotrexate is a disease-modifying antirheumatic drugs (DMARD) and antineoplastic drug that has dose-dependent antiproliferative effects. The basic mechanism of action of methotrexate is interference with various enzymes in folate metabolism, which causes a reduction in thymidine synthesis, DNA synthesis, and eventually cell death. It is indicated for several types of malignancies, severe, recalcitrant, disabling psoriasis, and severe, active rheumatoid arthritis. Methotrexate is discussed in Section 5.

There are several antibodies used for prevention and treatment of transplant rejection. These antibodies act in several ways: they block cytokines such as ILs and tumor necrosis factor (TNF), block lymphocyte surface receptors, and block specific signaling proteins between immune cells, e.g., T cells and antigen presenting cells (APCs), which causes interruption of immune activation. Basailixmab and daclizumab are anti-IL-2 receptor antibodies used for prophylaxis of acute organ transplant rejection. Abatacept and belatacept block costimulatory interaction between APCs and T cells needed to activate T lymphocytes.

SECTION 5: Disease-Modifying Antirheumatic Agents

Rheumatoid arthritis (RA) is a chronic, immunologic, inflammatory condition, often involving many peripheral joints, which can lead to progressive joint damage, deformities, and dysfunction. RA can have extraarticular manifestations including anemia, cutaneous, ocular, and/or oral dryness, and pulmonary involvement and systemic manifestations including morning stiffness, muscle weakness, weight loss, depression, and fatigue.

Drugs that can slow the progression of rheumatoid arthritis, induce clinical remission, and preserve joint function are called *DMARDS*. DMARDs are classified as nonbiologic (traditional or conventional) DMARDs, biologic DMARDs, which target specific cytokines or immune receptors, and targeted synthetic DMARDs. Mind Map 5.3 illustrates DMARDs and biologic drugs. Selection of pharmacotherapy should be discussed early in consultation with a rheumatologist. Drug choices are based on many factors including level of disease severity and activity, patient preferences, and comorbidities.[13] Pretreatment evaluation is comprehensive, including baseline complete blood count, serum creatinine, aminotransferases, erythrocyte sedimentation rate, and C-reactive protein, as well as screening for latent tuberculosis (TB) and, possibly, for hepatitis B and C viruses.[13]

Nonbiologic (traditional or conventional) DMARDs include methotrexate (MTX), hydroxychloroquine (HCQ), sulfasalazine (SSZ), and leflunomide (LEF). MTX is generally the initial therapy for most RA, and it is usually given in a single weekly dose, orally or occasionally subcutaneously. MTX is antiinflammatory and inhibits folic acid metabolism, which reduces purines and pyrimidines.

MTX is contraindicated in pregnancy and in women who may become pregnant and are not using adequate contraception, as well as persons with active severe liver and/or renal disease. The adverse effects of MTX are GI upset or stomatitis, but potential myelosuppression, especially macrocytic anemia, hepatotoxicity, and lung toxicity, requires regular monitoring. Folic acid (1 mg daily) is administered with MTX to reduce the risk of several common MTX toxicities.[14]

Other alternative traditional DMARDS include HCQ, SSZ, and LEF. LEF is administered orally, and its primary mode of action is inhibition of pyrimidine synthesis, which arrests cell phase progression and can trigger apoptosis.[15] It is contraindicated in pregnancy, nursing, and in patients with preexisting liver disease. The main adverse effects of LEF are diarrhea, increase in liver enzymes, rash with alopecia, and elevated blood pressure. LEF is contraindicated in pregnant and nursing women and in patients with liver disease. HCQ is an antimalarial drug, which is first-line alternative DMARD for patients with mild or limited disease. HCQ is well tolerated, although dose-related toxic retinopathy with macular damage can occur and requires routine eye testing. Other effects are nausea, rash and a prolonged QT interval.

Biologic agents for RA include TNF inhibitors (e.g., etanercept or adalimumab), abatacept, Janus kinases (JAK) inhibitors (tofacitinib, baricitinib), and anti–IL-6 antibodies (tocilizumab). These options maybe an alternative first line or used in combination with MTX for patients resistant to initial DMARD therapy.[13] Biologic agents are used to treat other systemic inflammatory diseases associated with autoimmunity and are discussed in Section 6.

SECTION 6: Biologic Agents and Kinase Inhibitors

Biologic agents are usually developed with molecular biologic techniques and designed to target specific immune functions, including interfering with cytokine function (TNF inhibitors, IL inhibitors), inhibiting cell signaling and T-cell activation (abatacept), and depleting or inactivating B cells (belimumab, rituximab). Kinase inhibitors (tofacitinib and baricitinib) are small molecules that target JAK, tofacitinib, and baricitinib and affect intracellular cell signaling in response to certain proinflammatory cytokines and growth factors. Biologic agents are used for a wide range of diseases including but not exclusive to inflammatory bowel diseases, certain autoimmune skin and joint diseases, asthma and atopic dermatitis, and those experienceds by organ transplant recipients. Biologic agents have descriptive nomenclature as follows: the ending "-cept" agents are formed by fusion of a receptor to the Fc part of human IgG1, and the ending "-mab" indicates a monoclonal antibody (mAb).[16]

There are five parenteral **TNF inhibitors**: etanercept, infliximab, adalimumab, certolizumab, and golimumab. The TNF inhibitors are used for inflammatory conditions, including RA, spondylarthritis, psoriasis, and inflammatory bowel disease. TNF has diverse immunologic effects including stimulation of inflammatory cytokine release, leukocyte migration, upregulation of cell adhesion molecules, activation of macrophages, and granuloma formation. The adverse effects of TNF inhibitors include injection site itching, pain, redness, irritation (common), and infusion reactions (with infliximab and mostly acute). There is an increased risk of infections including latent infections with TB and herpes zoster and opportunistic infections. There may be an increased risk for malignancies, especially nonmelanoma skin cancer and possibly certain lymphomas. There may be an increased risk for demyelinating disease, and TNF inhibitors should be avoided in patients with demyelinating diseases such as multiple sclerosis. Antidrug antibodies, which may reduce drug efficacy, and autoimmune antibodies are also associated with TNF inhibitors. TNF-alpha blockers may be continued in pregnancy and during lactation.[17]

IL inhibitors block the effects of IL-6 (tocilizumab and sarilumab), IL-17 (Secukinumab, Ixekizumab), and IL-12/23 (Ustekinumab and Guselkumab). Tocilizumab and sarilumab are subcutaneous or IV biologic agents for RA; adverse effects include a boxed warning about increased risk for developing serious infections including activation of latent TB and herpes zoster, injection site reactions, elevated liver enzymes, and potential demyelinating disease.[18]

IL-17 blockers (Secukinumab, Ixekizumab) are approved for severe psoriasis and psoriatic arthritis, as well as spondyloarthritis; they are administered subcutaneously. Secukinumab and Ixekizumab can increase the risk for infections including TB and may exacerbate inflammatory bowel disease.[19] IL-12/23 blockers (Ustekinumab [also IV] and Guselkumab) are approved for psoriatic arthritis; they are subcutaneously administered, and adverse effects include infections and injection site reactions and possibly nonmelanoma skin cancers.[20]

Other biologic agents include abatacept, which blocks costimulation signals between APCs and T cells; and B-cell depleters (rituximab) or inhibit factors that activate B cells (belimumab). Abatacept (IV or subcutaneous) is used for RA, juvenile idiopathic arthritis, and psoriatic arthritis. It is associated with infections, injection site and infusion reactions, nausea, and neutralizing drug antibodies. Rituximab (IV) depletes certain B cells, and it is used for non-Hodgkin lymphoma and chronic lymphocytic leukemia (see Chapter 10) and RA and granulomatosis with polyangiitis and microscopic polyangiitis. Adverse effects and warning associated with rituximab include hypersensitivity infusion reactions, infections including reactivation of latent TB and viral hepatitis, and severe skin and mucous membrane reactions. Belimumab is used parenterally for systemic lupus erythematosus, and it interferes with B-cell activation. Diarrhea, nausea, infections, and infusion reactions are most common adverse effects of belimumab.

Kinase inhibitors (tofacitinib and baricitinib) are orally administered small molecules that inhibit JAK, which are important for cell signaling and activation of immune cell function. Kinase inhibitors are an option for RA and severe ulcerative colitis. There are boxed warnings about increased cardiovascular risk, thrombosis, and cancer (lung and lymphoma) with the JAK inhibitors as well as increased risk for infections, increased liver enzymes, and hyperlipidemia.[21,22]

SECTION 7: Drugs for Anemia and Other Blood Disorders

Anemia is a deficiency in erythrocytes, which contain hemoglobin to carry oxygen to cells. Three primary nutrients—iron, vitamin B12, and folic acid, and hematopoietic growth factors such as erythropoietin are essential for regular growth and differentiation of hematopoietic cells. Anemias are diagnosed with a complete blood count: hemoglobin concentration, hematocrit, or red blood cell (RBC) count. A low hemoglobin concentration and/or low hematocrit generally indicates anemia. Causes of anemia are diverse including congenital anemias, e.g., sickle cell or thalassemia, iron deficiency (blood loss or dietary), megaloblastic anemias especially B12, folic acid deficiencies, as well as excessive alcohol and certain medications,

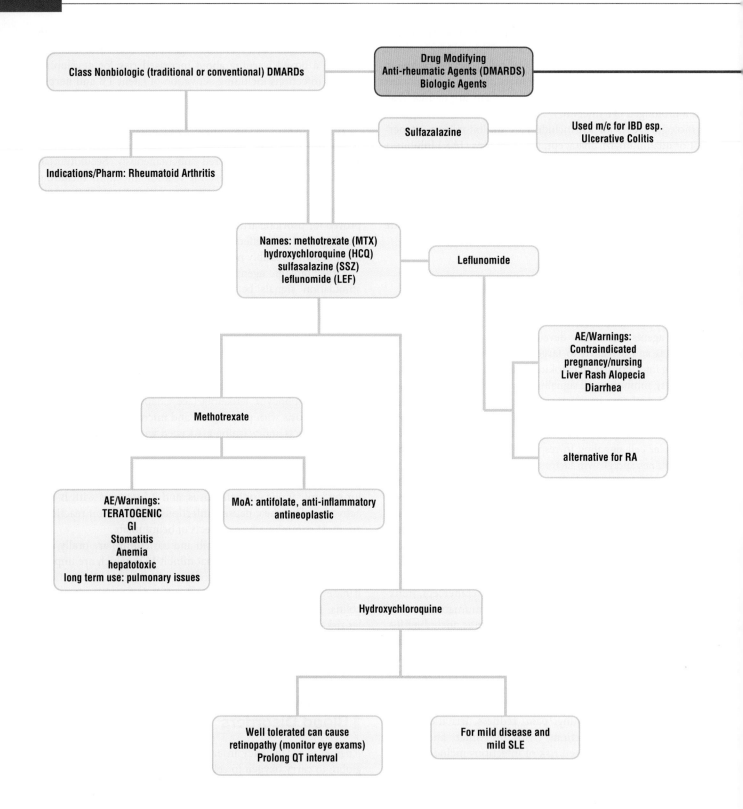

Class Nonbiologic (traditional or conventional) DMARDs

Drug Modifying
Anti-rheumatic Agents (DMARDS)
Biologic Agents

Sulfazalazine

Used m/c for IBD esp.
Ulcerative Colitis

Indications/Pharm: Rheumatoid Arthritis

Names: methotrexate (MTX)
hydroxychloroquine (HCQ)
sulfasalazine (SSZ)
leflunomide (LEF)

Leflunomide

AE/Warnings:
Contraindicated
pregnancy/nursing
Liver Rash Alopecia
Diarrhea

alternative for RA

Methotrexate

AE/Warnings:
TERATOGENIC
GI
Stomatitis
Anemia
hepatotoxic
long term use: pulmonary issues

MoA: antifolate, anti-inflammatory
antineoplastic

Hydroxychloroquine

Well tolerated can cause
retinopathy (monitor eye exams)
Prolong QT interval

For mild disease and
mild SLE

MIND MAP 5.3

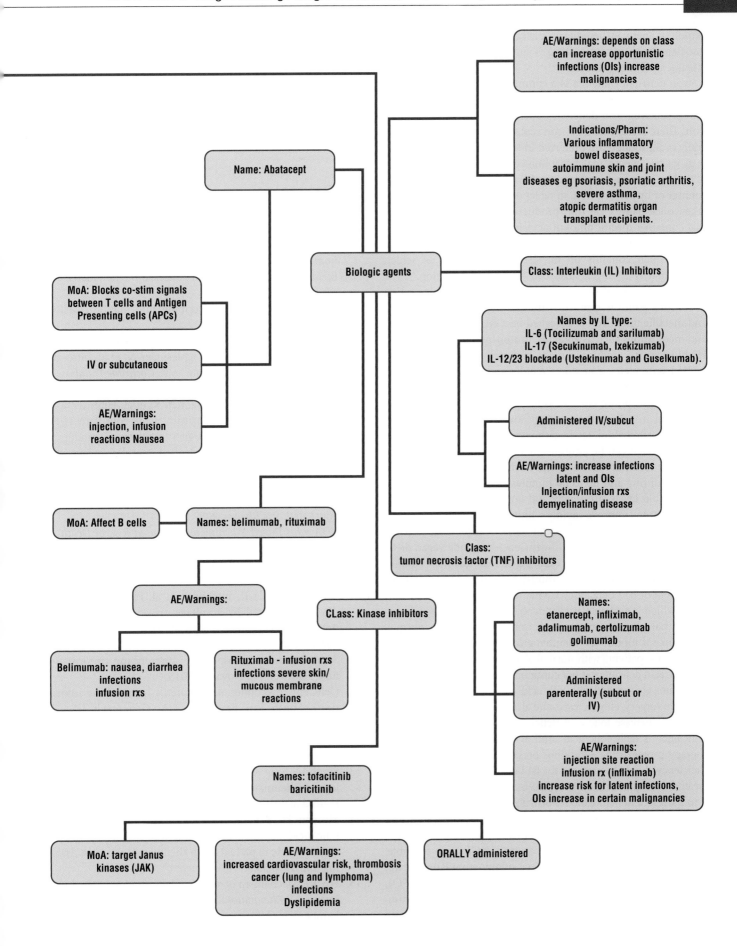

AE/Warnings: depends on class can increase opportunistic infections (OIs) increase malignancies

Indications/Pharm: Various inflammatory bowel diseases, autoimmune skin and joint diseases eg psoriasis, psoriatic arthritis, severe asthma, atopic dermatitis organ transplant recipients.

Name: Abatacept

Biologic agents

Class: Interleukin (IL) Inhibitors

MoA: Blocks co-stim signals between T cells and Antigen Presenting cells (APCs)

Names by IL type:
IL-6 (Tocilizumab and sarilumab)
IL-17 (Secukinumab, Ixekizumab)
IL-12/23 blockade (Ustekinumab and Guselkumab).

IV or subcutaneous

Administered IV/subcut

AE/Warnings: injection, infusion reactions Nausea

AE/Warnings: increase infections latent and OIs Injection/infusion rxs demyelinating disease

MoA: Affect B cells

Names: belimumab, rituximab

Class: tumor necrosis factor (TNF) inhibitors

AE/Warnings:

CLass: Kinase inhibitors

Names: etanercept, infliximab, adalimumab, certolizumab golimumab

Belimumab: nausea, diarrhea infections infusion rxs

Rituximab - infusion rxs infections severe skin/ mucous membrane reactions

Administered parenterally (subcut or IV)

AE/Warnings: injection site reaction infusion rx (infliximab) increase risk for latent infections, OIs increase in certain malignancies

Names: tofacitinib baricitinib

MoA: target Janus kinases (JAK)

AE/Warnings: increased cardiovascular risk, thrombosis cancer (lung and lymphoma) infections Dyslipidemia

ORALLY administered

hemolytic anemias (hereditary or acquired), and chronic anemia associated with systemic diseases such as cancer, autoimmune disease, and kidney disease.

Iron deficiency anemia is a common anemia that is usually treated with iron replacement therapy. Severe, symptomatic, or life-threatening iron deficiency anemia requires RBC transfusion. There are oral and IV iron replacement options, and generally oral products are preferred unless there is malabsorption (e.g., gastric bypass, malabsorption syndromes), poor tolerance of oral iron, or ongoing bleeding. Oral iron is available over the counter or by prescription, in tablet or liquid forms, and can be taken once daily. Oral iron products are usually ferrous salts that contain a specific amount of elemental iron; for example, a common recommendation is one tab of ferrous sulfate 325 mg tablet, which contains 65 mg elemental iron/tab of which approximately 25 mg is absorbed for RBC production.[23] The primary adverse effects of oral iron are GI upsets including abdominal pain/discomfort, nausea, constipation, dark stools, and metallic taste. Iron is absorbed best on an empty stomach, and medications such as antacids, proton-pump inhibitors, and H2 blockers may reduce iron absorption.

IV iron repletes iron stores rapidly and is used for patients with severe anemia, recent blood loss, poor tolerance to oral iron, malabsorption, chronic kidney disease. There are several parenteral iron formulations, e.g., low-molecular-weight iron dextran, ferumoxytol, ferric carboxymaltose, and iron sucrose, some of which can be administered as a single dose. IV irons can cause infusion reactions with flushing, fever, and myalgias; monitor during and up to 60 minutes after IV administration. Hemoglobin levels rise slowly and normalize by 6 to 8 weeks, and symptoms improve rapidly within a few days.[24]

B12 and folate deficiencies can cause megaloblastic anemia. Conditions that can cause B12 deficiencies include vegan diets, gastric or bariatric surgery, and pernicious anemia. Vitamin B12 and folic acid can be administered orally or parenterally. Treatment of B12 deficiency is vitamin B12 (also called *cobalamin*), which is available as cyanocobalamin and can be administered parenterally once a week until B12 levels are normal, then once a month for maintenance. Oral B12 once daily is effective for patients with normal absorption of B12.

Folic acid deficiency is not common in countries where cereals and grains are fortified with folic acid. Certain conditions such as bariatric surgery, chronic excessive alcohol, and severe malnutrition may increase folic acid deficiency. Treatment of folic acid deficiency is daily folic acid until anemia resolves and lifelong therapy if preexisting conditions persist. Patients with folic acid deficiency should be assessed for B12 deficiency and, if deficient, treated with appropriate B12 replacement. Anemias improve over 1 to 2 weeks and hemoglobin normalizes by 4 to 8 weeks.

Hematopoietic growth factors play a role in proliferation and differentiation of hematopoietic stem and progenitor cells. Several recombinant human growth factors (HGFs) are available, specifically granulocyte-macrophage colony-stimulating factor, granulocyte colony-stimulating factor, erythropoietin (EPO), thrombopoietin (TPO), and eltrombopag and romiplostim, which stimulate TPO receptors and increases platelets. These HGFs are administered parenterally and used in a variety of clinical settings including bone marrow failures, aplastic anemia, cytopenias with certain chemotherapy, and chronic anemia caused by chronic kidney disease. Adverse reactions include bone pain, flu-like symptoms, and transient leukopenia. Recombinant human EPO is associated with headache and hypertension, which can be severe. EPO can also increase the risk of thrombosis including myocardial infarction, stroke, and venous thromboembolism.[25]

REFERENCES

1. Bender BG, Berning S, Dudden R, et al. Sedation and performance impairment of diphenhydramine and second-generation antihistamines: a meta-analysis. *J Allergy Clin Immunol.* 2003;111:770.
2. Busse PJ. Allergic respiratory disease in the elderly. *Am J Med.* 2007;120:498.
3. Anjeso (meloxicam) [prescribing information]. Malvern, PA: Baudax Bio Inc; 2021.
4. Hill JB. Salicylate intoxication. *N Engl J Med.* 1973;288:1110.
5. Wechalekar MD, Vinik O, Schlesinger N, et al. Intra-articular glucocorticoids for acute gout. *Cochrane Database Syst Rev.* 2013:CD009920.
6. Terkeltaub RA, Furst DE, Bennett K, et al. High versus low dosing of oral colchicine for early acute gout flare: twenty-four-hour outcome of the first multicenter, randomized, double-blind, placebo-controlled, parallel-group, dose-comparison colchicine study. *Arthritis Rheum.* 2010;62:1060.
7. Perez-Ruiz F, Lioté F. Lowering serum uric acid levels: what is the optimal target for improving clinical outcomes in gout? *Arthritis Rheum.* 2007;57:1324.
8. *FDA adds Boxed Warning for Increased Risk of Death with Gout Medicine Uloric (febuxostat).* Available at: https://www.fda.gov/Drugs/DrugSafety/ucm631182.htm. Accessed on November 24, 2021.
9. Anzai N, Ichida K, Jutabha P, et al. Plasma urate level is directly regulated by a voltage-driven urate efflux transporter URATv1 (SLC2A9) in humans. *J Biol Chem.* 2008;283:26834.
10. Sandimmune (cyclosporine) [prescribing information]. East Hanover, NJ: Novartis; 2015.
11. CellCept (mycophenolate mofetil) [prescribing information]. South San Francisco, CA: Genentech USA Inc; 2019.
12. Cyclophosphamide injection, multi-dose vial [prescribing information]. Orlando, FL: Ingenus Pharmaceuticals; 2020.
13. Singh JA, Saag KG, Bridges SL Jr, et al. 2015 American College of Rheumatology Guideline for the treatment of rheumatoid arthritis. *Arthritis Rheumatol.* 2016;68:1.
14. Morgan SL, Baggott JE, Vaughn WH, et al. The effect of folic acid supplementation on the toxicity of low-dose methotrexate in patients with rheumatoid arthritis. *Arthritis Rheum.* 1990;33:9.
15. Fox RI. Mechanism of action of leflunomide in rheumatoid arthritis. *J Rheumatol Suppl.* 1998;53:20.
16. Lamberg L. A host of novel agents for treating psoriasis, psoriatic arthritis stir interest. *JAMA.* 2003;289:2779.

17. Adalimumab injection [product monograph]. Kirkland, Quebec, Canada: Pfizer Canada ULC; 2021.

18. Actemra (tocilizumab) [prescribing information]. South San Francisco, CA: Genentech Inc; 2021.

19. Cosentyx (secukinumab) [prescribing information]. East Hanover, NJ: Novartis; 2021.

20. Tremfya (guselkumab) [prescribing information]. Horsham, PA: Janssen Biotech Inc; 2020.

21. Xeljanz/Xeljanz XR (tofacitinib) [prescribing information]. New York, NY: Pfizer Inc; 2020.

22. Olumiant (baricitinib) [prescribing information]. Indianapolis, IN: Lilly USA LLC; 2020.

23. Schrier SL. So you know how to treat iron deficiency anemia. *Blood*. 2015;126:1971.

24. Rampton D, Folkersen J, Fishbane S, et al. Hypersensitivity reactions to intravenous iron: guidance for risk minimization and management. *Haematologica*. 2014;99:1671-1676.

25. Eprex (epoetin alfa) [product monograph]. Toronto, Ontario, Canada: Janssen Inc; 2021.

CHAPTER 6

Hormones and Endocrine Drugs

SECTION 1: Thyroid and Antithyroid Medications

Mind Map 6.1 illustrates thyroid medications. The thyroid gland synthesizes and secretes thyroid hormones, triiodothyronine (T3) and tetraiodothyronine (T4, thyroxine), which control metabolism, energy levels, body temperature, and growth and development. Iodide is reviewed for synthesis of T3 and T4, which is mainly ingested from food and concentrated in the thyroid for hormone biosynthesis. Control of thyroid is mainly via the hypothalamic pituitary thyroid axis via negative feedback. Thyrotropin-releasing hormone (TRH) from the hypothalamus stimulates thyroid-stimulating hormone (TSH) from the anterior pituitary, which in turn stimulates receptors on thyroid cells to increase the synthesis and release of T4 and T3. T3 inhibits TSH and TRH, and conversely low T3 stimulates TSH.

The primary pathologic conditions amenable to medications are hypothyroidism and hyperthyroidism. Hypothyroidism is mostly caused by chronic autoimmune hypothyroidism in iodine-sufficient regions of the world (Hashimoto thyroiditis). Signs and symptoms are variable but classically include weight gain; lethargy; menstrual irregularities; cold intolerance; constipation; dry skin, hair, and nails; periorbital edema; and myalgia. The laboratory tests that confirm primary hypothyroidism are a high serum TSH concentration and a low serum free thyroxine (T4) concentration. The treatment of choice for primary hypothyroidism is synthetic thyroxine (T4, levothyroxine), which is dosed in micrograms (mcg) once daily in tablet, soft gel, and liquid formulations. The average replacement dose of T4 in adults is approximately 1.6 mcg/kg body weight per day, which should be taken once daily on an empty stomach.[1] T4 therapy is monitored with clinical assessment and adjustment of T4 dose based on the serum TSH levels; initial adjustments of T4 dose are made every 6 weeks until the TSH is normal and patient's symptoms improve. Older patients and patients with coronary artery disease should start with lower initial dosages. Adverse effects of normal dosages of T4 are rare; overreplacement can cause cardiac arrhythmias and increase fracture risk.

There are other, less commonly used thyroid replacement formulations. T3 is available as 5- and 25-mcg tablets and is dosed orally twice daily. Desiccated thyroid extract (Thyroid USP) is a ratio mixture of T4 and T3 (approximately) of porcine and bovine origin. Most patients with hypothyroidism use T4 monotherapy, although certain patients with thyroidectomy or ablative therapy with radioiodine may benefit from combination therapy.

Hyperthyroidism is most often caused by Graves disease, which is an autoimmune disease more common in adult women. Other causes of hyperthyroidism include hyperfunctioning thyroid nodules (toxic adenomas) or thyroiditis. Clinical manifestations are variable and include heat intolerance, anxiety, weight loss despite a normal or increased appetite, hair and skin changes, eye changes such as lid lag, exophthalmos, menstrual irregularities, and increased frequency of bowel movements. Patients have a low serum TSH, and they may have elevated free T4 and T3 levels.

Medical treatment options for hyperthyroidism include thionamides, specifically methimazole or radioactive iodine therapy. Beta blockers such as atenolol are to improve symptoms. Thionamides are a class of two orally administered antithyroid medications: methimazole and propylthiouracil (PTU). Both thionamides block thyroid peroxidase activity, which prevents organification of iodine and coupling of iodotyrosines in the process of thyroid hormone synthesis. Methimazole is more commonly used because it is longer acting, more potent, and less toxic then PTU. PTU is generally not used except during the first trimester of pregnancy because it crosses the placenta less readily.[2] Adverse effects of the thionamides are nausea, rash, pruritus, and joint pain. Serious but less common adverse effects are agranulocytosis, especially within the 2 to 3 months of therapy, rarely hepatotoxicity (boxed warning and more common with PTU), and rarely antineutrophil cytoplasmic antibody–positive vasculitis, which is more common with PTU.[3-5]

Radioiodine is a highly effective treatment for Graves hyperthyroidism. It is administered orally as sodium iodide (131-I) in solution, or a capsule, and it is dosed based on thyroid gland size and 24-hour radioiodine uptake. Radioiodine concentrates in the thyroid and gradually damages and destroys the thyroid gland over several weeks to months. Pregnancy and breastfeeding are absolute contraindications to radioiodine and must be delayed 4 to 6 months after radioiodine therapy.[6] Posttreatment contact precautions to avoid exposure to household contacts include restrictions such as avoiding close contact, sleeping in same bed, sexual contact, and contact with utensils, with the period of restriction ranging from a few days to a few weeks.[7] The primary adverse effect of radioiodine is hypothyroidism requiring lifelong T4 therapy. Other adverse effects of radioactive iodine include thyroiditis, rebound hyperthyroidism, and worsening of orbitopathy with Graves disease. Laboratory values normalize by 4 to 10 weeks after treatment with radioiodine, and monitoring includes free T4, TSH, and sometimes total T3 levels.[7]

SECTION 2: Female Hormones

Mind Map 6.2 illustrates medications used in women's health. Estrogens and progestins, which are compounds with biologic activity like naturally occurring progesterone, are used for contraception and menopausal hormone therapy. Combined estrogen-progestin oral contraceptives (COCs) contain an estrogen component, usually ethynyl estradiol, and one of a several different progestins. COCs suppress follicular development, inhibit the luteinizing hormone surge, and prevent ovulation. The COCs vary in several ways including type and dosage (micrograms) of estrogen, type of progestin, cyclic versus extended-cycle versus continuous use and monophasic versus multiphasic (variable dosing of hormones throughout the cycle). The progestins are classified into generations and vary in their androgenic, estrogenic, and progestational effects. Cyclic pills are monthly packs of 21 active pills and 7 days placebo or 24 active days and 4 placebo; bleeding occurs during the placebo pills. Extended-cycle pills are generally 84 active pills with either 7 pill-free days or 7 days of very-low-dose estradiol. Continuous-cycle pills are taken daily with no pill-free interval. The progestins are grouped into first-generation progestins: norethindrone, norethindrone acetate, ethynodiol diacetate; second-generation progestins: levonorgestrel, norgestrel are more androgenic; third-generation progestins: norgestimate, desogestrel are less androgenic and more potent progestational; and fourth-generation progestins: drospirenone is antiandrogenic with some aldosterone antagonist effects.

Initiation of COCs and managing missed pills are important components to COC use. COCs can be started in a few different ways: quick start on the day that she is given the prescription, Sunday start pill on the first Sunday after her period begins, or start on the first day of menses. Patients should use a backup method for 7 days if the pill is started 5 days or more after the onset of menses.[8] Missed pills can lead to contraceptive failure and unscheduled bleeding. Patients who miss one pill can take the pill as soon as possible and continue the pack. Missing two or more pills requires backup contraception for 7 days, and patients should take one active pill as soon as possible and continue the pack. Emergency contraception can be considered

if unprotected intercourse occurred in the previous 5 days and/or three or more pills were missed.[9]

Other non-oral hormonal contraceptives include an intravaginal ring, transdermal patch, levonorgestrel intrauterine devices (IUDs), progestin subdermal implant, and injections of medroxyprogesterone. The combined estrogen and progestin vaginal ring is inserted and left in for 3 weeks and removed for 1 week. The combined estrogen and progestin contraceptive transdermal patch is applied weekly (for 3 weeks, then week 4 is patch-free).

Progestin-only contraceptive options include pills (POPs), implant, IUD, and injections. Patients who have contraindications to estrogen-containing contraceptives and postpartum breastfeeding women may elect progestin-only contraception. The progestin-only pills contain either norethindrone or drospirenone and generally are less effective then combined hormonal contraceptives (CHC). POPs should be taken at the same time every day with no pill-free intervals, and if the pill is taken more than 3 hours late or missed, backup contraception must be used. The etonogestrel implant is inserted subdermally in the upper arm and lasts for 3 years. Levonorgestrel-releasing IUDs are available in different formulations and can last from 3 to 7 years. Depot medroxyprogesterone acetate is an injectable progestin-only contraceptive administered every 3 months. Progestin-only contraceptives may cause more bleeding irregularities and acne flares, and increase ovarian follicular cysts. Depot medroxyprogesterone acetate can reversibly reduce bone mineral density, cause weight gain, and potentially exacerbate mood symptoms such as depression.[10] Patients taking POPs, the etonogestrel implant, and IUDs have a rapid return to fertility after discontinuation. There is a delay in fertility in patients taking depot medroxyprogesterone acetate.

There are noncontraceptive benefits of hormonal contraceptives. CHC are rapidly reversible, and they reduce menstrual and cycle-related problems including dysmenorrhea, irregular menstrual bleeding, heavy bleeding, and ovarian cysts. They also reduce endometrial and ovarian cancer. Certain extended- or continuous-cycle CHC and progestin-only contraceptives can reduce pelvic pain associated with endometriosis.

The primary adverse effects of hormonal contraceptives include unscheduled or breakthrough bleeding, nausea, and headaches are more common after initiation. Unscheduled bleeding that does not resolve but is related to the contraceptive may be managed by increasing the estrogen dose or increasing or changing to a more potent type of progestin. Amenorrhea occurs with continuous hormonal contraceptives and progestin-only contraceptives. Headaches may increase with hormonal contraceptives, especially during placebo periods. Patients with tension or cluster headaches and low-risk migraines without auras can take CHC. CHC increase relative risk of venous thromboembolism (VTE). Current data demonstrate little to no risk of breast cancer, although CHC are not recommended for women with personal history of breast cancer.[11]

The World Health Organization and the Centers for Disease Control and Prevention provide guidance to assess eligibility and contraindications to hormonal contraceptives.

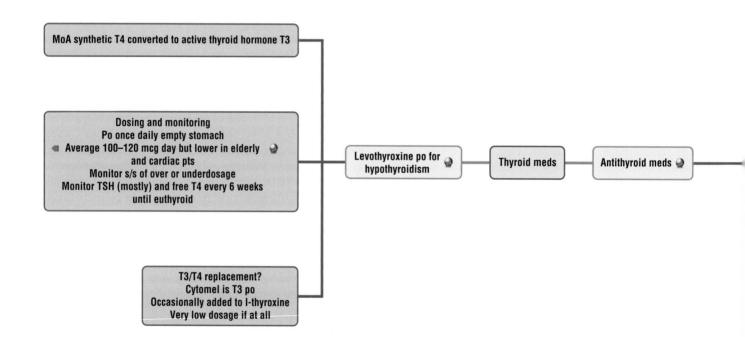

MoA synthetic T4 converted to active thyroid hormone T3

Dosing and monitoring
Po once daily empty stomach
Average 100–120 mcg day but lower in elderly
and cardiac pts
Monitor s/s of over or underdosage
Monitor TSH (mostly) and free T4 every 6 weeks
until euthyroid

Levothyroxine po for
hypothyroidism

Thyroid meds

Antithyroid meds

T3/T4 replacement?
Cytomel is T3 po
Occasionally added to l-thyroxine
Very low dosage if at all

MIND MAP 6.1

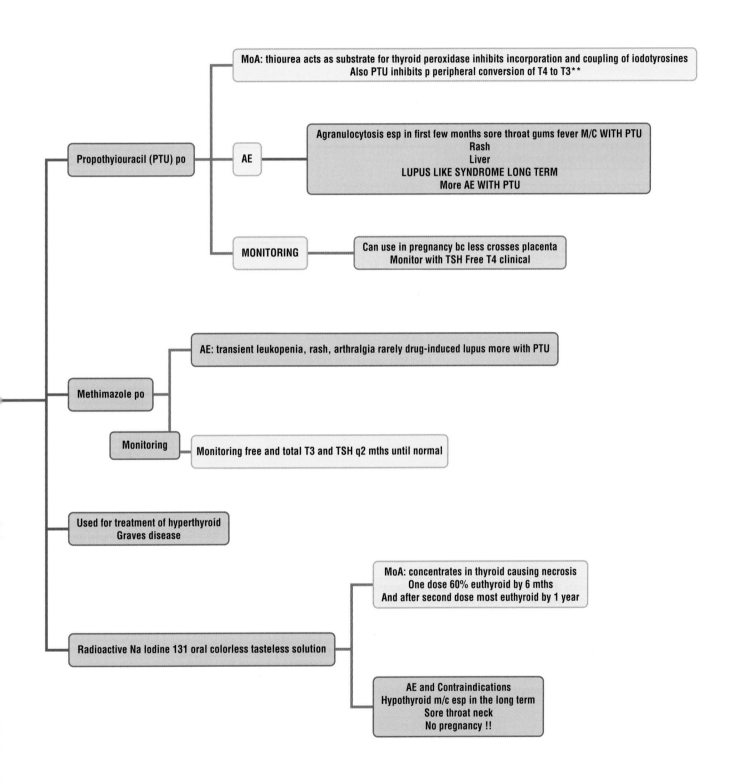

MoA: thiourea acts as substrate for thyroid peroxidase inhibits incorporation and coupling of iodotyrosines
Also PTU inhibits p peripheral conversion of T4 to T3**

Propothyiouracil (PTU) po

AE

Agranulocytosis esp in first few months sore throat gums fever M/C WITH PTU
Rash
Liver
LUPUS LIKE SYNDROME LONG TERM
More AE WITH PTU

MONITORING

Can use in pregnancy bc less crosses placenta
Monitor with TSH Free T4 clinical

AE: transient leukopenia, rash, arthralgia rarely drug-induced lupus more with PTU

Methimazole po

Monitoring

Monitoring free and total T3 and TSH q2 mths until normal

Used for treatment of hyperthyroid
Graves disease

MoA: concentrates in thyroid causing necrosis
One dose 60% euthyroid by 6 mths
And after second dose most euthyroid by 1 year

Radioactive Na Iodine 131 oral colorless tasteless solution

AE and Contraindications
Hypothyroid m/c esp in the long term
Sore throat neck
No pregnancy !!

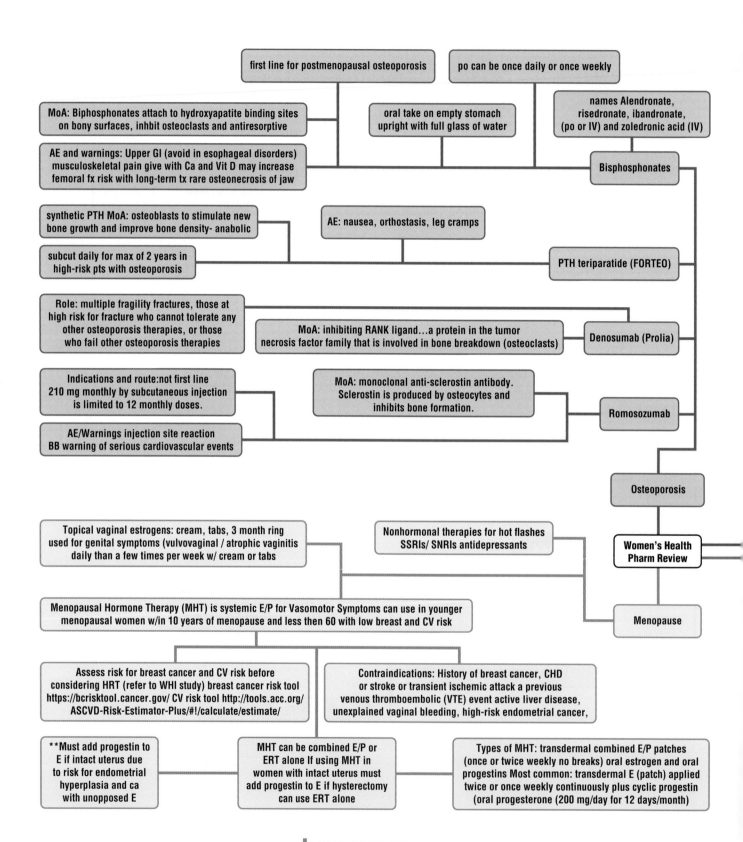

MIND MAP 6.2

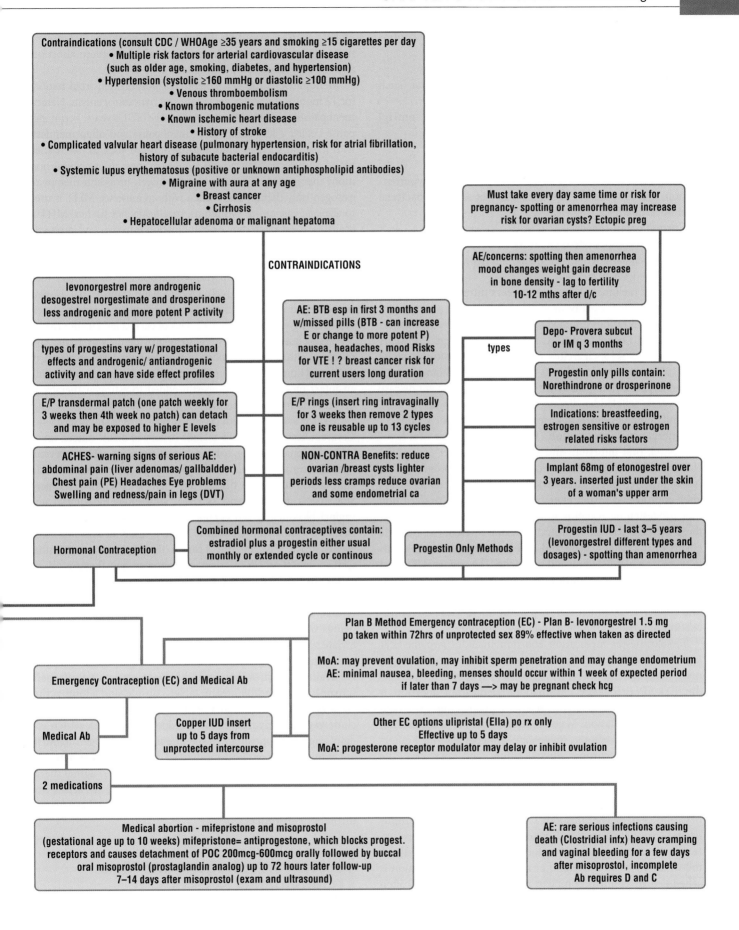

Contraindications (consult CDC / WHOAge ≥35 years and smoking ≥15 cigarettes per day
• Multiple risk factors for arterial cardiovascular disease
(such as older age, smoking, diabetes, and hypertension)
• Hypertension (systolic ≥160 mmHg or diastolic ≥100 mmHg)
• Venous thromboembolism
• Known thrombogenic mutations
• Known ischemic heart disease
• History of stroke
• Complicated valvular heart disease (pulmonary hypertension, risk for atrial fibrillation,
history of subacute bacterial endocarditis)
• Systemic lupus erythematosus (positive or unknown antiphospholipid antibodies)
• Migraine with aura at any age
• Breast cancer
• Cirrhosis
• Hepatocellular adenoma or malignant hepatoma

CONTRAINDICATIONS

Must take every day same time or risk for
pregnancy- spotting or amenorrhea may increase
risk for ovarian cysts? Ectopic preg

AE/concerns: spotting then amenorrhea
mood changes weight gain decrease
in bone density - lag to fertility
10-12 mths after d/c

levonorgestrel more androgenic
desogestrel norgestimate and drosperinone
less androgenic and more potent P activity

AE: BTB esp in first 3 months and
w/missed pills (BTB - can increase
E or change to more potent P)
nausea, headaches, mood Risks
for VTE ! ? breast cancer risk for
current users long duration

types

Depo- Provera subcut
or IM q 3 months

types of progestins vary w/ progestational
effects and androgenic/ antiandrogenic
activity and can have side effect profiles

Progestin only pills contain:
Norethindrone or drosperinone

E/P transdermal patch (one patch weekly for
3 weeks then 4th week no patch) can detach
and may be exposed to higher E levels

E/P rings (insert ring intravaginally
for 3 weeks then remove 2 types
one is reusable up to 13 cycles

Indications: breastfeeding,
estrogen sensitive or estrogen
related risks factors

ACHES- warning signs of serious AE:
abdominal pain (liver adenomas/ gallbaldder)
Chest pain (PE) Headaches Eye problems
Swelling and redness/pain in legs (DVT)

NON-CONTRA Benefits: reduce
ovarian /breast cysts lighter
periods less cramps reduce ovarian
and some endometrial ca

Implant 68mg of etonogestrel over
3 years. inserted just under the skin
of a woman's upper arm

Hormonal Contraception

Combined hormonal contraceptives contain:
estradiol plus a progestin either usual
monthly or extended cycle or continous

Progestin Only Methods

Progestin IUD - last 3–5 years
(levonorgestrel different types and
dosages) - spotting than amenorrhea

Plan B Method Emergency contraception (EC) - Plan B- levonorgestrel 1.5 mg
po taken within 72hrs of unprotected sex 89% effective when taken as directed

MoA: may prevent ovulation, may inhibit sperm penetration and may change endometrium
AE: minimal nausea, bleeding, menses should occur within 1 week of expected period
if later than 7 days —> may be pregnant check hcg

Emergency Contraception (EC) and Medical Ab

Medical Ab

Copper IUD insert
up to 5 days from
unprotected intercourse

Other EC options ulipristal (Ella) po rx only
Effective up to 5 days
MoA: progesterone receptor modulator may delay or inhibit ovulation

2 medications

Medical abortion - mifepristone and misoprostol
(gestational age up to 10 weeks) mifepristone= antiprogestone, which blocks progest.
receptors and causes detachment of POC 200mcg-600mcg orally followed by buccal
oral misoprostol (prostaglandin analog) up to 72 hours later follow-up
7–14 days after misoprostol (exam and ultrasound)

AE: rare serious infections causing
death (Clostridial infx) heavy cramping
and vaginal bleeding for a few days
after misoprostol, incomplete
Ab requires D and C

Category 4 contraindications to combined hormonal contraceptives include:

- Age ≥35 years and smoking ≥15 cigarettes per day
- Multiple risk factors for arterial cardiovascular disease (such as older age, smoking, diabetes, and hypertension)
- Hypertension (systolic ≥160 mmHg or diastolic ≥100 mmHg)
- VTE, unless on anticoagulation
- Known ischemic heart disease
- History of stroke
- Complicated valvular heart disease (pulmonary hypertension, risk for atrial fibrillation, history of subacute bacterial endocarditis)
- Current breast cancer
- Severe (decompensated) cirrhosis
- Hepatocellular adenoma or malignant hepatoma
- Migraine with aura
- Diabetes mellitus (DM) of >20 years duration or with nephropathy, retinopathy, or neuropathy[12,13]

Category 3 ratings are medical conditions where risk generally outweighs benefits of CHC use and include: age ≥35 years and smoking <15 cigarettes per day, hypertension (systolic 140–159 mmHg or diastolic 90–99 mmHg) or adequately controlled hypertension, past breast cancer with no current disease for 5 years, gallbladder disease, superficial venous thrombosis, and inflammatory bowel disease with risk factors for VTE.[12,13]

Emergency contraception (EC) options include oral levonorgestrel, oral ulipristal, and insertion of copper-containing IUD. Oral levonorgestrel is an over-the-counter progestin that is administered once, ideally within 72 hours but up to 5 days after unprotected sexual intercourse. Ulipristal is prescription oral progesterone receptor modulator that must be administered within 5 days of unprotected sexual intercourse. Adverse effects of ulipristal acetate and oral levonorgestrel-only products are irregular bleeding and headache. The copper IUD must be inserted by a healthcare provider within 5 days of unprotected sexual intercourse; it is the most effective method of EC. The copper IUD, which can provide up to 10 years of contraception, can cause cramping and heavy bleeding.[14]

First-trimester medication abortion includes two medications, mifepristone (a progesterone and glucocorticoid antagonist), in combination with misoprostol (a synthetic prostaglandin E1) for pregnancy termination. Medication abortion is highly effective, and it can be used in pregnancies up to 77 days (11 weeks) of gestation. Major contraindications to medication abortion include ectopic pregnancy, anticoagulation, hemorrhagic disorders, chronic adrenal failure, and porphyria. The basic steps of the medication abortion are as follows: confirm pregnancy and gestational age, and assess contraindications in the initial outpatient visit. Oral mifepristone is administered first, and 24 to 48 later misoprostol 800 mcg can be self-administered buccally (placed and dissolved in the buccal space between the cheek and the gum for 30 minutes) or vaginally. A follow-up visit 1 to 2 weeks after misoprostol administration is scheduled to confirm complete pregnancy termination often with transvaginal ultrasound or serial serum human chorionic gonadotropin (hCG). Common side effects are vaginal bleeding often heavier than menses and within a few hours of misoprostol, and abdominal cramping and pain. Other side effects include nausea, vomiting, diarrhea, and headache. Complications include heavy bleeding, infection, incomplete abortion, and unrecognized ectopic pregnancy.[15,16]

Menopause is the permanent cessation of menstrual periods for 12 months, follicular depletion, and hypoestrogenism. Natural menopause usually occurs at a median age of 51.4 years. Perimenopause begins a few years before menopause and often manifests with irregular menses, vasomotor symptoms such as hot flashes, mood and sleep changes, and vaginal dryness. Menopausal hormone therapy (MHT) is combined estrogen-progestin therapy or estrogen-only therapy for women without a uterus. MHT is used to alleviate vasomotor symptoms, specifically hot flashes. MHT is available as estrogen only or combination estrogen and progestin in multiple systemic transdermal (patches, gels, lotion, spray) and oral formulations. MHT is indicated for symptomatic, healthy, younger women within 10 years of menopause or younger than age 60 years. Common regimens are daily transdermal 17-beta estradiol and cyclic administration of oral micronized progesterone (200 mg/day for the first 12 days of each calendar month) for 5 years or less. Continuous regimens provide daily systemic hormones of either estrogen alone in women with a hysterectomy or combined hormones in women with an intact uterus. Women with an intact uterus require progestin added to estrogen therapy to prevent endometrial hyperplasia and potentially cancer.[17]

MHT is associated with certain adverse effects and health risks. Contraindications to MHT include history of breast cancer, unexplained vaginal bleeding, coronary heart disease (CHD), a previous venous thromboembolic (VTE) event or stroke or transient ischemic attack, active liver disease, and high-risk endometrial cancer. Side effects include breast soreness, sometimes moodiness, and vaginal bleeding, which occurs frequently with cyclic regimens. Risks associated with combined MHT include increases in CHD events, stroke, VTE, and breast cancer; there is no increase in either CHD or breast cancer risk seen with estrogen-only therapy.[17,18]

Genitourinary syndrome of menopause (GSM) manifests as vaginal atrophy and causes vaginal dryness, burning, dyspareunia, and sometimes urinary symptoms. Treatment of GSM beings with vaginal moisturizers and lubricants, which can alleviate symptoms but do not affect vaginal tissue. Vaginal estrogen therapy is used for persistent symptoms. Vaginal estrogens are available by prescription and include conjugated estrogens (cream) and estradiol (cream, tablet, capsule, and a long-acting 90 days vaginal ring). Other medications available for GSM include vaginal dehydroepiandrosterone (prasterone), which is a daily vaginal suppository. Ospemifene is an estrogen agonist/antagonist that is orally administered daily for GSM and may be useful for women who do not want or cannot use vaginal therapies. Ospemifene can increase hot flashes, and it carries box warnings for potential increased risk of endometrial cancer and thrombotic disorders.

SECTION 3: Androgens and Male Reproductive System

Mind Map 6.3 illustrates medications used in men's health. Testosterone therapy is used to treat male hypogonadism from either primary hypogonadism (disease of testes) or disease of the hypothalamus or pituitary (secondary hypogonadism). Testosterone is synthesized by the testes, binds to androgen receptors, and exerts its effects on multiple tissues to cause virilization, increase muscle, maintain bone density, and increase libido and energy. Symptoms and signs of androgen deficiency in adult males include decreased sex drive (libido), decreased morning erections, difficulty building muscle, decreased energy, and depressed mood. Low morning serum testosterone levels in conjunction with clinical manifestations confirm the diagnosis of male hypogonadism. Testosterone replacement therapy (TRT) is a highly effective primary treatment for male hypogonadism, although in males desiring fertility other options are available. In males with hypogonadism who desire fertility subcutaneous injections of gonadotropins such as hCG and human menopausal gonadotropin can increase testosterone and spermatogenesis.

TRT is available in a variety of dosing preparations and regimens. Topical/transdermal testosterone delivery systems are gels, or a solution applied daily, which may cause skin irritation, absorption issues, are costly, and can transfer to other people including women, pregnant women, and children. Parenteral testosterone includes intramuscular long-acting testosterone enanthate and testosterone cypionate (injected every 1–2 weeks), and extralong-acting testosterone undecanoate (injected by a trained healthcare professional every 10–14 weeks). There is also a nasal testosterone gel administered three times per day and subcutaneous testosterone pellets implanted every 3 to 6 months.

Certain contraindications, adverse effects, and risks are associated with TRT. Possible contraindications include prostate cancer, breast cancer, severe untreated sleep apnea, and erythrocytosis, e.g., hematocrit >50%. Potential adverse effects include erythrocytosis, which requires monitoring of hematocrit and potential reduction of dose or therapeutic phlebotomy. There is a potential but inconclusive risk of venous thromboembolism and inconclusive data on cardiovascular risk.[19,20] There are recommendations to monitor for prostate cancer during testosterone therapy. Testosterone gels may transfer to another person, and patients should follow instructions such as washing hands and keeping application site covered with clothing to minimize secondary exposure.

Erectile dysfunction (ED) is a common type of male sexual dysfunction with many underlying causes. ED is defined as the inability to achieve and/or maintain an erection sufficient for satisfactory sexual intercourse.[21] The most commonly used and highly effective class of medications for ED treatment are the oral phosphodiesterase type 5 inhibitors (PDE5 inhibitors). The PDE5 inhibitors act to increase cyclic guanosine monophosphate (GMP) by competitively inhibiting the PDE5 enzyme. Cyclic GMP increases vasodilation, which is important in initiating and maintaining penile erections. PDE5 inhibitors are also indicated in men with benign prostatic hyperplasia (BPH) symptoms and erectile dysfunction.

The PDE5 inhibitor medications include sildenafil, vardenafil, tadalafil, and avanafil. Tadalafil is longest acting, can last up to 36 hours, and can be taken daily or as needed. Sildenafil and vardenafil last for up to 4 hours and are taken 1 hour before sexual activity. Avanafil is the most rapid acting and can be taken 30 to 45 minutes before sexual activity. Food can delay and affect the absorption of vardenafil and sildenafil.

There are important adverse effects, contraindications, and drug interactions with the PDE5 inhibitors. **PDE5 inhibitors are contraindicated in patients taking any form of nitrates because of potential life-threatening hypertension.** Alpha-adrenergic antagonists can also cause vasodilation and symptomatic hypotension when taken with PDE5 inhibitors. PDE5 inhibitors cause vasodilation, and the most common related side effects are flushing, headaches, dyspepsia, and sometimes nasal congestion. Visual side effects can occur, specifically temporary and reversible blue vision with sildenafil and, rarely, nonarteritic anterior ischemic optic neuropathy.[22] Sudden, short-term, and unilateral hearing loss is rare side effect of sildenafil, vardenafil, and tadalafil.

Alprostadil is another medication for ED, which is indicated for men who cannot use or fail therapy with oral PDE5 inhibitors. Alprostadil is a prostaglandin E1 analog, which causes vascular smooth muscle relaxation and vasodilation. It is available as intracavernosal penile injection or as an intraurethral gel, which is delivered by applicator into the urethral meatus. Priapism, which is penile erection lasting more than 4 to 6 hours, is an uncommon but serious effect of injectable alprostadil. Priapism is an emergency and requires immediate urologic attention. Penile pain was the most common adverse effect.

BPH is a common problem in aging men, which can be asymptomatic or cause lower urinary tract symptoms (LUTS). LUTS include irritative symptoms such as urinary frequency, urgency, nocturia, and incontinence and/or voiding symptoms such as slow urinary stream, straining to void, urinary intermittency or hesitancy, splitting of the voiding stream, and terminal dribbling. Medical therapy for BPH include two primary classes: alpha-1 adrenergic antagonist for initial treatment and 5-alpha reductase inhibitors (5-ARIs). Selective alpha-1 adrenergic receptor antagonists include terazosin, doxazosin, tamsulosin, alfuzosin, and silodosin. The selective alpha-1 adrenergic receptor antagonists block alpha-1 receptors on prostatic smooth muscle causing relaxation of the smooth muscle of the bladder neck and the prostatic urethra. The adverse effects of the alpha-1 adrenergic receptor antagonists include dizziness and hypotension, although these effects are less common with tamsulosin and silodosin because they are more selective for prostatic alpha-1a receptors. Tamsulosin and silodosin may cause retrograde ejaculation. Intraoperative floppy iris syndrome may be associated with alpha-1 adrenergic blockers in men taking alpha-1 adrenergic blockers and undergoing cataract surgery.[23]

The 5-ARIs finasteride and dutasteride block the conversion of testosterone to dihydrotestosterone (DHT), which decreases the progression of BPH. The 5-alpha reductase inhibitors take several months to work and are often added to alpha-1 antagonists. Adverse effects of the 5-alpha reductase inhibitors include sexual dysfunction, that is, impotence, ejaculatory dysfunction, and decreased libido. 5-ARIs may be associated with an increase in the incidence of high-grade prostate cancers.[24] 5-ARIs are contraindicated in pregnancy because of potential adverse effects on a developing male fetus.

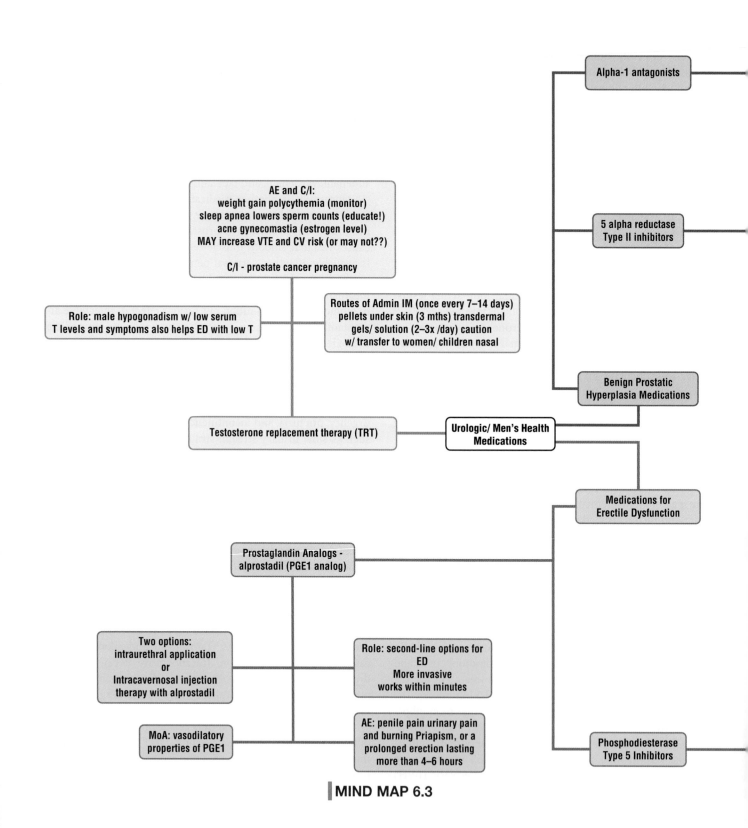

MIND MAP 6.3

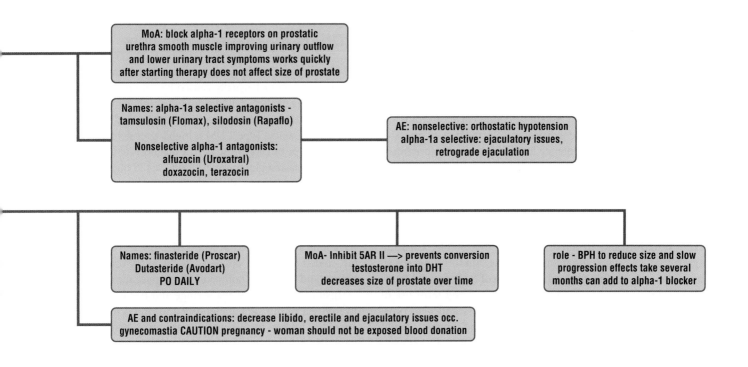

MoA: block alpha-1 receptors on prostatic urethra smooth muscle improving urinary outflow and lower urinary tract symptoms works quickly after starting therapy does not affect size of prostate

Names: alpha-1a selective antagonists - tamsulosin (Flomax), silodosin (Rapaflo)

Nonselective alpha-1 antagonists: alfuzocin (Uroxatral) doxazocin, terazocin

AE: nonselective: orthostatic hypotension alpha-1a selective: ejaculatory issues, retrograde ejaculation

Names: finasteride (Proscar) Dutasteride (Avodart) PO DAILY

MoA- Inhibit 5AR II —> prevents conversion testosterone into DHT decreases size of prostate over time

role - BPH to reduce size and slow progression effects take several months can add to alpha-1 blocker

AE and contraindications: decrease libido, erectile and ejaculatory issues occ. gynecomastia CAUTION pregnancy - woman should not be exposed blood donation

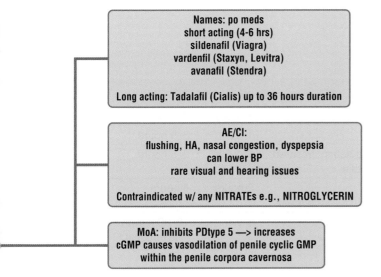

Names: po meds
short acting (4-6 hrs)
sildenafil (Viagra)
vardenfil (Staxyn, Levitra)
avanafil (Stendra)

Long acting: Tadalafil (Cialis) up to 36 hours duration

AE/CI:
flushing, HA, nasal congestion, dyspepsia
can lower BP
rare visual and hearing issues

Contraindicated w/ any NITRATEs e.g., NITROGLYCERIN

MoA: inhibits PDtype 5 —> increases cGMP causes vasodilation of penile cyclic GMP within the penile corpora cavernosa

SECTION 4: Adrenal Hormones: Glucocorticosteroids

Natural and synthetic glucocorticoids or corticosteroids have cortisol-like activity and include systemic, topical, inhaled, and intranasal preparations. Glucocorticoids are used for a variety of endocrine conditions, that is, evaluation of the hypothalamic-pituitary-adrenal (HPA) axis and treatment of adrenal insufficiency, inflammatory, allergic, and immunologic disorders. The corticosteroids can be compared and classified by potency of antiinflammatory activity and duration of action. The short-acting and least potent systemic corticosteroids include hydrocortisone and cortisone, intermediate-acting steroids with intermediate potency include prednisone, prednisolone, and methylprednisolone, and the longest-acting and most potent corticosteroid is dexamethasone.

Major side effects of corticosteroids involve multiple organs and can result from short-term or chronic therapy. Complications of chronic corticosteroid use are related to **suppression of HPA function** and hypercortisolism, for example, **Cushing syndrome**. Dermatologic changes include skin thinning, striae, bruising, acne, Cushingoid redistribution of body fat with truncal obesity, buffalo hump, and moon facies. Long-term use of corticosteroids increases the risk of cataracts and glaucoma. Glucocorticoids can suppress immunity and impair wound healing, which can then increase risk for infections. Osteoporosis and osteonecrosis (avascular or ischemic necrosis of bone and, less commonly, proximal muscle myopathy) are associated with chronic corticosteroid use. Gastrointestinal (GI) irritation, ulceration, and bleeding can occur, especially with concomitant nonsteroidal antiinflammatory drugs. Neuropsychiatric effects include insomnia, elevated or dysphoric mood, hypomania, and sometimes psychosis. Hyperglycemia is a common side effect of glucocorticoids, which can worsen DM. HPA axis suppression with adrenal insufficiency can result from abrupt cessation of systemic corticosteroids. This is the primary reason for gradual tapering of systemic corticosteroids when they are administered for 3 or more weeks.

SECTION 5: Endocrine Pancreas and Drugs for Diabetes Mellitus

DM is characterized by persistent hyperglycemia and is generally divided into types 1 usually caused by autoimmune destruction of the pancreatic beta cells, leading to absolute insulin deficiency, and type 2 DM related to insulin resistance and variable relative insulin deficiency. Type 2 DM is highly prevalent and is the most common type of DM in adults. The diagnosis of DM is confirmed by fasting plasma glucose (FPG) FPG ≥126 mg/dL (7 mmol/L), 2-hour plasma glucose during a 75-g oral glucose tolerance test (OGTT) ≥200 mg/dL (11.1 mmol/L) during an OGTT, or glycated hemoglobin (A1C) A1C ≥6.5%.[25] Medications used to treat diabetes, achieve glycemic goals, and decrease diabetic complications are illustrated in Mind Map 6.4 and insulins in Table 6.1, and they can be divided into insulins, oral hypoglycemic agents, and injectable noninsulin hypoglycemic agents.

Insulins are injected via syringe and needles or pens or delivered via pump subcutaneously and dosed in units. Insulins are either human insulin analogs or human insulin of recombinant deoxyribonucleic acid origin and they are characterized by onset, peak, and duration of action as follows: rapid, short, intermediate, long, and ultralong acting (see Table 6.1). Rapid- and short-acting insulins are designated as "prandial" insulins and are injected before meals to provide "bolus" coverage of meal related glucose increases. Basal insulins are generally intermediate, long- or ultralong-acting insulins and injected once daily. All patients with type 1 DM and many patients with type 2 DM require insulin therapy. Insulin therapy requires self blood glucose monitoring to detect hypoglycemia and monitor

TABLE 6.1	Insulins		
Type and name of insulin	Onset	Peak	Duration
Rapid-acting insulin analog (insulin lispro)	5–15 min	1–1.5 h	3–5 hours
Rapid-acting insulin analog insulin aspart	5–15 min	1–1.5 h	3–5 hours
Rapid-acting insulin glulisine	5–15 min (most rapid acting, injected directly before meals)	1–1.5 h	3–5 hours
Short-acting regular human insulin (*also available for IV administration*)	30–60 min Inject about 30 min before the meal	2 hours	8 hours
Intermediate-acting neutral protamine hagedorn (NPH)	2–4 h	6–7 h	10–20 h (may require 2 daily injections)
Long-acting analog Insulin glargine	0.5–1 h	Flat	~24 h
Long-acting analog Insulin detemir	0.5–1 h	Flat	17 hours
Ultralong-acting analog Insulin degludec	0.5–1.5 h	Flat	>42 h

for hyperglycemia. The most serious risk of insulin is hypoglycemia, which is more common in type 1 DM and can be fatal. Symptomatic hypoglycemia can be managed by ingesting 15 to 20 grams of fast-acting carbohydrate such as glucose tablets, sugar, hard candies, fruit juice, or soda. Severe hypoglycemia requires IV dextrose or administration of glucagon (subcutaneous, intramuscular, or nasal). Other adverse effects of insulin include weight gain and changes in subcutaneous fatty tissue at injection sites specifically lipoatrophy or lipohypertrophy.

Noninsulin oral and injectable medications for type 2 diabetes are classified by class/name and mechanism of action. There are several classes of noninsulin hypoglycemics including: (1) biguanides specifically metformin, (2) sulfonylureas, (3) meglitinides, (4) thiazolidinediones, (5) α-glucosidase inhibitors, (6) glucagon-like peptide 1 (GLP-1) receptor agonists, (7) dipeptidyl peptidase 4 (DPP-4) inhibitors, and (8) sodium-glucose cotransporter inhibitors (SGLTs). **Metformin** is an oral biguanide and is the first-line initial therapy for most patients with type 2 DM. Metformin has multiple actions but primarily reduces hepatic gluconeogenesis. The most common adverse effects of metformin are dose-related GI distress, mild loss of appetite, which can cause modest weight loss, nausea, abdominal cramps, and loose stools. Metformin has a boxed warning about rare but potentially fatal lactic acidosis, which is more likely in patients with hypoperfusion and hypoxemia. Metformin is contraindicated in patients with impaired kidney function, estimated glomerular filtration rate <30 mL/min/1.73 m^2, active liver disease, tissue hypoperfusion from any cause, and history of lactic acidosis during metformin therapy.[26]

Sulfonylureas are oral hypoglycemics that bind to receptors on beta cells in the pancreas causing inhibition potassium influx, which leads to depolarization, increased calcium influx, and increases insulin release from the pancreas. Second-generation sulfonylureas currently used in practice are glyburide, glipizide, and glimepiride, which can be added to other agents in patients who fail to achieve glycemic goals. Hypoglycemia, which is more common with glyburide and weight gain, is the most common adverse effect of the sulfonylureas.

The oral **meglitinides,** repaglinide and nateglinide, work similarly to sulfonylureas and cause insulin secretion by pancreatic beta cells. Repaglinide and nateglinides are rapid acting with short duration of action and are usually dosed before each meal. Repaglinide may have better efficacy and can be used in patients with chronic kidney disease. Weight gain and, less often, hypoglycemia are adverse effects of meglitinides.[27]

Oral **thiazolidinediones (TZD),** pioglitazone and rosiglitazone, act as peroxisome proliferator-activated receptors agonists affecting gene transcription, which regulates glucose and lipid metabolism and increases insulin sensitivity in adipose tissue and muscle.[28] Pioglitazone is the primary TZD used, and rosiglitazone use is restricted because of potential increased risk of acute myocardial infarction (MI) and cardiovascular deaths.[29] There are several contraindications to TZDs including active liver disease, fracture risk, heart failure, active or history of bladder cancer, and pregnancy. Adverse effects and risks of TZDs include weight gain, fluid retention, worsening heart failure, decreased bone density and increase fracture risk, possible bladder cancer, and potential hepatotoxicity.

The oral **α-glucosidase inhibitors**, acarbose and miglitol, inhibit alpha-glucosidase GI enzymes to slow the breakdown of dietary carbohydrates into monosaccharides. They are dosed orally three times a day with meals. GI adverse effects are very common and dose related and include flatulence, diarrhea, and abdominal discomfort.

The **GLP-1 receptor agonists** include exenatide (twice-daily injection), lixisenatide (once-daily injection), liraglutide (once-daily injection), extended-release exenatide (once weekly), dulaglutide (once weekly), and semaglutide (once-weekly injection or once-daily oral tablet). GLP-1 agonists lower blood glucose by increasing insulin release, delaying gastric emptying, decreasing postmeal glucagon release and reducing food intake.[30] In addition to improving glycemic control, evidence suggests GLP-1 agonists can reduce cardiovascular disease (CVD) outcomes in patients with type 2 DM and CVD.[31,32] The most common adverse effects of GLP-1 agonists are GI related, particularly nausea, vomiting, and diarrhea. Pancreatitis can occur with GLP-1 agonists, and patients with a history of pancreatitis should not use this class of medications. GLP-1 agonists should not be used in patients with a personal or family history of medullary thyroid cancer or multiple endocrine neoplasia 2A or 2B.

The oral **DPP-4 inhibitors** include sitagliptin, saxagliptin, linagliptin, and alogliptin. The DPP-4 inhibitors reduce blood glucose by inhibiting the breakdown of glucose-dependent insulinotropic polypeptide andGLP-1 via dipeptidyl peptidase 4 enzyme inhibition. The adverse effects and potential concerns of the DPP-4 inhibitors are headache and upper respiratory tract infection. Long-term safety is not established, and the DPP-4 inhibitors have been associated with pancreatitis and should not be used in patients with a history of pancreatitis.[33]

The oral SGLTs or flozins include canagliflozin, dapagliflozin, empagliflozin, and ertugliflozin. The SGLTs reduce plasma glucose by blocking reabsorption of filtered glucose in the proximal tubules of the nephrons. In addition to reducing blood glucose, certain SGLTs may reduce atherosclerotic cardiovascular morbidity and mortality in patients with type 2 diabetes and overt CVD, and in patients with type 2 diabetes and heart failure they can reduce the risk of major cardiovascular events.[34,35] The SGLTs are also associated with blood pressure reduction and modest weight loss. The primary adverse effects of SGLTs are an increase in genitourinary infections. Other risks associated with the SGLTs include hypotension, acute kidney injury, and increased risk of diabetic ketoacidosis. In patients with risk factors for amputation, certain SGLTs increased the risk for lower limb amputations.[36]

SECTION 6: Osteoporosis

Osteoporosis is a skeletal disorder characterized by low bone mass, increased bone fragility, decreased bone strength, and increased risk of fracture. Postmenopausal osteoporosis is a primary cause of osteoporosis, although other risk factors include cigarette smoking, excessive alcohol, low body weight, personal and family history of fracture, and glucocorticoid use. Dual-energy X-ray absorptiometry bone density tests define

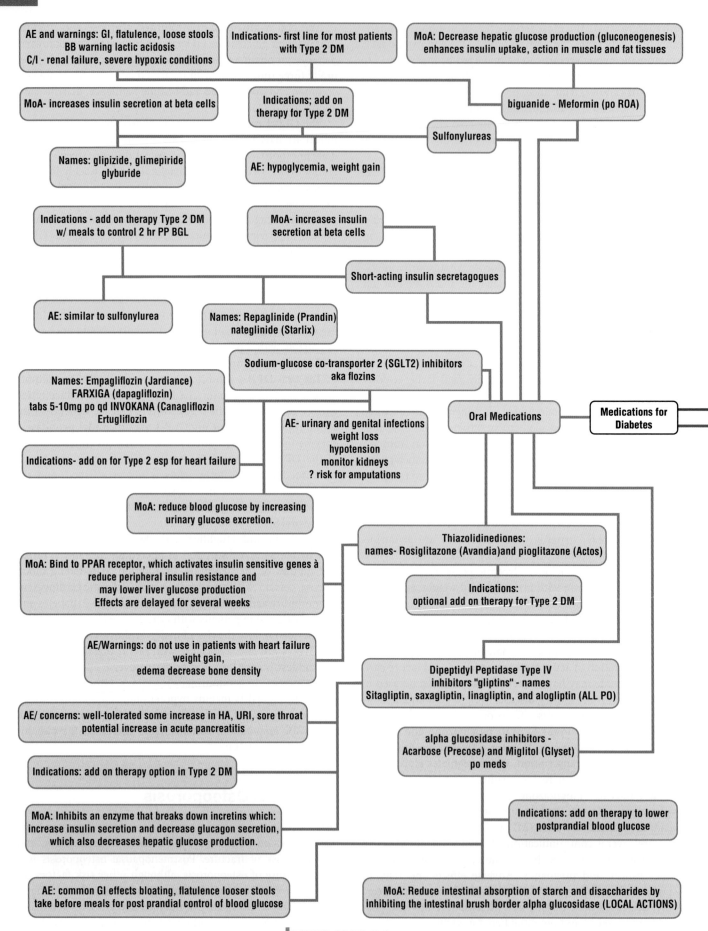

MIND MAP 6.4

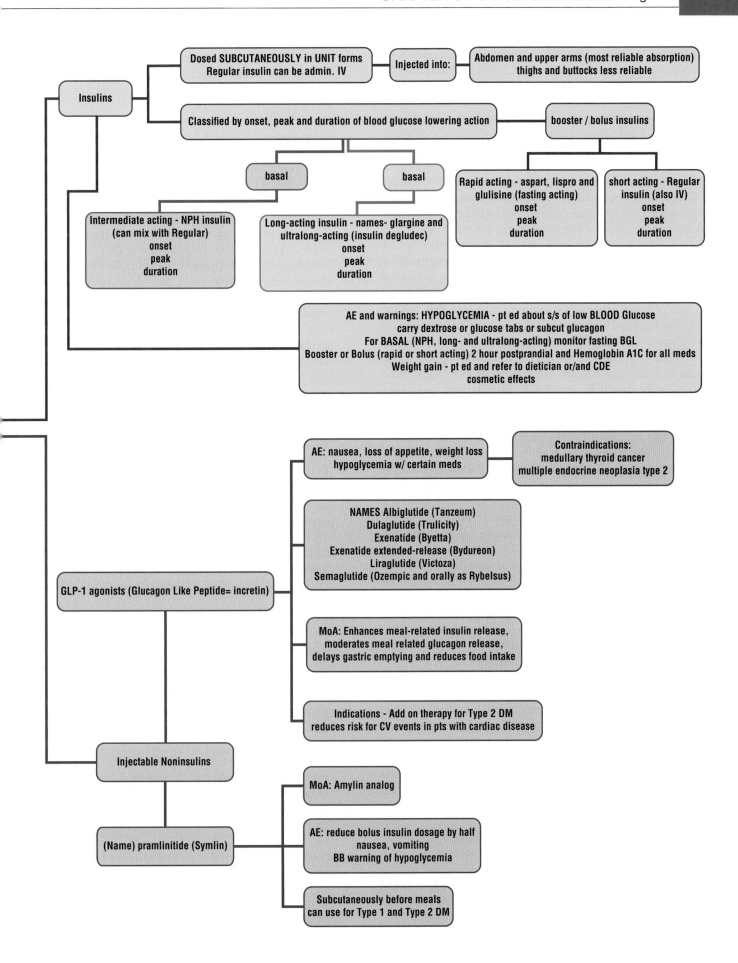

Insulins

Dosed SUBCUTANEOUSLY in UNIT forms
Regular insulin can be admin. IV

Injected into:

Abdomen and upper arms (most reliable absorption)
thighs and buttocks less reliable

Classified by onset, peak and duration of blood glucose lowering action

booster / bolus insulins

basal

basal

Rapid acting - aspart, lispro and glulisine (fasting acting)
onset
peak
duration

short acting - Regular insulin (also IV)
onset
peak
duration

Intermediate acting - NPH insulin (can mix with Regular)
onset
peak
duration

Long-acting insulin - names- glargine and ultralong-acting (insulin degludec)
onset
peak
duration

AE and warnings: HYPOGLYCEMIA - pt ed about s/s of low BLOOD Glucose
carry dextrose or glucose tabs or subcut glucagon
For BASAL (NPH, long- and ultralong-acting) monitor fasting BGL
Booster or Bolus (rapid or short acting) 2 hour postprandial and Hemoglobin A1C for all meds
Weight gain - pt ed and refer to dietician or/and CDE
cosmetic effects

AE: nausea, loss of appetite, weight loss
hypoglycemia w/ certain meds

Contraindications:
medullary thyroid cancer
multiple endocrine neoplasia type 2

NAMES Albiglutide (Tanzeum)
Dulaglutide (Trulicity)
Exenatide (Byetta)
Exenatide extended-release (Bydureon)
Liraglutide (Victoza)
Semaglutide (Ozempic and orally as Rybelsus)

GLP-1 agonists (Glucagon Like Peptide= incretin)

MoA: Enhances meal-related insulin release,
moderates meal related glucagon release,
delays gastric emptying and reduces food intake

Indications - Add on therapy for Type 2 DM
reduces risk for CV events in pts with cardiac disease

Injectable Noninsulins

MoA: Amylin analog

AE: reduce bolus insulin dosage by half
nausea, vomiting
BB warning of hypoglycemia

(Name) pramlinitide (Symlin)

Subcutaneously before meals
can use for Type 1 and Type 2 DM

osteoporosis as a T-score (bone density compared with what is normally expected in a healthy young adult of the same sex) of -2.5 standard deviations and below. Classes of medications for osteoporosis include bisphosphonates, parathyroid hormone and parathyroid hormone-related protein (PTHrP) analogs (teriparatide, abaloparatide), romosozumab, and denosumab. Vitamin D3 and calcium (dietary and supplemental) are generally advised in addition to medications.

The names and routes of administration of the bisphosphonates are alendronate (po once-daily or once-weekly dosing), risedronate (po once-daily or once-weekly dosing), ibandronate (po or IV every 3 months), and zoledronic acid (IV infusion once a year). The oral bisphosphonates are the generally preferred initial therapy for most cases of osteoporosis. The oral bisphosphonates should be taken on an empty stomach without any other medications first thing in the morning with a full 8-ounce (240-mL) glass of water and in an upright position. The action of bisphosphonates is antiresorptive, and they bind to bony surfaces and inhibit osteoclastic mediated bone resorption.

There are adverse effects and contraindications of bisphosphonates. Oral bisphosphonates can irritate the upper GI mucosa and may cause reflux, esophagitis, or esophageal ulceration. They should be avoided in patients with esophageal disorders and in severe renal disease.[37] IV bisphosphonates may cause acute infusion reactions, which respond to ibuprofen or acetaminophen. Other adverse effect are hypocalcemia and musculoskeletal pain. There have been reports of bone-related issues, specifically osteonecrosis of the jaw, especially in patients with certain cancers on IV bisphosphonates and related to dental procedures. The other rare bone issue is atypical femur fracture with long-term therapy. Duration of therapy with bisphosphonates depends on fracture risk and can range from 3 to 10 years.

Another treatment for osteoporosis includes denosumab, which is an antiresorptive medication. Denosumab inhibits receptor activator of nuclear factor kappa-B ligand, which inhibits osteoclasts. Denosumab is injected subcutaneously once every 6 months indefinitely. Adverse effects and risks include rapid bone loss and an increase in vertebral fracture after discontinuation, back pain, and musculoskeletal pain.[38]

PTHrP analogs (teriparatide, abaloparatide) are anabolic agents used subcutaneously daily for severe osteoporosis for up to 2 years.[39,40] Teriparatide and abaloparatide are well tolerated with hypercalcemia and hypercalciuria as primary adverse effects. Contraindications to teriparatide and abaloparatide are primary or secondary hyperparathyroidism, hypercalcemia, and risks for osteosarcoma. Maximum duration of treatment with teriparatide and abaloparatide is 2 years because of potential risk for osteosarcoma.[41]

Romosozumab is an anabolic agent that enhances osteoblast function and reduces fractures. It is administered subcutaneously once monthly for 12 months for patients with severe osteoporosis, fragility fractures, and patients who cannot tolerate other therapies. Romosozumab is associated with a boxed warning of serious cardiovascular events (cardiac, ischemic, and cerebrovascular accidents).[42]

REFERENCES

1. Roos A, Linn-Rasker SP, van Domburg RT, et al. The starting dose of levothyroxine in primary hypothyroidism treatment: a prospective, randomized, double-blind trial. *Arch Intern Med.* 2005;165:1714.
2. Alexander EK, Pearce EN, Brent GA, et al. 2017 Guidelines of the American Thyroid Association for the diagnosis and management of thyroid disease during pregnancy and the postpartum. *Thyroid.* 2017;27:315.
3. Andersohn F, Konzen C, Garbe E. Systematic review: agranulocytosis induced by nonchemotherapy drugs. *Ann Intern Med.* 2007;146:657.
4. FDA Drug Safety Communication. *New Boxed Warning on Severe Liver Injury with Propylthiouracil.* 2010. Available at: http://www.fda.gov/Drugs/DrugSafety/PostmarketDrug SafetyInformationforPatientsandProviders/ucm209023.htm.
5. Balavoine AS, Glinoer D, Dubucquoi S, Wémeau JL. Antineutrophil cytoplasmic antibody-positive small-vessel vasculitis associated with antithyroid drug therapy: how significant is the clinical problem? *Thyroid.* 2015;25:1273.
6. Safa AM, Schumacher OP, Rodriguez-Antunez A. Long-term follow-up results in children and adolescents treated with radioactive iodine (131I) for hyperthyroidism. *N Engl J Med.* 1975;292:167.
7. American Thyroid Association Taskforce on Radioiodine Safety, Sisson JC, Freitas J, et al. Radiation safety in the treatment of patients with thyroid diseases by radioiodine 131I: practice recommendations of the American Thyroid Association. *Thyroid.* 2011;21:335.
8. Curtis KM, Jatlaoui TC, Tepper NK, et al. U.S. Selected practice recommendations for contraceptive use, 2016. *MMWR Recomm Rep.* 2016;65:1.
9. Black A, Guilbert E, Costescu D, et al. No. 329-Canadian Contraception Consensus part 4 of 4 chapter 9: combined hormonal contraception. *J Obstet Gynaecol Can.* 2017;39:229-268.
10. Committee Opinion No. 602: Depot medroxyprogesterone acetate and bone effects. *Obstet Gynecol.* 2014;123:1398. Reaffirmed 2021.
11. Marchbanks PA, McDonald JA, Wilson HG, et al. Oral contraceptives, and the risk of breast cancer. *N Engl J Med.* 2002;346:2025.
12. Curtis KM, Tepper NK, Jatlaoui TC, et al. U.S. medical eligibility criteria for contraceptive use, 2016. *MMWR Recomm Rep.* 2016;65:1.
13. Department of Reproductive Health, World Health Organization. *Medical Eligibility Criteria for Contraceptive Use.* 5th ed. Geneva: World Health Organization; 2015.
14. The American College of Obstetricians and Gynecologists. Practice bulletin summary no. 152: emergency contraception. *Obstet Gynecol.* 2015;126:685-686. A pregnancy test should be administered if menses is delayed by a week of more than expected.
15. Kulier R, Kapp N, Gülmezoglu AM, et al. Medical methods for first trimester abortion. *Cochrane Database Syst Rev.* 2011:CD002855.

16. Cleland K, Creinin MD, Nucatola D, et al. Significant adverse events, and outcomes after medical abortion. *Obstet Gynecol.* 2013;121:166.

17. Stuenkel CA, Davis SR, Gompel A, et al. Treatment of symptoms of the menopause: an Endocrine Society Clinical Practice Guideline. *J Clin Endocrinol Metab.* 2015;100:3975.

18. The NAMS 2017 Hormone Therapy Position Statement Advisory Panel. The 2017 hormone therapy position statement of The North American Menopause Society. *Menopause.* 2017;24:728.

19. Fernández-Balsells MM, Murad MH, Lane M, et al. Clinical review 1: adverse effects of testosterone therapy in adult men: a systematic review and meta-analysis. *J Clin Endocrinol Metab.* 2010;95:2560.

20. Glueck CJ, Wang P. Testosterone therapy, thrombosis, thrombophilia, cardiovascular events. *Metabolism.* 2014;63:989.

21. Burnett AL, Nehra A, Breau RH, et al. Erectile dysfunction: AUA guideline. *J Urol.* 2018;200:633.

22. *Sudden, Short Term and Unilateral Hearing Loss is Rare Side Effect of Sildenafil, Vardenafil, and Tadalafil.* Available at: http://www.accessdata.fda.gov/drugsatfda_docs/label/2014/20895s039s042lbl.pdf.

23. Chatziralli IP, Sergentanis TN. Risk factors for intraoperative floppy iris syndrome: a meta-analysis. *Ophthalmology.* 2011;118:730.

24. Proscar (finasteride) [prescribing information]. Jersey City, NJ: Organon LLC; 2021.

25. American Diabetes Association. Standards of medical care in diabetes–2014. *Diabetes Care.* 2014;37(suppl 1):S14.

26. Glucophage (metformin) [prescribing information]. Princeton, NJ: Bristol-Myers Squibb; 2018.

27. Prandin (repaglinide) [prescribing information]. Bridgewater, NJ: Amneal Specialty; 2019.

28. Hauner H. The mode of action of with thiazolidinediones. *Diabetes Metab Res Rev.* 2002;18(suppl 2):S10.

29. US Food and Drug Administration. *Q&A: Avandia (rosiglitazone).* Available at: http://www.fda.gov/Drugs/DrugSafety/PostmarketDrugSafetyInformationforPatientsandProviders/ucm226976.htm.

30. Lee YS, Jun HS. Anti-diabetic actions of glucagon-like peptide-1 on pancreatic beta-cells. *Metabolism.* 2014;63:9.

31. Holman RR, Bethel MA, Mentz RJ, et al. Effects of once-weekly exenatide on cardiovascular outcomes in type 2 diabetes. *N Engl J Med.* 2017;377:1228.

32. Kristensen SL, Rørth R, Jhund PS, et al. Cardiovascular, mortality, and kidney outcomes with GLP-1 receptor agonists in patients with type 2 diabetes: a systematic review and meta-analysis of cardiovascular outcome trials. *Lancet Diabetes Endocrinol.* 2019;7:776.

33. US Food and Drug Administration. *Information for Healthcare Professionals - Acute Pancreatitis and Sitagliptin (marketed as Januvia and Janumet).* Available at: http://www.fda.gov/Drugs/DrugSafety/PostmarketDrugSafetyInformationforPatientsandProviders/DrugSafetyInformationforHeathcareProfessionals/ucm183764.htm.

34. Zinman B, Wanner C, Lachin JM, et al. Empagliflozin, cardiovascular outcomes, and mortality in type 2 diabetes. *N Engl J Med.* 2015;373:2117.

35. Zelniker TA, Wiviott SD, Raz I, et al. SGLT2 inhibitors for primary and secondary prevention of cardiovascular and renal outcomes in type 2 diabetes: a systematic review and meta-analysis of cardiovascular outcome trials. *Lancet.* 2019;393:31.

36. Chang HY, Singh S, Mansour O, et al. Association between sodium-glucose cotransporter 2 inhibitors and lower extremity amputation among patients with type 2 diabetes. *JAMA Intern Med.* 2018;178:1190.

37. Reid IR. Bisphosphonates in the treatment of osteoporosis: a review of their contribution and controversies. *Skeletal Radiol.* 2011;40:1191–1196. doi:10.1007/s00256-011-1164-9.

38. Cummings SR, San Martin J, McClung MR, et al. Denosumab for prevention of fractures in postmenopausal women with osteoporosis. *N Engl J Med.* 2009;361:756.

39. Miller PD, Hattersley G, Riis BJ, et al. Effect of abaloparatide vs placebo on new vertebral fractures in postmenopausal women with osteoporosis: a randomized clinical trial. *JAMA.* 2016;316:722.

40. Neer RM, Arnaud CD, Zanchetta JR, et al. Effect of parathyroid hormone (1-34) on fractures and bone mineral density in postmenopausal women with osteoporosis. *N Engl J Med.* 2001;344:1434.

41. Tashjian AH Jr, Chabner BA. Commentary on clinical safety of recombinant human parathyroid hormone 1-34 in the treatment of osteoporosis in men and postmenopausal women. *J Bone Miner Res.* 2002;17:1151.

42. Evenity (romosozumab-aqqg) [prescribing information]. Thousand Oaks, CA: Amgen Inc; 2020.

CHAPTER 7

Gastrointestinal Pharmacology

Gastroesophageal reflux disease (GERD) is a common condition in which reflux of stomach contents causes clinical symptoms and/or injury to the esophageal mucosa. Classic symptoms are heartburn and regurgitation of acidic contents, although other symptoms include chest pain, dysphagia, and sometimes chronic cough and hoarseness. GERD can be associated with erosive esophagitis or can be symptomatic without esophageal mucosa injury. Complications of untreated GERD include Barrett esophagus, esophageal adenocarcinoma, or worsening of asthma.

The medical treatment of GERD and erosive esophagitis includes antacids, sucralfate, histamine 2 receptor antagonists (H2RAs), and proton-pump inhibitors (PPIs). Mind Map 7.1 highlights these medications.

Antacids are orally administered short-acting medications used for intermittent relief of reflux symptoms generally after meals. Antacids are weak bases that contain magnesium trisilicate, aluminum hydroxide, or calcium carbonate alone or combination. Antacids react with stomach acid to neutralize gastric pH. Antacids have a rapid onset of action of approximately 5 minutes, and their action lasts for 30 to 60 minutes. The effects of antacids are prolonged when there is food in the stomach. Calcium carbonate containing antacids can cause carbon dioxide formation, which can cause gas and belching. Magnesium-containing antacids may cause diarrhea, and aluminum antacids may cause constipation; both are excreted by kidney, so use caution in patients with renal disease.

H2RAs (e.g., cimetidine, famotidine, and nizatidine) are used for GERD and peptic ulcer disease (PUD). They work by blocking histamine type 2 receptors on the parietal cells in the stomach, which reduces stomach acid secretion. Oral H2RAs are usually administered twice daily usually for up to 12 weeks. H2RAs are generally well tolerated; adverse effects are most common with cimetidine. Long-term cimetidine use has been associated with gynecomastia and impotence. Cimetidine is also more commonly associated with drug interactions. Long-term use of H2RAs can cause B12 deficiency.[1]

PPIs (e.g., omeprazole, lansoprazole, dexlansoprazole, rabeprazole, pantoprazole, and esomeprazole) are the most efficacious

acid suppressants and have faster control of symptoms and better healing rates than H2RAs. PPIs irreversibly bind to the H-K-ATPase pumps on the parietal cells blocking gastric acid secretion. PPIs are indicated for PUD including nonsteroidal antiinflammatory drug (NSAID) induced, *Helicobacter pylori* induced, GERD, erosive esophagitis, and Barrett esophagus. They are most effective after a prolonged fast and should be administered orally once daily, 30 minutes to 60 minutes before breakfast. All the PPIs are available orally, and pantoprazole and esomeprazole are also available as intravenous (IV) formulations.

The PPIs are associated with certain clinically important adverse effects and drug interactions. Some of the gastrointestinal adverse effects include increased risk of *Clostridium difficile* infection, increase in enteric infections, and increase in colonization by multi drug-resistant organisms; long-term use may cause atrophic gastritis.[2-5]

There are other adverse effects and drug interactions associated with PPIs. PPIs can cause malabsorption of certain minerals and vitamins with long-term use. Hypomagnesaemia can occur with long-term use (>1 year) because of intestinal malabsorption. PPIs may reduce calcium absorption, and the US Food and Drug Administration (FDA) assigned safety information about a possible increased risk of fractures of the hip, wrist, and spine with PPIs. Vitamin B12 deficiency can occur with long-term PPI use and may require periodic monitoring of serum vitamin B12 levels.[6] Kidney disease and drug-induced lupus have also been reported with PPIs. All PPIs are metabolized by phase I hepatic cytochrome P450 enzymes, primarily CYP2C19. There are some drug interactions, including decreased activation of clopidogrel, which may reduce the efficacy of clopidogrel.[7]

TREATMENT OF PEPTIC ULCER DISEASE

PUD are defects in the gastric and/or duodenal mucosa that extend through the muscularis mucosae. The most common causes of PUD are *H. pylori* infection and NSAIDs and aspirin use. Many patients with PUD are asymptomatic, but classic clinical presentation is recurrent upper abdominal pain. Complications from PUD include most commonly upper gastrointestinal (GI) bleeding as well as perforation and obstruction. Treatment of PUD includes healing and prevention of recurrence of ulcers. Patients with NSAID- or aspirin-induced ulcers should discontinue NSAIDs if possible and start PPIs for 4 to 8 weeks depending on the size of the ulcer. Patients who cannot discontinue NSAIDs or aspirin need daily maintenance PPI therapy.

Patients with *H. pylori* positive ulcers are treated with an eradication regimen including a PPI (e.g., omeprazole 20 mg twice daily) with two antibiotics for 14 days. First-line antibiotic regimens for *H. pylori* eradication are bismuth quadruple therapy, which consists of bismuth subsalicylate, metronidazole, tetracycline, and a PPI given for 14 days OR clarithromycin triple therapy, which consists of clarithromycin, amoxicillin, and a PPI for 14 days. Metronidazole can be used instead of amoxicillin patients who are allergic to penicillin. Eradication rates are lower with clarithromycin due to increased resistance. Adverse effects of each antibiotic are discussed in Chapter 9, but the regimens are well tolerated. Other regimens for eradication include concomitant therapy with clarithromycin, amoxicillin, a nitroimidazole (tinidazole or metronidazole), and a PPI administered together for 14 days or hybrid therapy with amoxicillin and a PPI for 7 days followed by amoxicillin, clarithromycin, a nitroimidazole, and a PPI for 7 days.[8] Confirmation of eradication of *H. pylori* with either urea breath test or a fecal antigen test should be performed 4 or more weeks after completion of the eradication regimens.

ANTIEMETIC DRUGS (MIND MAP 7.2)

Nausea and vomiting are clinical manifestations of a variety of disorders including GI infections, medications, for example, chemotherapy-induced nausea and vomiting, postoperative nausea/vomiting, metabolic disorders, inner ear, and central nervous system disorders. The physiology of nausea and especially vomiting is complex and involves several neurotransmitters and their interaction between the gut, inner ear, and parts of the brain, especially the chemoreceptor trigger zone and the emetic center in the medulla. The primary receptors and neurotransmitters involved in the vomiting reflex include M1—muscarinic, acetylcholine, D2—dopamine, H1—histamine, 5-hydroxytryptamine (HT-3)—serotonin, and Neurokinin 1 (NK1) receptor—substance P.[9]

Table 7.1 and Mind Map 7.2 detail the common characteristics of antiemetic drugs that target various signaling pathways in nausea and vomiting. Specific indications for each antiemetic class are also detailed in this table.[10]

DRUGS FOR CONSTIPATION (MIND MAP 7.3)

Constipation is a common problem with several underlying causes. Functional constipation is defined as chronic infrequent, hard stools, straining with defecation, sensation of incomplete evacuation, or anorectal blockage with defecation. Medications for chronic constipation are generally classified by their mechanism of action and onset of action to produce a bowel movement. Table 7.2[13,14] and Mind Map 7.3 highlight laxatives used to treat constipation.

Initial management of chronic constipation includes patient education to increase fluid intake and increase dietary fiber up to 20 to 35 g/day from bran, citrus fruits, and legumes. Bulk-forming laxative supplements, especially psyllium with increase in fluids, can be added to improve bowel habits. If fiber and bulk-forming laxatives are not effective, osmotic laxatives such as polyethylene glycol (PEG) powder can be added once daily with water. Stimulant laxatives such as bisacodyl should not be used daily. Patients with chronic idiopathic constipation that does not respond to usual treatments may require one of the guanylate cyclase-C receptor agonists, lubiprostone, or the serotonin 5-HT4 receptor agonist, prucalopride. Constipation caused by opioid medications can be managed with daily stool softeners, PEG powder, and stimulant laxatives. Severe constipation caused by opioid medications may require a mu opioid receptor antagonist, e.g., subcutaneous methylnaltrexone, or oral naloxegol or oral naldemedine.[15]

ANTIDIARRHEAL MEDICATIONS

Diarrhea is passage of frequent loose or watery stools and has variable causes. Acute diarrhea lasts less than 2 weeks and chronic diarrhea is more than 30 days duration. Infectious diarrhea may be managed symptomatically or, in certain cases, with a course of antimicrobial medication. Symptomatic treatment is rehydration preferably with oral solutions containing water, electrolytes, and sugar. Antimotility agents include loperamide (two tablets [4 mg] initially, then 2 mg after each unformed stool for ≤2 days) and diphenoxylate (two tablets [5 mg] 4 times daily for ≤2 days), which are opioids that act on the muscle layers of the intestines to inhibit peristalsis and decrease the frequency of loose or watery bowel movements. Diphenoxylate is formulated with atropine and may have anticholinergic effects, e.g., dry mouth, flushing, blurry vision, and tachycardia. These antidiarrheals should be avoided in patients with fever or bloody diarrhea. Bismuth salicylate (30 mL or two tablets every 30 minutes for eight doses) is an alternative antidiarrheal agent, which has antisecretory and antimicrobial effects and is also approved for relief of traveler's diarrhea.[16] Bismuth subsalicylate contains salicylate, which is contraindicated with aspirin allergies and can cause darkening of stool and tongue.

INFLAMMATORY BOWEL DISEASE (CROHN DISEASE AND ULCERATIVE COLITIS)

Inflammatory bowel disease (IBD) is a chronic immune-mediated inflammatory disease of the GI tract. There are two types of IBD: Crohn disease (CD), which can affect any portion of the GI tract with transmural inflammation; and ulcerative colitis (UC), which affects the colon and rectum, and the inflammation is limited to the mucosal layer of the colon. Treatment of IBD includes induction and remission, and there are multiple classes of medications including biologic agents for UC and CD. The 5-aminosalicylates (5-ASA) are mostly effective for induction and maintenance of remission in UC and play less of a role in CD. The 5-ASA have multiple antiinflammatory and immunosuppressant effects on the intestinal mucosa, all of which are not specifically identified. Names of the 5-ASA are sulfazalasine, olsalazine, balsalazide, and mesalamine, and routes of administration include oral and topical enemas and suppositories.

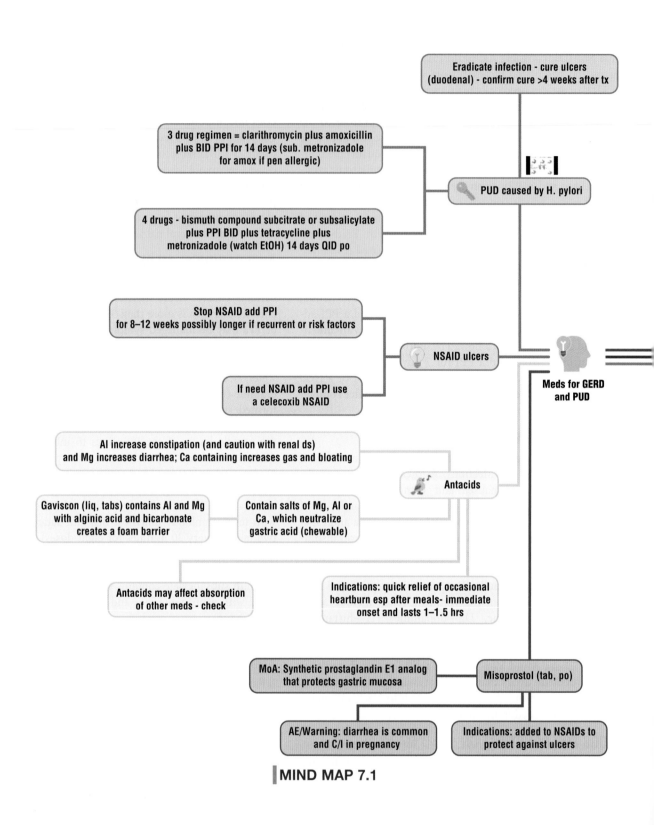

MIND MAP 7.1

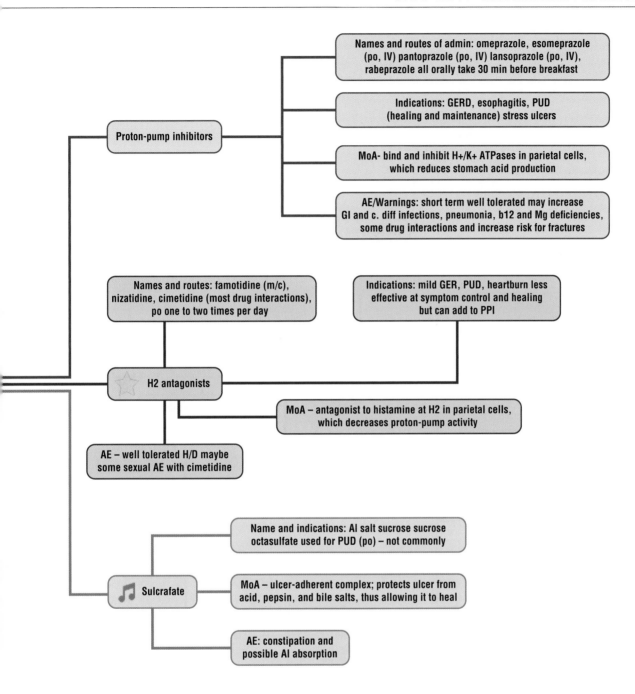

Proton-pump inhibitors

Names and routes of admin: omeprazole, esomeprazole (po, IV) pantoprazole (po, IV) lansoprazole (po, IV), rabeprazole all orally take 30 min before breakfast

Indications: GERD, esophagitis, PUD (healing and maintenance) stress ulcers

MoA- bind and inhibit H+/K+ ATPases in parietal cells, which reduces stomach acid production

AE/Warnings: short term well tolerated may increase GI and c. diff infections, pneumonia, b12 and Mg deficiencies, some drug interactions and increase risk for fractures

H2 antagonists

Names and routes: famotidine (m/c), nizatidine, cimetidine (most drug interactions), po one to two times per day

Indications: mild GER, PUD, heartburn less effective at symptom control and healing but can add to PPI

MoA – antagonist to histamine at H2 in parietal cells, which decreases proton-pump activity

AE – well tolerated H/D maybe some sexual AE with cimetidine

Sulcrafate

Name and indications: Al salt sucrose sucrose octasulfate used for PUD (po) – not commonly

MoA – ulcer-adherent complex; protects ulcer from acid, pepsin, and bile salts, thus allowing it to heal

AE: constipation and possible Al absorption

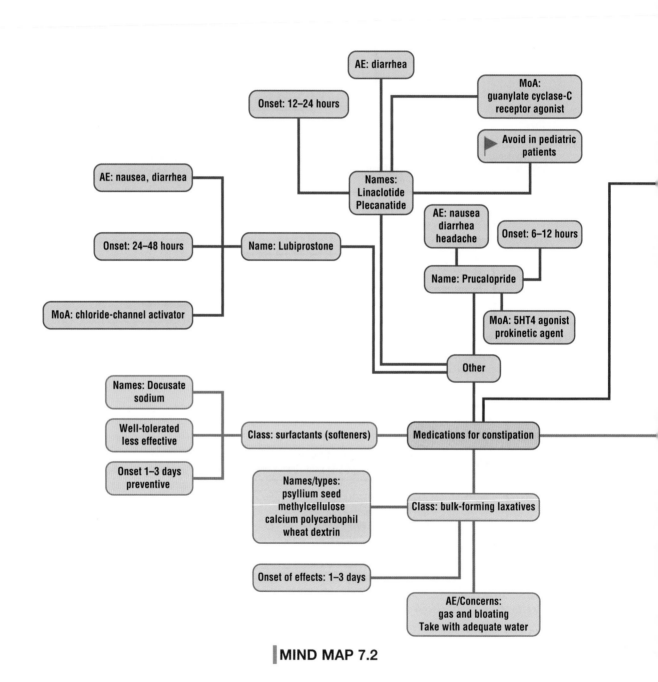

MIND MAP 7.2

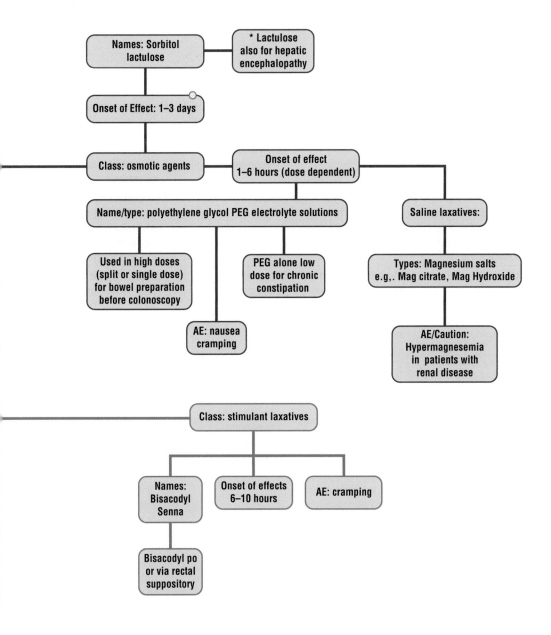

Names: Sorbitol lactulose

* Lactulose also for hepatic encephalopathy

Onset of Effect: 1–3 days

Class: osmotic agents

Onset of effect 1–6 hours (dose dependent)

Name/type: polyethylene glycol PEG electrolyte solutions

Used in high doses (split or single dose) for bowel preparation before colonoscopy

PEG alone low dose for chronic constipation

AE: nausea cramping

Saline laxatives:

Types: Magnesium salts e.g,. Mag citrate, Mag Hydroxide

AE/Caution: Hypermagnesemia in patients with renal disease

Class: stimulant laxatives

Names: Bisacodyl Senna

Onset of effects 6–10 hours

AE: cramping

Bisacodyl po or via rectal suppository

TABLE 7.1 Antiemetic Drugs

Class of drugs and Mechanism of action	Names and Administration	Indications	Adverse Effects	Warnings/ Contraindications
5HT3 receptor antagonists Block 5HT3 type receptors on vagus nerve, and in the CNS especially the CTZ and emetic center	Ondansetron (dosage varies, oral tabs, oral disintegrating tabs, oral film and IV) Granisetron (oral, IV, subcutaneous, transdermal) Dolasetron (po) Palonosetron (IV)	Acute emesis with chemotherapy (CINV) agents with moderate to high emetogenic potential usually in combination with other medications Acute severe nausea and vomiting	Headache Constipation Prolong QT interval	Prolong QT interval Serotonin syndrome: use caution with other serotonergic agents
Centrally acting dopamine receptor antagonists Block D2-dopamine receptors in the area postrema	Prochlorperazine is in the phenothiazine class of dopamine receptor antagonists Formulations: po, IV, IM and rectal, dosages vary)	Acute nausea vomiting Migraine-related nausea vomiting	Extrapyramidal reactions such as dystonia Drowsiness, restlessness	Prochlorperazine: Black box warning: increased mortality in elderly patients with dementia-related psychosis
	Metoclopramide is in the benzamide class of dopamine receptor antagonists (Formulations: po, IV, and nasal, dosages vary)	FDA indication for metoclopramide is mainly diabetic gastroparesis		Metoclopramide: black box warning risks of irreversible tardive dyskinesia with higher dosing and long-term use
Neurokinin receptor antagonists Block effects of substance P in brainstem nucleus tractus solitarius and the area postrema[11]	Aprepitant (po, IV) Fosaprepitant (IV) Netupitant (combination with palonosetron, po) Rolapitant (po)	Acute and delayed emesis in patients treated with highly emetogenic chemotherapy drugs (CINV)	Dizziness Hiccups Fatigue asthenia	Aprepitant, fosaprepitant, and netupitant are moderate inhibitors of CYP3A4 → potential for drug interactions Rolapitant inhibits CYP2D6→ potential for drug interactions
Cannabinoid receptor agonists activates cannabinoid receptors CB1 and CB2	Dronabinol 5–10 mg orally every 6–8 hours nabilone 1–2 mg every 12 hours	Adjunctive to other antiemetics	Vertigo, xerostomia, hypotension, dysphoria increased appetite	
Histamine H1 antagonists Histamine, acetylcholine plays a role in motion sickness Promethazine also blocks dopaminergic receptors	Dimenhydrinate 50 mg po every 4 hours Meclizine, 25–50 mg po every 24 hours Promethazine (oral, rectal, IV, IM)	Motion sickness Promethazine is also used to control acute nausea and vomiting	Sedation	Promethazine has boxed warning to avoid in pediatric patients younger than 2 years because of the potential for fatal respiratory depression Promethazine warning about severe chemical irritation and damage to tissues with parenteral administration[12]
Muscarinic receptor antagonists Histamine, acetylcholine plays a role in motion sickness	Scopolamine transdermal, 1 mg every 72 hours	Motion sickness	Dry mouth, drowsiness, blurry vision	Caution with BPH, narrow angle glaucoma, GU obstruction
Glucocorticoids Antiemetic action unknown	Dexamethasone oral dosage varies on regimen	Adjunctive to other antiemetics for CINV	Insomnia, increased energy, and elevated mood Increased appetite	

5HT3, 5-Hydroxytryptamine 3; BPH, benign prostatic hyperplasia; CINV, chemotherapy-induced nausea and vomiting; CNS, central nervous system; CTZ, chemoreceptor trigger zone; FDA, US Food and Drug Administration; GU, genitourinary; IM, intramuscular; IV, intravenous; PO, oral.
Adapted from: Singh P, Yoon SS, Kuo B. Nausea: a review of pathophysiology and therapeutics. Therap Adv Gastroenterol 2016;9:98.

Sulfasalazine is a prodrug of 5-ASA complexed to sulfapyridine; sulfasalazine is split by bacteria in the colon into 5-ASA, which has the antiinflammatory effects, and sulfapyridine is absorbed systemically and causes adverse effects. The other 5-ASAs include olsalazine, balsalazide, and mesalamine that are not bound to sulfapyridine and are better tolerated.

Glucocorticoids are indicated for moderate-to-severe IBD for induction of remission. Some of the glucocorticoids used for IBD include oral prednisone and budesonide, which are initiated at high dosages and tapered over several weeks. Oral budesonide is formulated for local release in the distal small bowel with minimal systemic effects. IV methylprednisolone may be given for serious exacerbations in hospitalized patients. Topical glucocorticoids in enemas, foams, and suppositories are useful for distal colorectal disease. Glucocorticoids are limited to short-term use and induction of remission because of multiple adverse effects, which are discussed in Chapter 6.[17]

Immunomodulating drugs (e.g., azathioprine and 6-mercaptopurine, both of which are thiopurines) or methotrexate are options for maintenance of remission in patients with CD. The onset of action of these medications is delayed by about 3 to 6 months. The details of immunomodulating medications, including adverse effects and toxicities, are discussed in Chapter 6.

Several classes of biologic agents are used for IBD, which include anti-tumor necrosis factor agents (i.e., infliximab, adalimumab, or certolizumab pegol), ustekinumab, an antiinterleukin 12/23 antibody, and the antiintegrin monoclonal antibodies (vedolizumab, which is a humanized anti-alpha-4-beta-7 integrin monoclonal antibody; and natalizumab, which is a humanized monoclonal antibody directed against alpha-4 integrin). These agents are used for induction and maintenance in IBD, especially CD. Most biologic agents are administered as subcutaneous injections or IV infusions.[18] Biologic agents and their associated adverse effects and toxicities are discussed in detail in Chapter 5.

Medications Used to Treat Irritable Bowel Syndrome

IBS is a functional GI disorder characterized by various symptoms including chronic abdominal discomfort and altered bowel habits.[11] The medical treatment for IBS depends in part on the primary symptom, constipation (IBS-C) or diarrhea (IBS-D), and symptom severity.[19] Patients with constipation-predominant IBS can use over-the-counter osmotic laxatives such as PEG. Lubiprostone, linaclotide, or plecanatide are also approved for constipation (IBS-C), but they are expensive.

There are over-the-counter and prescription medications for patients with diarrhea-predominant IBS. The antidiarrheal loperamide is available over the counter as needed for loose stools. The main FDA-approved prescription medications for IBS-D include eluxadoline (100 mg orally BID with food), which is a mixed opioid receptor agonist/antagonist, and rifaximin (550 mg PO TID for 14 days), which is an antibiotic that alters the intestinal microbiome.[20] Adverse effects of eluxadoline are nausea and constipation, and it is contraindicated in patients with pancreatic, biliary, and severe liver disease. Adverse effects of rifaximin are nausea and increased alanine transaminase, and it is contraindicated in patients who are allergic to any of the rifamycin antimicrobials.

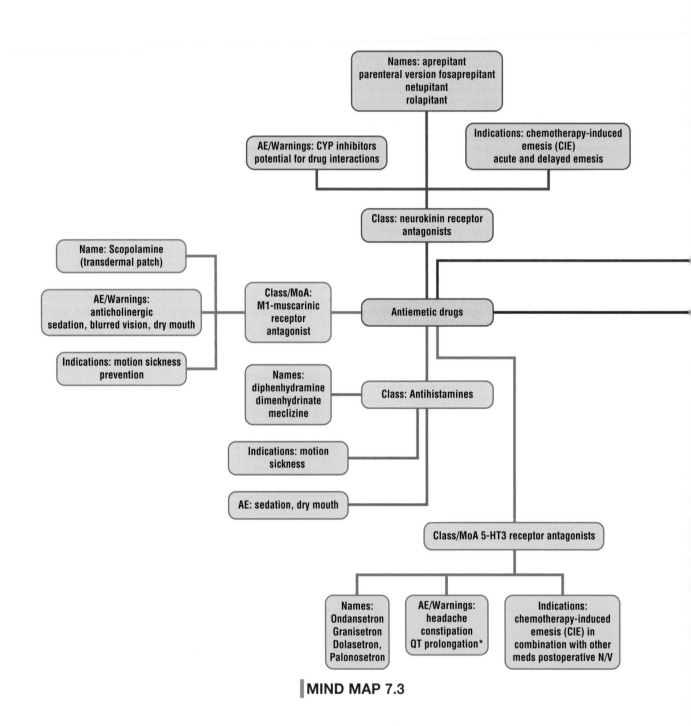

Names: aprepitant
parenteral version fosaprepitant
netupitant
rolapitant

AE/Warnings: CYP inhibitors
potential for drug interactions

Indications: chemotherapy-induced
emesis (CIE)
acute and delayed emesis

Class: neurokinin receptor
antagonists

Name: Scopolamine
(transdermal patch)

AE/Warnings:
anticholinergic
sedation, blurred vision, dry mouth

Class/MoA:
M1-muscarinic
receptor
antagonist

Antiemetic drugs

Indications: motion sickness
prevention

Names:
diphenhydramine
dimenhydrinate
meclizine

Class: Antihistamines

Indications: motion
sickness

AE: sedation, dry mouth

Class/MoA 5-HT3 receptor antagonists

Names:
Ondansetron
Granisetron
Dolasetron,
Palonosetron

AE/Warnings:
headache
constipation
QT prolongation*

Indications:
chemotherapy-induced
emesis (CIE) in
combination with other
meds postoperative N/V

MIND MAP 7.3

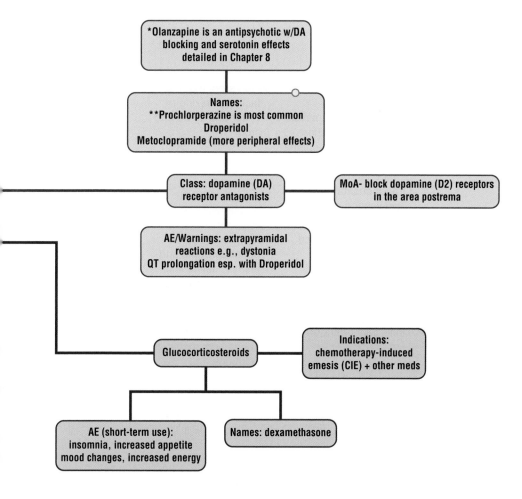

*Olanzapine is an antipsychotic w/DA
blocking and serotonin effects
detailed in Chapter 8

Names:
**Prochlorperazine is most common
Droperidol
Metoclopramide (more peripheral effects)

Class: dopamine (DA)
receptor antagonists

MoA- block dopamine (D2) receptors
in the area postrema

AE/Warnings: extrapyramidal
reactions e.g., dystonia
QT prolongation esp. with Droperidol

Glucocorticosteroids

Indications:
chemotherapy-induced
emesis (CIE) + other meds

AE (short-term use):
insomnia, increased appetite
mood changes, increased energy

Names: dexamethasone

TABLE 7.2	Medications Used For Constipation			
Drug class	Names and Administration	Onset of action	Mechanism of action	Adverse effects/ Contraindications
Bulk-forming laxatives	Psyllium Up to 1 tablespoon (≅3.5 grams fiber) 3 times per day Methylcellulose Up to 1 tablespoon (≅2 grams fiber) or 4 caplets (500 mg fiber per caplet) 3 times per day Synthetic fibers polycarbophil 2–4 tabs (500 mg fiber per tab) per day	Slow onset 12–72 hours Add water to reduce gas and bloating	Indigestible materials draw water and increase fecal mass	Abdominal bloating or flatulence
Stool softeners/ surfactants	Docusate salts (oral or enema) 100 mg 2 times per day Glycerin suppository One suppository (2 or 3 grams) per rectum for 15 minutes 1 time per day	Slow onset for oral docusate of 24–72 hours used for prevention of constipation Rapid onset with enema or suppository (15–30 minutes) Oral docusate used for prevention of constipation	Soften stool material facilitate mixing of water and lipids into stool	
Osmotic laxatives	Nonabsorbable sugars: Sorbitol 30 grams (120 mL of 25% solution) 1 time per day Lactulose: 10–20 grams (15–30 mL) every other day. May increase up to 2 times per day	sorbitol and lactulose 24–48 hours	Poorly absorbed or nonabsorbable sugars and saline laxatives which increase intestinal fluid secretion and frequency	Nausea, bloating, cramping and flatulence
	Magnesium salts magnesium citrate 200 mL (11.6 grams) 1 time per day Magnesium sulfate solution 2–4 level teaspoons (approximately 10–20 grams) of granules dissolved in 8 ounces (240 mL) of water; may repeat in 4 hours. Do not exceed 2 doses per day	Dose dependent onset of action 0.5–3 hours	Poorly absorbed and act as hyperosmolar solutions	Watery stools and urgency Magnesium can accumulate with renal insufficiency
	Polyethylene glycol (PEG)-electrolyte solutions Dose for bowel cleansing: 1–2 L of solution should be ingested rapidly (over 1–2 hours) on the evening before the procedure and again 4–6 hours before the procedure	Large volume PEG-electrolyte onset within an hour	Nonabsorbable, osmotically active sugar (PEG) some combined with sodium sulfate, sodium chloride, sodium bicarbonate, and potassium chloride	Nausea, bloating, cramping
	PEG powder for chronic constipation 17–34 g of powder dissolved in 8 oz of water once daily	PEG powder onset 1–3 days		
Stimulant laxatives	Bisacodyl 10–30 mg orally daily senna 15–30 mg	Orally produce a softer bowel movement in 6–12 hours	Irritate intestinal lining and smooth muscle and stimulate fluid, electrolyte secretion, and motility	Nausea and vomiting and abdominal cramping Limit long-term use

TABLE 7.2 Medications Used For Constipation—cont'd

Drug class	Names and Administration	Onset of action	Mechanism of action	Adverse effects/ Contraindications
Chloride secretion activators	Lubiprostone 24 mcg orally twice daily	Onset within 24 hours	Small intestinal chloride channel activator that enhances chloride-rich intestinal fluid secretion and increases transit	Nausea in up to 30% and diarrhea Known or suspected mechanical gastrointestinal (GI) obstruction
	Linaclotide 145 mcg orally once daily Plecanatide 3 mg orally once daily	Within a week	Guanylate cyclase-C receptor agonist which stimulate intestinal chloride secretion and increases transit	Common side effect is diarrhea Boxed warning: contraindicated in pediatric patients
Serotonin 5-hydroxytryptamine (5-HT4)-receptor agonists	Prucalopride dose of 2 mg orally once daily		5-HT4 receptors activation in GI tract leads to increased release of acetylcholine, which stimulates motility throughout the GI tract	Nausea, abdominal pain, and diarrhea

Adapted from: Mearin F, Lacy BE, Chang L, et al. Bowel disorders. *Gastroenterology* 2016;18:S0016-5085(16)00222-5 and Longstreth GF, Thompson WG, Chey WD, et al. Functional bowel disorders. *Gastroenterology* 2006;130:1480.

REFERENCES

1. Burget DW, Chiverton SG, Hunt RH. Is there an optimal degree of acid suppression for healing of duodenal ulcers? A model of the relationship between ulcer healing and acid suppression. *Gastroenterology*. 1990;99:345.
2. Howell MD, Novack V, Grgurich P, et al. Iatrogenic gastric acid suppression and the risk of nosocomial Clostridium difficile infection. *Arch Intern Med*. 2010;170:784.
3. Aseeri M, Schroeder T, Kramer J, Zackula R. Gastric acid suppression by proton pump inhibitors as a risk factor for clostridium difficile-associated diarrhea in hospitalized patients. *Am J Gastroenterol*. 2008;103:2308.
4. Willems RPJ, van Dijk K, Ket JCF, Vandenbroucke-Grauls CMJE. Evaluation of the association between gastric acid suppression and risk of intestinal colonization with multidrug-resistant microorganisms: a systematic review and meta-analysis. *JAMA Intern Med*. 2020;180:561.
5. Klinkenberg-Knol EC, Nelis F, Dent J, et al. Long-term omeprazole treatment in resistant gastroesophageal reflux disease: efficacy, safety, and influence on gastric mucosa. *Gastroenterology*. 2000;118:661.
6. Lam JR, Schneider JL, Zhao W, Corley DA. Proton pump inhibitor and histamine 2 receptor antagonist use and vitamin B12 deficiency. *JAMA*. 2013;310:2435.
7. FDA's MedWatch Safety Alerts. *Plavix and Prilosec Drug Interaction*. 2009. Available at: http://www.fda.gov/For Consumers/ConsumerUpdates/ucm192103.htm#Plavixand PrilosecDrugInteractions.
8. Fallone CA, Chiba N, Van Zanteri, et al. The Toronto Consensus for treatment of Helicobacter pylori infection in Adults. *Gastro*. 2016;15:51.
9. Miller AD. Central mechanisms of vomiting. *Dig Dis Sci*. 1999;44:39S.
10. Singh P, Yoon SS, Kuo B. Nausea: a review of pathophysiology and therapeutics. *Therap Adv Gastroenterol*. 2016;9:98.
11. Saito R, Takano Y, Kamiya HO. Roles of substance P and NK(1) receptor in the brainstem in the development of emesis. *J Pharmacol Sci*. 2003;91(2):87-94.
12. Wishart DS, Knox C, Guo AC, et al. DrugBank: a knowledgebase for drugs, drug actions and drug targets. *Nucleic Acids Res*. 2008;36(Database issue):D901-D906. doi:10.1093/nar/gkm958
13. Mearin F, Lacy BE, Chang L, et al. Bowel disorders. *Gastroenterology*. 2016;S0016-5085(16)00222-00225.
14. Longstreth GF, Thompson WG, Chey WD, et al. Functional bowel disorders. *Gastroenterology*. 2006;130:1480.
15. Crockett SD, Greer KB, Heidelbaugh JJ, et al. American Gastroenterological Association Institute Guideline on the medical management of opioid-induced constipation. *Gastroenterology*. 2019;156:218.
16. Pepto-Bismol (bismuth subsalicylate) suspension [prescribing information]. Cincinnati, OH: Procter & Gamble;

2021. Bismuth subsalicylate contains salicylate which is contraindicated with aspirin allergies, and it can cause darkening of stool and tongue.

17. Benchimol EI, Seow CH, Steinhart AH, Griffiths AM. Traditional corticosteroids for induction of remission in Crohn's disease. *Cochrane Database Syst Rev.* 2008:CD006792.

18. Lichtenstein GR, Loftus EV, Issacs KL, et al. ACG clinical guideline: management of Crohn's disease in adults. *Am J Gastroenterol.* 2018;113:481-517.

19. Moayyedi P, Andrews CN, MacQueen G, et al. Canadian Association of Gastroenterology clinical practice guideline for the management of irritable bowel syndrome (IBS). *J Can Assoc Gastroenterol.* 2019;2:6-29.

20. Lacy BE, Pimentel M, Brenner DM, et al. ACG clinical guideline: management of irritable bowel syndrome. *Am J Gastroenterol.* 2021;116:17-44.

CHAPTER 8

Drugs Affecting Central Nervous System

This chapter reviews a diverse group of medications affecting the central nervous system (CNS) ranging from sedative/hypnotics, anesthetics, opioids, and opioid use disorder to antiepileptics, migraine medications, and medications for Parkinson and Alzheimer. There is also a section dedicated to psychopharmacology.

SECTION 1: Sedative Hypnotics
(Mind Map 8.1)

Sedative/hypnotic agents work to cause a calming feeling and reduce anxiety (sedatives), and hypnotics cause drowsiness and facilitate sleep onset and maintenance. Hypnotics have more CNS depressant effects, and sedative dosages can be increased for hypnotic effects. Medications in the sedative hypnotic class are used clinically for acute anxiety, panic, premedication before surgery, or certain unpleasant procedures and for short-term treatment of insomnia.

Medications approved for the treatment of **insomnia** disorder fall into four categories based on mechanism of action:

- **Benzodiazepine (BZ) receptor agonists (BZRAs)**: BZ BZRAs and non-BZ BZRAs.

   There are five older **BZ** hypnotics (estazolam, flurazepam, temazepam, triazolam, and quazepam) approved for short-term treatment of insomnia. The BZs facilitate the **inhibitory** activity of gamma-aminobutyric acid (GABA) by binding to sites on the GABA-A receptor complex, which is found on neurons in the CNS; this causes an increase in the frequency of chloride channel-opening events. There are other BZs, specifically alprazolam, clonazepam, and lorazepam, which are mainly used for acute anxiety and panic attacks. Some BZs have anticonvulsant and muscle-relaxing effects. The differences in BZs are mainly related to their duration of action and half-lives. The primary adverse effects of BZs are sleepiness, drowsiness, and dizziness. BZs can impair psychomotor performance and cause anterograde amnesia, rebound anxiety, dependence, and withdrawal with long-term chronic use.

Long-term use of BZs is also associated with tolerance. Boxed warnings for BZs include the risks of misuse, abuse and addiction, physical dependence, and withdrawal. Patients who are taking BZs on a chronic basis require **gradual tapering** to avoid potentially life-threatening withdrawal reactions including **seizures**. The use of BZs and opioids can increase the risk for profound CNS depression and potential life-threatening respiratory depression. BZs are schedule IV-controlled substances.[1]

There are three oral **non-BZ BZRAs** (eszopiclone, zaleplon, and zolpidem or Z drugs), which act similarly to BZ but are more selective for certain types of GABA-A receptors. Eszopiclone has the longest half-life and is used for sleep onset and sleep maintenance insomnia. Zaleplon has the shortest half-life and is used for sleep onset insomnia. Zolpidem has multiple formulations that vary in duration of action including a rapid-release middle-of-the-night use sublingual tablet and an extended-release formulation. Adverse effects and warnings with the non-BZ BZRAs include sleepiness, drowsiness, and dysgeusia with eszopiclone.[2]

Patients should have several hours of sleep before performing tasks that require mental alertness such as driving or operating heavy machinery. There is a boxed warning about serious complex sleep-related behaviors such as sleepwalking, sleep-driving, and engaging in other activities while not fully awake.[3]

BZs and non-BZ receptor agonists are high-risk medications in geriatric patients. Non-BZRAs are also schedule IV controlled substances.

- **Dual orexin receptor antagonists (DORAs) (lemborexant, suvorexant, and daridorexant)** are oral sedatives indicated for short-term treatment of sleep onset and/or sleep maintenance types of insomnia. The DORAs, lemborexant, and suvorexant act by antagonizing the wake-promoting effects of orexins (also called *hypocretin*) by blocking orexin A and orexin B to receptors OX1R and OX2R in the hypothalamus and cortex and suppress the wake drive.[4] They are administered before bedtime with at least 7 hours of sleep before

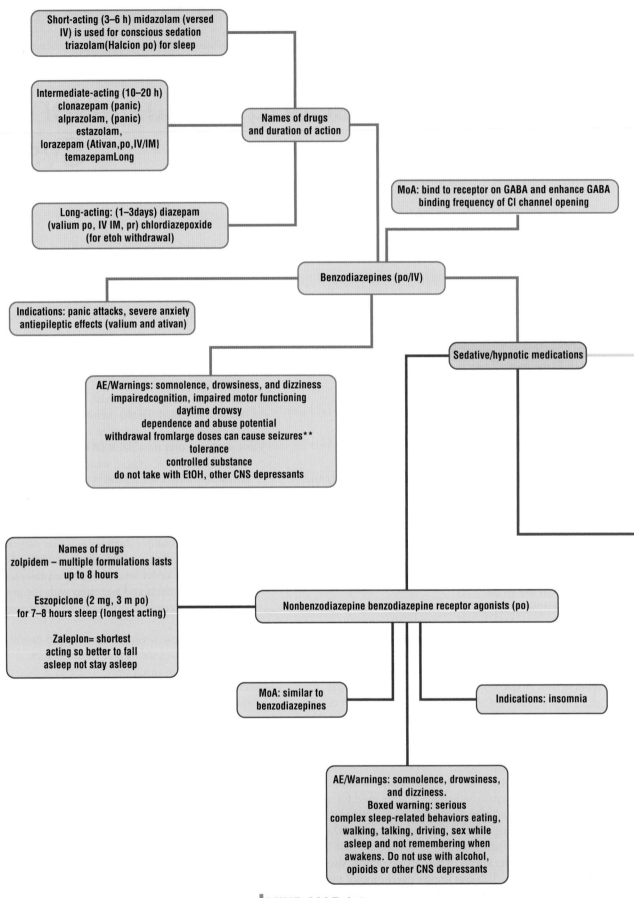

MIND MAP 8.1

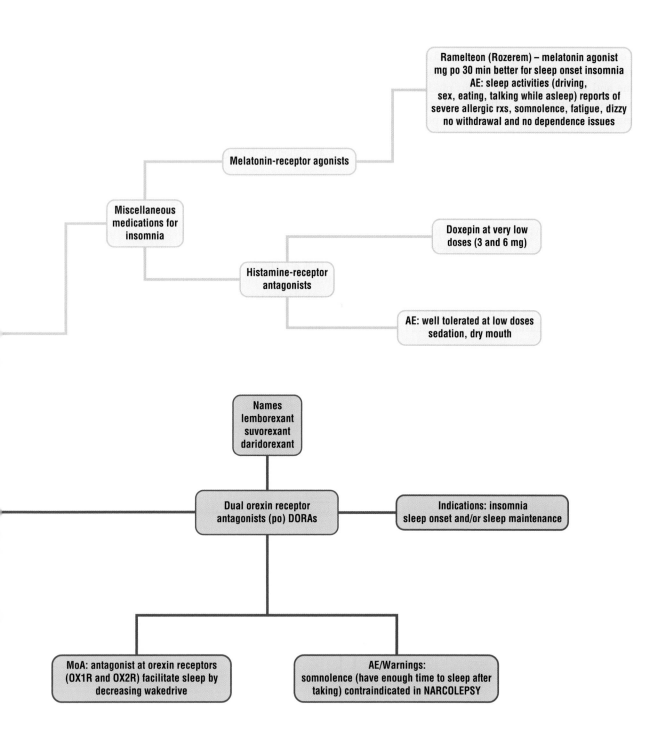

awakening. The primary adverse effects of DORAs are drowsiness, abnormal dreams, and headaches. DORAs are contraindicated in narcolepsy.

- **Histamine-receptor antagonists (low-dose doxepin).** The mechanism of doxepin was discussed in Chapter 5 and in the psychopharmacology section of this chapter. Doxepin is an antihistamine and is classified as a tricyclic antidepressant (TCA). Low-dose doxepin is an option for sleep maintenance insomnia in adults and is taken orally near bedtime on an empty stomach. The adverse effects of low-dose doxepin are sedation, upper respiratory tract infection, and nausea. Doxepin is contraindicated in urinary retention and glaucoma.[5]

- **Melatonin-receptor agonists (ramelteon)** are orally administered for sleep onset insomnia. Ramelteon works as an agonist at melatonin MT1 and MT2 receptors, which are prominent in the hypothalamic suprachiasmatic nucleus, which inhibits wakefulness, promotes sleepiness, and regulates circadian rhythm.[6] Ramelteon is well tolerated, with primary adverse effects of somnolence, dizziness, fatigue, and nausea. Ramelteon's efficacy is moderate, but it does not have issues with dependence or abuse. **Tasimelteon**, also an MT1 and

MT2 agonist, is used for certain circadian rhythm disorders and non-24-hour sleep-wake disorder.

- **Barbiturates** are an older class of sedative/hypnotics that also bind to GABA receptors but increase the duration of the GABA-gated chloride channel openings and have other pharmacologic effects. Barbiturates have a lower margin of safety compared to BZs and can cause profound and potentially fatal cardiac and respiratory depression. Certain barbiturates are occasionally used for general anesthesia, e.g., methohexital (Brevital), and as an antiepileptic drug (phenobarbital).

SECTION 2: Anesthetics

Local anesthetics (LAs) (Mind Map 8.2) are used to produce loss of sensation to a specific body part or region. LAs are weak bases that are chemically classified as either esters or amides. LAs work by blocking voltage-gated sodium channels (Nav) in the nerve plasma membrane, which inhibits action potentials.[7]

Clinical uses of the LAs include topical, local infiltration into skin, subcutaneous, and soft tissue; peripheral nerve blocks;

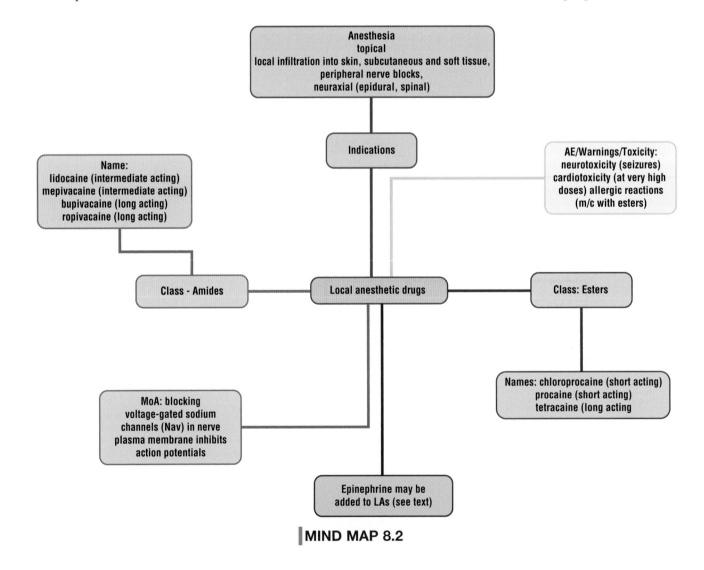

MIND MAP 8.2

and neuraxial (epidural, which is injected into the epidural space often with catheter introduced; and spinal, which is injected into the subarachnoid space).

The commonly used **ester** LAs include **chloroprocaine, procaine,** and **tetracaine;** the amides are **lidocaine, bupivacaine, ropivacaine,** and **mepivacaine.**

The LAs can also be grouped by onset and duration of action generally as follows:

Chloroprocaine and procaine are short-acting LAs. Lidocaine, mepivacaine, and prilocaine are intermediate acting (2–5 hours for anesthesia). Bupivacaine, ropivacaine, levobupivacaine, tetracaine, and etidocaine are long-acting LAs (variable 4–15 hours). The onset of action of LAs depends on site of injection, concentration of anesthetic, and, in some cases, alkalinization, which affects the fraction of nonionized LA molecules and increases permeability in nerves. The order of sequence of nerve function blockade after administration of LAs is loss of sympathetic function first, then loss of sensation to sharp pain, temperature, then pressure, and last reduced motor function.

Epinephrine may be added to LAs, especially to lidocaine, for several reasons. Epinephrine causes vasoconstriction, which reduces systemic absorption. It localizes the action of the LA, prolongs the duration of analgesia, reduces systemic toxicity, and increases the maximum safe dose. For example, for lidocaine without epinephrine, the maximum dose is approximately 4 mg/kg, and for lidocaine with epinephrine, the maximum dose is 7 mg/kg.

Adverse effects and toxicity of LAs include **neurotoxicity, cardiotoxicity,** and allergic reactions. LA systemic toxicity (LAST) refers to seizures or cardiac arrest associated with LAs. The CNS is sensitive to LAs and toxic clinical manifestations begin with certain premonitory signs including restlessness, circumoral numbness, tongue paresthesia, agitation, metallic taste, and nervousness. Increasing doses can cause seizures and eventually coma and respiratory depression. Cardiotoxicity occurs at much higher doses than neurotoxicity and has variable presentations of bradycardia, heart blocks, hypotension, ventricular arrhythmias, and ultimately cardiac arrest. Local allergic contact dermatitis can occur more often with **ester LAs.**[8]

General anesthetics (Mind Map 8.3) use intravenous (IV) and inhaled medications to establish a reversible state of:
- Hypnosis
- Amnesia
- Analgesia
- Akinesia
- Autonomic and sensory block.

Stages of anesthesia depth are described as the following:

Stage I Analgesia state: Patient is conscious and rational, with decreased perception of pain.

Stage II Delirium stage: Patient is unconscious; body responds reflexively; irregular breathing pattern with breath holding.

Stage III Surgical anesthesia: Increasing degrees of muscle relaxation; unable to protect airway.

Stage IV Medullary depression: There is depression of cardiovascular and respiratory centers.[9]

General anesthesia occurs when a patient does not respond to noxious surgical stimuli. General anesthetic agents produce a dose-response level of sedation and anesthesia, with higher doses causing **respiratory depression**. Airway management including endotracheal intubation for ventilation and oxygenation is a critical component of general anesthesia. Neuromuscular blocking agents (NMBA) are administered to facilitate endotracheal intubation during induction of general anesthesia.

Propofol, etomidate, and **ketamine** are the primary IV sedative/hypnotic agents used to induce a state of surgical anesthesia. Propofol is the most used IV anesthetic, and it is administered for conscious sedation, short duration ambulatory procedures, and general anesthesia. Propofol is lipophilic IV anesthetic, which activates GABA receptors, and it is an antagonist of the N-methyl-D-aspartate (NMDA) receptor.[10,11] Propofol is rapid acting with rapid recovery from anesthesia, antiemetic, and has anticonvulsant properties. Disadvantages of propofol are pain with injection, **dose-dependent respiratory depression**, and hypotension. **Etomidate** is used for patients with hemodynamic instability because it does not affect blood pressure or cause myocardial depression. Etomidate causes postoperative nausea and vomiting, pain during injection, involuntary jerking movements, and may cause adrenal sufficiency.[12]

Ketamine is a glutamate NMDA receptor antagonist with analgesic properties, and can be used in hypotensive patients because it increases sympathetic tone. Ketamine also causes bronchodilation and minimal respiratory depression. Ketamine causes unpleasant emergence reactions including vivid dreams, hallucinations, and out-of-body experiences. **Methohexital** is a less commonly used IV barbiturate anesthetic administered for electroconvulsive therapy. It causes dose-dependent **respiratory depression** and hypotension and pain on injection.

Other agents used during induction of anesthesia include opioids such as fentanyl (to supplement analgesia, reduce respiratory reflexes during intubation) and BZs such as midazolam as an anxiolytic.

Inhaled anesthetics are volatile gases used to induce or maintain surgical anesthesia. The potent volatile anesthetic agents include sevoflurane (most common in the United States), desflurane, and isoflurane; nitrous oxide is a low-potency anesthetic gas. The inhaled anesthetics are inspired, reach the alveoli, and pass into the pulmonary capillary blood for distribution to the brain, spinal cord, and body. The blood:gas partition coefficient of an inhalation agent affects the onset of its effect. Anesthetics with a low blood:gas partition coefficient are poorly soluble in blood and require less agent to saturate the blood, which causes more rapid onset of anesthesia. The main measure of potency of the inhaled anesthetics is minimum alveolar concentration (MAC), which is the concentration of the inhaled gas in the alveoli required to prevent movement in response to a noxious stimulus in 50% of subjects.[13] The MAC is inversely related to potency of the inhaled anesthetic.

Clinical effects of the inhaled anesthetics include sedation and anesthesia, skeletal muscle relaxation, bronchodilation with dose-dependent **respiratory depression,** vasodilation and

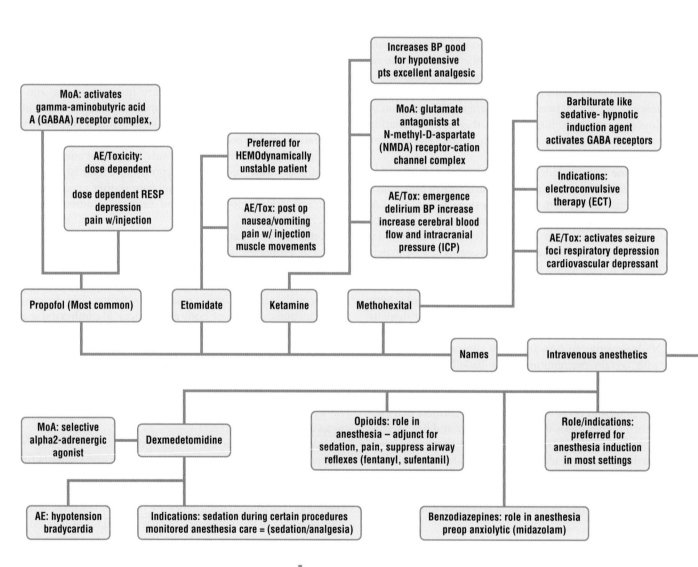

MIND MAP 8.3

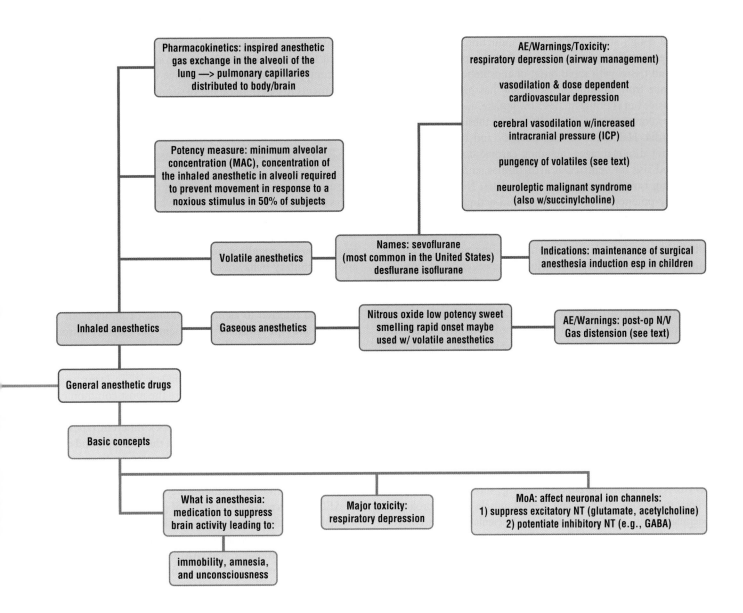

Pharmacokinetics: inspired anesthetic gas exchange in the alveoli of the lung —> pulmonary capillaries distributed to body/brain

AE/Warnings/Toxicity:
respiratory depression (airway management)

vasodilation & dose dependent cardiovascular depression

cerebral vasodilation w/increased intracranial pressure (ICP)

pungency of volatiles (see text)

neuroleptic malignant syndrome (also w/succinylcholine)

Potency measure: minimum alveolar concentration (MAC), concentration of the inhaled anesthetic in alveoli required to prevent movement in response to a noxious stimulus in 50% of subjects

Volatile anesthetics

Names: sevoflurane (most common in the United States) desflurane isoflurane

Indications: maintenance of surgical anesthesia induction esp in children

Inhaled anesthetics

Gaseous anesthetics

Nitrous oxide low potency sweet smelling rapid onset maybe used w/ volatile anesthetics

AE/Warnings: post-op N/V Gas distension (see text)

General anesthetic drugs

Basic concepts

What is anesthesia: medication to suppress brain activity leading to:

Major toxicity: respiratory depression

MoA: affect neuronal ion channels:
1) suppress excitatory NT (glutamate, acetylcholine)
2) potentiate inhibitory NT (e.g., GABA)

immobility, amnesia, and unconsciousness

dose-dependent cardiovascular depression, and cerebral vasodilation with increased intracranial pressure.

Specific inhaled anesthetics include sevoflurane, desflurane, isoflurane, and the gas nitrous oxide. Halothane is not available in North America or Europe and has generally been replaced by safer options such as sevoflurane. **Sevoflurane** is the most used general anesthetic with rapid onset, less pungent, sweet smelling, bronchodilatory effects but less cardiac depressant effects, and less effects on cerebral blood flow. Desflurane is the most pungent inhaled volatile anesthetic, which causes airway irritation and cough and is not used for induction. Desflurane has low potency and causes tachycardia, but it is poorly soluble in blood and tissue with rapid onset of anesthetic effects and fast emergence from anesthesia. Isoflurane has high potency and inexpensive but is pungent, has slow uptake, accumulates in fat, which prolongs time to emerge from anesthesia, and can cause tachycardia. Halothane is high potency and low cost but has significant disadvantages including cardiac depressant effects, increased risk for ventricular arrhythmias, and **hepatotoxicity including rare but acute severe hepatitis.** Nitrous oxide is a very-low-potency, sweet-smelling, rapid-acting gas that is often coadministered with volatile anesthetics as a "second gas" to speed onset and depth of anesthesia. Nitrous oxide gas is associated with postoperative nausea and vomiting, and it can diffuse and distend gas-filled spaces including bowel, increased middle ear pressure, pneumothorax, pneumoperitoneum, pneumocephalus, intraocular gas, or venous air embolism.[14]

Malignant hyperthermia (MH) is a rare but serious autosomal dominant disorder that can be triggered by volatile anesthetic agents alone or in combination with the neuromuscular blocker succinylcholine. MH begins during anesthesia with hypercarbia, tachypnea, tachycardia, hyperthermia, and jaw and generalized muscle rigidity, which can progress to rhabdomyolysis, disseminated intravascular coagulation, and death. **The antidote for MH is IV dantrolene** as well as supportive care with oxygenation, ventilation, and discontinuation of triggering events.

Neuromuscular blockers are used intravenously to facilitate intubation and cause muscle relaxation during general anesthesia. NMBAs are classified as depolarizing, e.g., succinylcholine, which binds to nicotinic receptors on skeletal muscle causing prolonged depolarization with desensitization, fasciculations, and flaccid paralysis; and nondepolarizing NMBAs, which are competitive antagonists of acetylcholine at skeletal muscle nicotinic receptors. Succinylcholine is a depolarizing NMBA used for intubation due to its rapid and reliable onset and shortest duration of effect. Adverse effects of succinylcholine include myalgias, increased intracranial pressure, hyperkalemia, bradycardia, allergic reactions, and it is a trigger for MH. Nondepolarizing, competitive NMBAs are classified structurally as either steroidal or benzylisoquinoliniums and by duration of action (short, intermediate, or long acting). Some characteristics of the nondepolarizing NMBAs are:

Steroidal compounds
- Rocuronium and vecuronium are intermediate acting, commonly used for endotracheal intubation and during surgery.
- Pancuronium is a long-acting steroidal NMDA and is rarely used.

Benzylisoquinolinium compounds
- Mivacurium is short acting, low potency, and associated with histamine release at high doses.
- Cisatracurium and atracurium are intermediate-acting NMBAs; cisatracurium is more potent and does not cause histamine release.

Reversal of neuromuscular blockade can occur spontaneously or with the use of acetylcholinesterase inhibitor, **neostigmine IV to reverse succinylcholine,** and **sugammadex IV to inactivate steroidal NMBAs, e.g., rocuronium.**

Monitoring of neuromuscular function (response of the muscle to the neurostimulation) with administration of NMBAs is accomplished by using qualitative observation of muscular movements to a peripheral nerve stimulator, or quantitative and objective monitors such as electromyography.[15]

SECTION 3: Antiepileptics (Mind Map 8.4)

Seizure types are usually classified as generalized, focal, or unknown. Generalized seizures involve both hemispheres and can be motor and nonmotor (absence) seizures. Focal seizures involve one hemisphere and can be motor or nonmotor and may involve certain cognitive, autonomic, emotional, sensorimotor, and involuntary behaviors. Epilepsy is a neurologic condition with several underlying causes and is characterized by recurrent seizures, usually two or more, 24 hours apart. Seizure medications, also referred to as *anticonvulsants* or *antiepileptic drugs* (*AEDs*), are the primary treatment for seizure disorders/epilepsy.[16]

Antiepileptic drugs are generally classified by their mechanism of action, although several AEDs work in many ways:
- **Sodium channel modulators** are the most common type of AEDs.
- The **calcium channel blockers** block different types of calcium channels in neurons, both in the thalamus and calcium channels, which regulate neurotransmitter release.[17]
- Another class of AEDs **increases the supply or activity of GABA,** which is an inhibitory neurotransmitter.
- AED can **decrease the activity of glutamate,** which is an excitatory neurotransmitter, by blocking certain glutamate receptors, e.g., NMDA and alpha-amino-3-hydroxy-5-methyl-4-isoxazole-propionic acid (AMPA) receptors.
- Drugs with other mechanisms of action alter the fusion of synaptic vesicles and modulate neurotransmitter release.[18]

Many antiepileptic drugs have a narrow therapeutic index and require serum drug monitoring. Several AEDs are cytochrome P450 enzyme inducers and are associated with **drug interactions.** Several AEDs are teratogenic, especially **valproic acid/valproate,** phenytoin, phenobarbital, and topiramate.[19] AEDs may be associated with **suicidal ideation** and **suicidal tendencies.**

Carbamazepine and structurally similar drugs oxcarbazepine and eslicarbazepine prolong the inactivation state of sodium channels and block rapidly firing sodium channels. Carbamazepine is used for the treatment of focal and generalized seizures. Carbamazepine is a potent inducer of CYP system, is an autoinducer, and is associated with several drug interactions. Common side effects are nausea, drowsiness, dizziness, blurry or double vision, and sometimes hyponatremia. Serious and potentially life-threatening adverse events (AEs) with labeling warning include risk of Stevens-Johnson syndrome (SJS), toxic epidermal necrolysis (TEN), and bone marrow suppression. SJS/TEN is more common in patients of Asian ancestry with the **human leukocyte antigen-B*1502 allele.** Carbamazepine can cause leukopenia, especially in the first 3 months, and, rarely, aplastic anemia (pancytopenia). Carbamazepine is associated with teratogenic effects and should not be used during pregnancy. Nonhormonal or long-acting reversible contraceptive choices of intrauterine devices or intramuscular depot medroxyprogesterone acetate should be used to prevent pregnancy.[20]

Oxcarbazepine and **eslicarbazepine** are indicated for treatment of focal seizures. Oxcarbazepine minimally affects the CYP system and has fewer drug interactions than carbamazepine. The adverse effects of oxcarbazepine are like those of carbamazepine, but oxcarbazepine may have a greater risk of **hyponatremia** due to an effect on antidiuretic hormone. Eslicarbazepine is a prodrug with similar adverse effects to carbamazepine, including hyponatremia. These medications are not recommended during pregnancy.

Phenytoin (oral) and **IV fosphenytoin** also block voltage-dependent neuronal sodium channels. Phenytoin is an older antiepileptic, but it is still used for focal and generalized seizures and for status epilepticus. Phenytoin is a potent inducer of CYP and phase II Uridine 5'-diphospho-glucuronosyltransferaseglucuronidation, and it has many drug interactions. The major side effects of phenytoin are confusion, slurred speech, double vision, and ataxia. Long-term effects include gingival hypertrophy, hirsutism, folic acid depletion, and decreased bone density (supplement with vitamin D and calcium). There is also a risk of SJS and TEN with phenytoin.

Lamotrigine inactivates voltage-gated sodium channels but may have other mechanisms affecting glutamate and aspartate. It is indicated for adjunctive treatment of focal-onset seizures and generalized tonic-clonic seizures. Drug levels of lamotrigine are increased by an interaction with valproate, which requires dosage adjustment. Adverse effects are mainly nausea, dizziness, and somnolence. Lamotrigine can be associated with a **rash,** especially in the first 4 to 8 weeks of therapy. Lamotrigine should be discontinued immediately in patients who develop a **rash** because of the risk of SJS or TEN. Lamotrigine should be avoided in patients with certain **cardiac conditions,** e.g., heart blocks, arrhythmias, structural heart disease, Brugada syndrome, or other sodium channelopathies.[21]

Valproate is a broad-spectrum AED with multiple mechanisms of action including blockade of rapid-firing sodium channels and increasing GABA levels. Valproate is indicated for generalized tonic-clonic, absence, and focal seizures, and it is also used in bipolar disorder. Valproate has several adverse effects and potentially serious labeling warnings. AEs of valproate include nausea, vomiting, tremors, thrombocytopenia, and hair loss. Some patients experience drowsiness while others have insomnia. Weight gain, obesity, and metabolic syndrome are also associated with valproate. Labeled warnings include **acute hepatocellular injury** with jaundice, especially in the first 6 months of therapy, and rarely acute **pancreatitis.** Valproate-related hyperammonemic encephalopathy can occur within the first week of therapy. Valproate is **contraindicated in pregnancy** and is associated with the highest rate of teratogenicity of AEDs.[22]

Ethosuximide is a narrow-spectrum AED that blocks thalamic calcium currents and is indicated for **generalized absence seizures only.** The main AE of ethosuximide is nausea, sometimes vomiting, sleep disturbance, drowsiness, and hyperactivity.[23]

Gabapentin and pregabalin inhibit calcium currents that affect neurotransmitter release and reduce neuronal excitability. They are used for focal seizures, and they are also used for neuropathic pain. Gabapentin is dosed three times daily, and pregabalin is usually twice daily, orally. The primary adverse effects are sedation, ataxia, tremor, and sometimes weight gain. Gabapentin can cause CNS and respiratory depression, especially in conjunction with opioids. Pregabalin is classified as a schedule V controlled substance because it can cause euphoria.

Topiramate is a broad-spectrum AED that acts as a sodium channel blocker, enhances GABA activity, and blocks glutamate at NMDA receptors. It is indicated for focal-onset or primary generalized tonic-clonic seizures. The primary adverse effects of topiramate are **significant cognitive impairment** (attention, memory, language), sedation, dizziness, and mood changes. Additional adverse effects of topiramate include short-term paresthesia, **weight loss** (it is used for obesity treatment), metabolic acidosis because of inhibition of carbonic anhydrase, decreased sweating, and increased risk of **kidney stones.**

Zonisamide blocks calcium channels and sodium channels and is broad-spectrum AED. It is indicated as an add-on therapy for focal and generalized seizures. The primary adverse effects of zonisamide are dizziness, drowsiness, anorexia with weight loss, kidney stones, and, less commonly, decreased sweating. A range of neuropsychiatric effects including agitation, cognitive dysfunction, and confusion, are also related to zonisamide.

Levetiracetam and brivaracetam are related AEDs. The mechanism of action of both AEDs is probably related to binding to synaptic vesicle protein 2A, which affects neurotransmitter vesicle fusion and release into the synaptic cleft.[18] Levetiracetam is a broad-spectrum AED and is indicated for focal, myoclonic, and generalized tonic-clonic seizures. Brivaracetam is approved for focal seizures. Levetiracetam and brivaracetam are well tolerated, and the most common adverse effects are fatigue, sedation, dizziness, and upper respiratory infections with levetiracetam. Behavioral changes, especially irritability, may be more common in children.[24]

Perampanel is a noncompetitive AMPA-type glutamate receptor antagonist. It is an option for focal seizures and adjunctive for generalized tonic-clonic seizures. Perampanel has a boxed warning of serious neuropsychiatric effects including aggression, hostility, and homicidal ideations, especially in the initial 6 weeks of therapy. Perampanel is classified as a Schedule III controlled substance because of potential for dependence, withdrawal, and tolerance.[25]

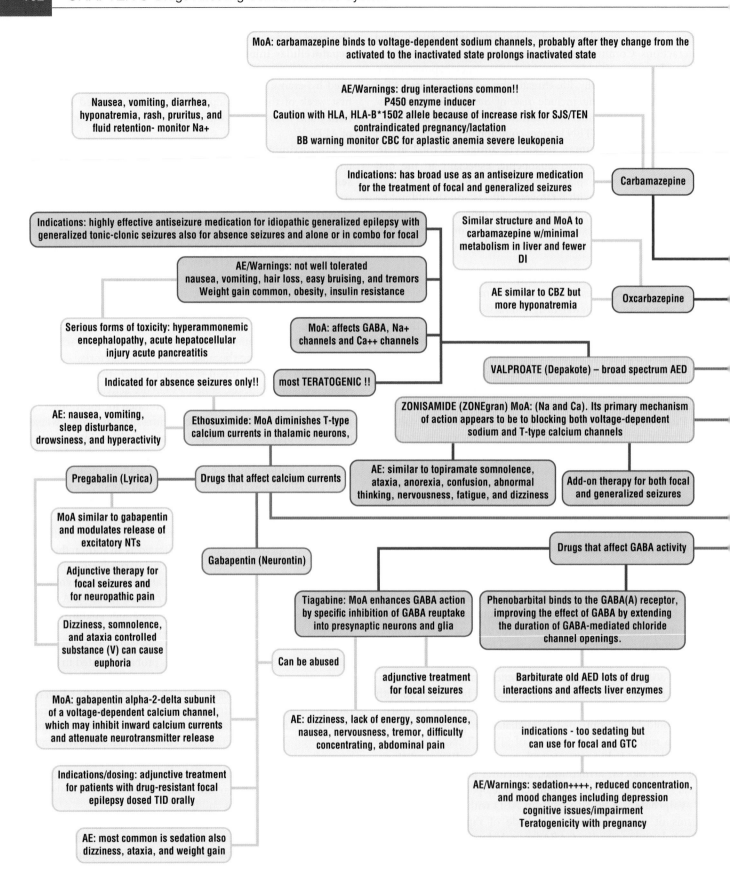

MoA: carbamazepine binds to voltage-dependent sodium channels, probably after they change from the activated to the inactivated state prolongs inactivated state

Nausea, vomiting, diarrhea, hyponatremia, rash, pruritus, and fluid retention- monitor Na+

AE/Warnings: drug interactions common!!
P450 enzyme inducer
Caution with HLA, HLA-B*1502 allele because of increase risk for SJS/TEN
contraindicated pregnancy/lactation
BB warning monitor CBC for aplastic anemia severe leukopenia

Indications: has broad use as an antiseizure medication for the treatment of focal and generalized seizures

Carbamazepine

Indications: highly effective antiseizure medication for idiopathic generalized epilepsy with generalized tonic-clonic seizures also for absence seizures and alone or in combo for focal

Similar structure and MoA to carbamazepine w/minimal metabolism in liver and fewer DI

AE/Warnings: not well tolerated
nausea, vomiting, hair loss, easy bruising, and tremors
Weight gain common, obesity, insulin resistance

AE similar to CBZ but more hyponatremia

Oxcarbazepine

Serious forms of toxicity: hyperammonemic encephalopathy, acute hepatocellular injury acute pancreatitis

MoA: affects GABA, Na+ channels and Ca++ channels

Indicated for absence seizures only!!

most TERATOGENIC !!

VALPROATE (Depakote) – broad spectrum AED

AE: nausea, vomiting, sleep disturbance, drowsiness, and hyperactivity

Ethosuximide: MoA diminishes T-type calcium currents in thalamic neurons,

ZONISAMIDE (ZONEgran) MoA: (Na and Ca). Its primary mechanism of action appears to be to blocking both voltage-dependent sodium and T-type calcium channels

Pregabalin (Lyrica)

Drugs that affect calcium currents

AE: similar to topiramate somnolence, ataxia, anorexia, confusion, abnormal thinking, nervousness, fatigue, and dizziness

Add-on therapy for both focal and generalized seizures

MoA similar to gabapentin and modulates release of excitatory NTs

Gabapentin (Neurontin)

Drugs that affect GABA activity

Adjunctive therapy for focal seizures and for neuropathic pain

Tiagabine: MoA enhances GABA action by specific inhibition of GABA reuptake into presynaptic neurons and glia

Phenobarbital binds to the GABA(A) receptor, improving the effect of GABA by extending the duration of GABA-mediated chloride channel openings.

Dizziness, somnolence, and ataxia controlled substance (V) can cause euphoria

Can be abused

adjunctive treatment for focal seizures

Barbiturate old AED lots of drug interactions and affects liver enzymes

MoA: gabapentin alpha-2-delta subunit of a voltage-dependent calcium channel, which may inhibit inward calcium currents and attenuate neurotransmitter release

AE: dizziness, lack of energy, somnolence, nausea, nervousness, tremor, difficulty concentrating, abdominal pain

indications - too sedating but can use for focal and GTC

Indications/dosing: adjunctive treatment for patients with drug-resistant focal epilepsy dosed TID orally

AE/Warnings: sedation++++, reduced concentration, and mood changes including depression cognitive issues/impairment
Teratogenicity with pregnancy

AE: most common is sedation also dizziness, ataxia, and weight gain

MIND MAP 8.4

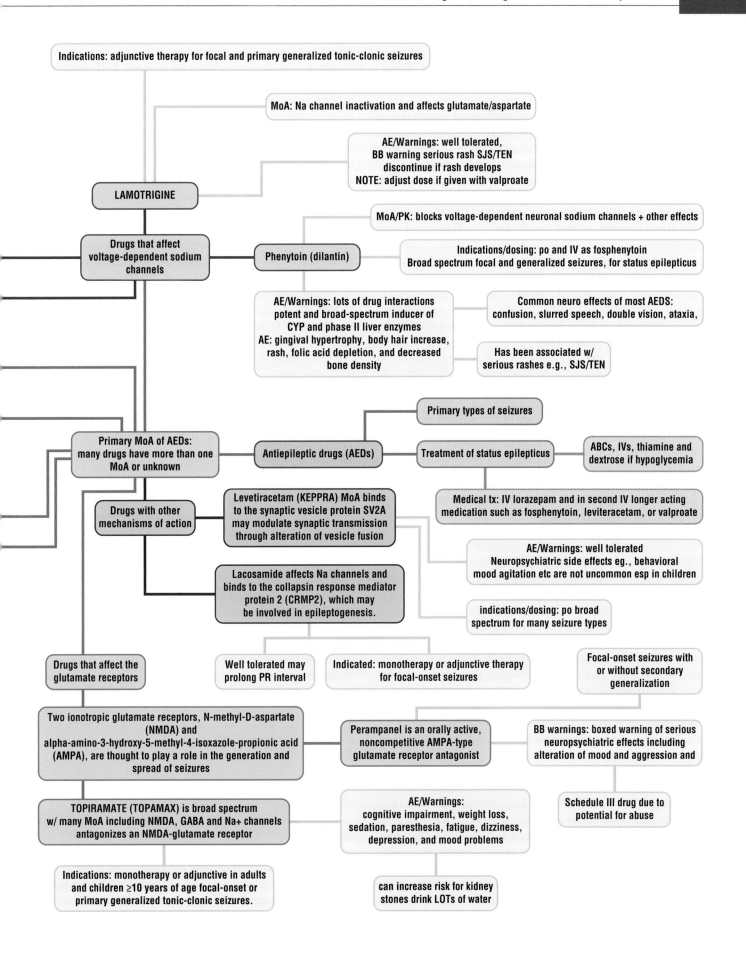

Indications: adjunctive therapy for focal and primary generalized tonic-clonic seizures

MoA: Na channel inactivation and affects glutamate/aspartate

AE/Warnings: well tolerated,
BB warning serious rash SJS/TEN
discontinue if rash develops
NOTE: adjust dose if given with valproate

LAMOTRIGINE

Drugs that affect
voltage-dependent sodium
channels

Phenytoin (dilantin)

MoA/PK: blocks voltage-dependent neuronal sodium channels + other effects

Indications/dosing: po and IV as fosphenytoin
Broad spectrum focal and generalized seizures, for status epilepticus

AE/Warnings: lots of drug interactions
potent and broad-spectrum inducer of
CYP and phase II liver enzymes
AE: gingival hypertrophy, body hair increase,
rash, folic acid depletion, and decreased
bone density

Common neuro effects of most AEDS:
confusion, slurred speech, double vision, ataxia,

Has been associated w/
serious rashes e.g., SJS/TEN

Primary types of seizures

Primary MoA of AEDs:
many drugs have more than one
MoA or unknown

Antiepileptic drugs (AEDs)

Treatment of status epilepticus

ABCs, IVs, thiamine and
dextrose if hypoglycemia

Drugs with other
mechanisms of action

Leveteiracetam (KEPPRA) MoA binds
to the synaptic vesicle protein SV2A
may modulate synaptic transmission
through alteration of vesicle fusion

Medical tx: IV lorazepam and in second IV longer acting
medication such as fosphenytoin, leviteracetam, or valproate

AE/Warnings: well tolerated
Neuropsychiatric side effects eg., behavioral
mood agitation etc are not uncommon esp in children

Lacosamide affects Na channels and
binds to the collapsin response mediator
protein 2 (CRMP2), which may
be involved in epileptogenesis.

indications/dosing: po broad
spectrum for many seizure types

Drugs that affect the
glutamate receptors

Well tolerated may
prolong PR interval

Indicated: monotherapy or adjunctive therapy
for focal-onset seizures

Focal-onset seizures with
or without secondary
generalization

Two ionotropic glutamate receptors, N-methyl-D-aspartate
(NMDA) and
alpha-amino-3-hydroxy-5-methyl-4-isoxazole-propionic acid
(AMPA), are thought to play a role in the generation and
spread of seizures

Perampanel is an orally active,
noncompetitive AMPA-type
glutamate receptor antagonist

BB warnings: boxed warning of serious
neuropsychiatric effects including
alteration of mood and aggression and

TOPIRAMATE (TOPAMAX) is broad spectrum
w/ many MoA including NMDA, GABA and Na+ channels
antagonizes an NMDA-glutamate receptor

AE/Warnings:
cognitive impairment, weight loss,
sedation, paresthesia, fatigue, dizziness,
depression, and mood problems

Schedule III drug due to
potential for abuse

Indications: monotherapy or adjunctive in adults
and children ≥10 years of age focal-onset or
primary generalized tonic-clonic seizures.

can increase risk for kidney
stones drink LOTs of water

Lacosamide inhibits neuronal firing by enhancing the slow inactivation of sodium channels. It is approved for focal-onset seizures. In addition to the usual CNS effects such as dizziness, drowsiness, headache, and ataxia, lacosamide may cause cardiac arrhythmias and heart blocks.

Tiagabine and stiripentol affect GABA neurotransmission at GABA receptors and by inhibiting GABA reuptake, respectively. Tiagabine is an adjunctive treatment for focal seizures, and stiripentol is approved as adjunct therapy for seizures associated with Dravet syndrome. The adverse effects of tiagabine are mainly dizziness, drowsiness, nervousness, and decreased concentration. Tiagabine has been associated with new-onset seizures in patients using it for off-label psychiatric and pain indications.

Rufinamide prolongs the inactive state of sodium channels, and it is US Food and Drug Administration (FDA) approved as an adjunctive treatment for seizures associated with Lennox-Gastaut syndrome. Rufinamide is well tolerated with mainly somnolence and nausea as adverse effects, but it can shorten the QT interval on electrocardiogram.

BZs bind to the GABA(A) receptor, enhance GABA binding, and increase the frequency of GABA chloride channel opening. Lorazepam, diazepam, and nasal midazolam are used for status epilepticus. Clonazepam is an anxiolytic and sedative, which is indicated as adjunctive therapy for myoclonic and atonic seizures. The BZs were discussed in the sedative hypnotic section of this chapter.

SECTION 4: Drugs for Migraines and Cluster headaches

Medications used for the acute treatment of migraines include nonsteroidal antiinflammatory drugs (NSAIDs) or acetaminophen, triptans, antiemetics, calcitonin gene-related peptide (CGRP) antagonists, lasmiditan, and occasionally dihydroergotamine. NSAIDs and acetaminophen, which were discussed in Chapter 5, are used for mild to moderate migraine attacks. Moderate to severe migraine attacks are generally treated with migraine-specific agents, usually **triptans.** Triptans (sumatriptan, zolmitriptan, naratriptan, rizatriptan, almotriptan, eletriptan, and frovatriptan) are serotonin 1b/1d agonists that cause vasoconstriction in pain-sensitive dural blood vessels, decrease the release of vasoactive inflammatory peptides, and inhibit transmission of pain in certain ascending and descending brain pathways.[26,27]

Most of the triptans are administered orally; sumatriptan is rapid acting and can also be given as a subcutaneous injection, a nasal spray, or a nasal powder. Zolmitriptan is also available for both nasal and oral use. Triptans are generally well tolerated, and the most common adverse effects include nausea, dizziness, drowsiness, weakness, and chest discomfort. Sumatriptan injections can cause short-term chest pressure or heaviness, flushing, weakness, dizziness, a feeling of warmth, and paresthesia. Triptans should not be used with monoamine oxidase inhibitors (MAOIs) or ergot preparations. They should be avoided in patients with hemiplegic migraine, basilar migraine, ischemic

stroke, ischemic heart disease, Prinzmetal's angina, uncontrolled hypertension, and pregnancy.[28]

Other drugs for acute migraines include **CGRP antagonists** (rimegepant and ubrogepant), lasmiditan, and ergots, which may be alternatives for patients who cannot tolerate triptans. CGRP antagonists were initially approved for prevention of episodic migraines (discussed later). Oral CGRP antagonists, rimegepant and ubrogepant, are approved for acute migraine treatment. The most common adverse effects of peptide (CGRP) antagonists (rimegepant and ubrogepant) are nausea, somnolence, and dry mouth.

Lasmiditan is an oral selective serotonin 1F receptor agonist approved for acute migraine. Although it is a serotonin agonist, lasmiditan does not cause vasoconstriction and can be used as an alternative to triptans in patients with cardiovascular risk factors. The main adverse effect is dizziness, which can impair driving or other related activities; patients should be counseled to wait at least 8 hours between dosing and operating heavy machinery or driving.[29]

Ergots (ergotamine and dihydroergotamine) are an older class of medications for migraine headaches, which are less commonly used. The ergots have multiple pharmacologic actions including 5HT1, 5HT2 agonist effects, alpha-1, and dopamine receptors, and they are more likely to cause vasospasm than triptans. **Dihydroergotamine** is available parenterally (subcutaneous and IV) and intranasally for acute migraine. Adverse effects, especially nausea, vomiting, and diarrhea, are more common with ergot derivatives. Ergots are contraindicated in pregnancy, breastfeeding, and in patients with hypertension or ischemic heart disease.[30]

Antiemetics are also used for acute migraines accompanied by nausea and vomiting. Parenteral prochlorperazine or metoclopramide are dopamine antagonists and antiemetics, which also reduce headache for acute migraines. These antiemetics may be given with IV diphenhydramine to reduce dystonic reactions. The antiemetics are discussed in Chapter 7.

Migraine prophylaxis may be indicated for migraine headaches that are frequent and/or long-lasting (e.g., ≥ 12 hours), increase the risk of medication overuse headaches, and cause significant disability or impair quality of life.[31]

There are several classes of medications for migraine prevention: beta-blockers (e.g., propranolol or metoprolol), certain antidepressants (amitriptyline, venlafaxine), certain antiepileptics, e.g., valproate or topiramate, and oral or parenteral CGRP antagonists. The beta-blockers are discussed in Chapter 3, the antidepressants in Section 7 and antiepileptics in Section 3 in this chapter. In general, patients begin with one of the antidepressants either amitriptyline or venlafaxine, or one of the beta blockers (metoprolol or propranolol), or topiramate.[32]

CGRP is a neuropeptide in the peripheral and CNS, which increases trigeminovascular pain transmission from trigeminal nerves to the CNS and causes cerebral vasodilation and neurogenic inflammation.[33] The CGRP antagonist class of drugs, which are approved for migraine prevention, includes two oral: **rimegepant** and **atogepant** and four parenteral: antagonist monoclonal antibodies **erenumab** subcutaneous injection, **fremanezumab** subcutaneous, **galcanezumab** subcutaneous, and **eptinezumab**

IV. Adverse effects of the oral CGRP-antagonists are nausea, constipation, and abdominal discomfort.[34] Adverse effects of the injectable CGRP-antagonists are injection site reactions and constipation.[35] The CGRP-antagonists are currently expensive and do not have long-term safety data.

Cluster headaches are less common primary headaches that occur most commonly in young adult males. They are severe, unilateral, and usually occur with ipsilateral autonomic symptoms such as eye tearing, eye redness, miosis, and nasal congestion or rhinorrhea. The treatment for acute cluster headaches is **inhaled oxygen at high-flow rates** for at least 15 minutes. Alternatively, a triptan, usually **subcutaneous sumatriptan** or intranasal sumatriptan or zolmitriptan, can be used for acute cluster headaches.[36] Verapamil, a calcium channel blocker, is the preventive treatment of choice for cluster headaches. A short, tapered course of glucocorticosteroids such as prednisone for a brief episode of cluster headaches is another option. Galcanezumab, a human monoclonal antibody that binds to the CGRP, is also approved for chronic cluster headaches.

SECTION 5: Drugs for Parkinson Disease (Mind Map 8.5)

Parkinson disease (PD) is a neurodegenerative disease that primarily causes degeneration of dopamine-producing neurons in the basal ganglia, especially the substantia nigra pars compacta and in the pontine locus ceruleus.[37]

PD generally affects older adults and is characterized by motor symptoms, e.g., progressive tremor, bradykinesia, and rigidity, followed by later-onset postural instability and cognitive dysfunction. The primary drugs that have antiparkinsonian activity are levodopa, dopamine agonists (DAs), monoamine oxidase type B (MAO B) inhibitors, and amantadine. Catechol-O-methyltransferase (COMT) inhibitors are used to manage motor fluctuations associated with levodopa therapy. Drugs used to treat PD are illustrated in Mind Map 8.5.

Levodopa, which is the precursor to dopamine, is formulated with **carbidopa,** which is a peripheral decarboxylase inhibitor, which blocks conversion of L-dopa into dopamine before it crosses the blood-brain barrier; this decreases certain dopamine-related adverse effects. The combination drug is a ratio of carbidopa-levodopa, and it has immediate- and controlled-release oral formulations. Levodopa is the most effective drug for symptomatic treatment of PD. Levodopa is generally preferred for patients with moderate to severe PD.[38]

The most common adverse effects of levodopa are nausea, somnolence, lightheadedness, and headache. Confusion, hallucinations, and delirium may occur later in therapy and more commonly in elderly patients. Motor fluctuations such as "wearing off" with the reemergence of Parkinson symptoms and abnormal, involuntary movements, e.g., dyskinesias, can occur with chronic L-dopa therapy. Treatment of **wearing off** includes adjustment of levodopa dosing and the use of adjunctive medications including COMT inhibitors, e.g., entacapone and opicapone or a MAO B inhibitor (rasagiline, safinamide, or selegiline) or a non-ergot DA, such as pramipexole or ropinirole.

The **non-ergot DA** used for PD are oral pramipexole, ropinirole, and transdermal rotigotine, which can be used as monotherapy for mild PD or add-on therapy for PD. Apomorphine is another DA available as a sublingual film or subcutaneous injection parenteral DA, which is used for rescue therapy for certain motor fluctuations such as sudden wearing off; nausea is a common adverse effect.[39] The most common adverse effects of DA are nausea, vomiting, sleepiness, orthostatic hypotension, confusion, and peripheral edema. Confusion and hallucinations can occur, especially in older patients. Pramipexole has a labeled warning about sudden drowsiness and sleep attacks that can occur without warning.[40] Patients who suddenly stop DA without tapering can develop withdrawal symptoms including craving, anxiety, panic, depression, pain, fatigue, and nausea.[41]

There are three oral **MAO B inhibitors** available for patients with PD: selegiline (also as a transdermal patch), rasagiline, and safinamide. They are indicated as adjunctive therapy for PD or for very-early-stage mild PD. The MAO B inhibitors inhibit monoamine oxidase type B, which catalyzes the catabolism of mainly dopamine. They are contraindicated with other drugs that are potent inhibitors of monoamine oxidase such as linezolid, tramadol, and certain tricyclic and selective serotonin reuptake inhibitors. The most common adverse effects of the MAO B inhibitors are nausea and headache and possibly confusion with selegiline.

COMT inhibitors are used to manage motor fluctuations associated with levodopa therapy. The COMT inhibitors include entacapone and opicapone, which inhibit COMT and increase levels of levodopa. The most common AE of COMT inhibitors are similar to levodopa: dyskinesia, psychiatric effects, nausea, orthostatic hypotension, and somnolence.

Amantadine is an oral medication primarily useful for mild PD with tremor as a predominant symptom. The mechanism of action of amantadine is not clear, but it may affect dopamine reuptake, dopamine release, and stimulate dopamine receptors. The main adverse effects of amantadine are livedo reticularis and ankle edema; some people experience lightheadedness, confusion, and nightmares.[42]

SECTION 6: Alzheimer Disease

Alzheimer disease (AD) is a neurodegenerative disorder that is a common cause of dementia in older patients, typically after the age of 65 years. It is associated with progressive memory impairment; deficits in problem solving, judgment, and insight; and gradual progressive decline in other cognitive domains with later-onset behavioral and psychiatric symptoms. Treatments can help symptoms but do not stop the progression of the disease. **Cholinesterase inhibitors (donepezil oral, rivastigmine oral, and galantamine oral and transdermal)** increase acetylcholine and may modestly improve cognition and global functioning in patients with AD. The main adverse effects of cholinesterase inhibitors are diarrhea, nausea, and sometimes loss of appetite and vomiting. Cholinergic activity can also decrease heart rate and blood pressure. They are contraindicated in patients with baseline bradycardia or known cardiac conduction system abnormalities.

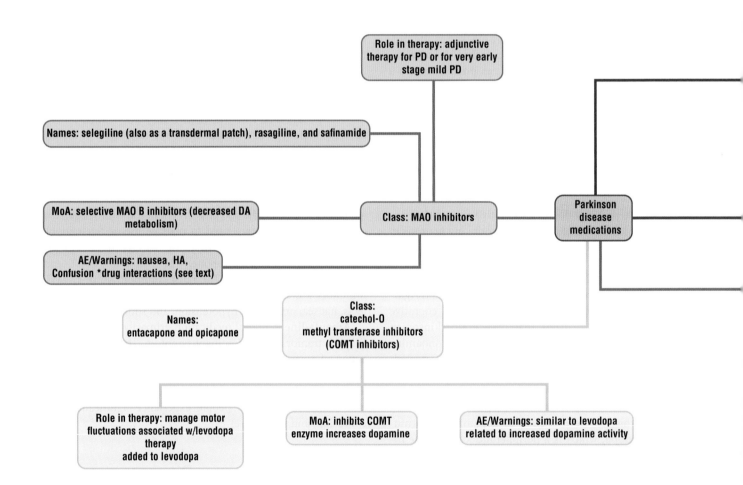

Role in therapy: adjunctive therapy for PD or for very early stage mild PD

Names: selegiline (also as a transdermal patch), rasagiline, and safinamide

MoA: selective MAO B inhibitors (decreased DA metabolism)

Class: MAO inhibitors

AE/Warnings: nausea, HA, Confusion *drug interactions (see text)

Parkinson disease medications

Names: entacapone and opicapone

Class: catechol-O methyl transferase inhibitors (COMT inhibitors)

Role in therapy: manage motor fluctuations associated w/levodopa therapy
added to levodopa

MoA: inhibits COMT enzyme increases dopamine

AE/Warnings: similar to levodopa related to increased dopamine activity

MIND MAP 8.5

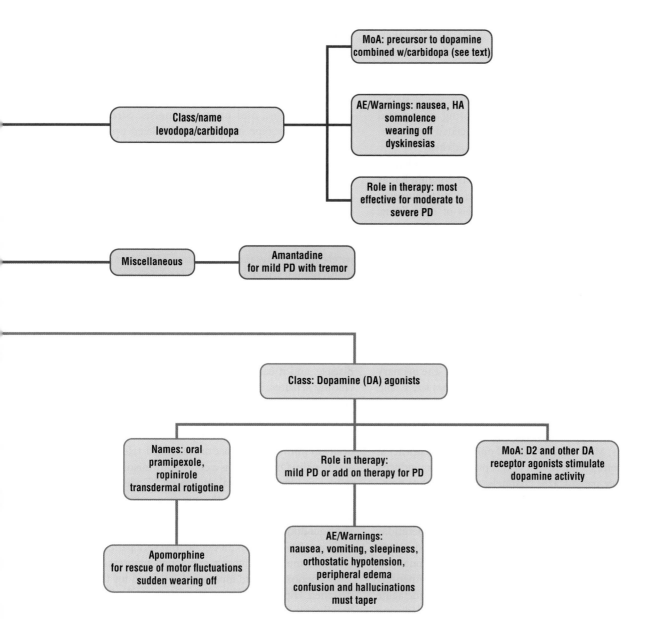

Memantine is an oral NMDA receptor antagonist that is used in combination with a cholinesterase inhibitor for moderate to severe AD. Memantine inhibits activation of NMDA receptors by the excitatory neurotransmitter glutamate and modestly improves cognition and global functioning.[43] Memantine is well tolerated, with dizziness as the main side effect; confusion and hallucinations can occur less commonly.

Aducanumab is an intravenously administered recombinant monoclonal antibody directed against amyloid beta approved for mild AD in patients with documented amyloid pathology. Aducanumab reduces brain beta amyloid levels, but clinical effectiveness is unclear. Amyloid-related imaging abnormalities, which cause either cerebral edema or hemorrhage in variable degrees of severity, are the dose-related adverse effect of aducanumab. Regular clinical assessments for neurologic symptoms and magnetic resonance imaging monitoring are required during therapy.[44] Other adverse effects associated with aducanumab are headache, confusion, falls, and diarrhea.

Vitamin E 1000 international units twice daily is well tolerated and may be added to therapy in patients with AD. Vitamin E may have a modest benefit in patients with AD by delaying progression to negative outcomes such as loss of activities of daily living, progression to severe dementia, or institutionalization.[45]

SECTION 7: Opioids (Mind Map 8.6)

Opioids are the most effective analgesic for moderate to severe acute pain treatment. Opiates are compounds structurally related to products found in opium derived from the seed pod of the poppy plant. Opioids include all-natural, semisynthetic, and synthetic opioids, which bind to opioid receptors. The primary opiate receptors are mu, kappa, and delta receptors (μ, κ, and δ), which are distributed in the peripheral and CNS and in peripheral sites, particularly the gastrointestinal tract. Opioids are classified as opioid receptor agonists, antagonists, or mixed agonist-antagonists. Most clinically useful opioid analgesics act at the **mu (μ)** receptors. Opioids act at receptors causing reduced opening of voltage-gated Ca2+ channels, which inhibits pain-activating neurotransmitter release and stimulation of K+ currents causing hyperpolarization of postsynaptic neurons.

There are important clinical pharmacologic considerations related to opioids. Opioids are used for analgesia in moderate to severe acute pain, and in conjunction with other modalities, opioids are used for pain associated with cancer and other terminal illnesses. Other clinical uses of the opioids include acute pulmonary edema, cough suppressant, diarrhea, and during general and regional anesthesia. Opioids can be administered orally, rectally, intranasally, parenterally, and regionally via epidural or spinal administration. Opioids are illustrated in Mind Map 8.6.

The toxicity and undesirable effects of opioids are significant. The most common adverse effects of opioids are nausea, vomiting, sedation, **constipation**, pruritus, and miosis (pupil constriction). IV opioids, especially fentanyl, can cause truncal rigidity. Opioids can cause increased sphincter of Oddi pressure, which may exacerbate biliary colic or pancreatitis.

The dose-limiting toxicity of opioids is respiratory depression, which can be life-threatening. Opioids are associated with tolerance and dependence (withdrawal). Tolerance, which is a diminished therapeutic effect leading to an increase in dose requirements, can occur after a few weeks of continuous dosing. Dependence leads to withdrawal syndrome when the opioid is stopped. The timing, intensity, and duration of withdrawal symptoms depend on the opioid. Physical opioid withdrawal is manifested by rhinorrhea, excessive lacrimation, yawning, chills, goosebumps, hyperventilation, tachycardia, hyperthermia, mydriasis, myalgias, nausea vomiting, and diarrhea. Psychologic withdrawal manifestations include anxiety, irritability, insomnia, restlessness, and hostility.

The most used opioids are classified by their effects on opioid receptors as **strong agonists, mild to moderate agonists, mixed receptor actions, and pure antagonists. Strong agonists** include the prototype morphine and related opioids hydromorphone and oxymorphone. **Morphine** is available parenterally, rectally, and in various oral formulations with short, intermediate, or long durations of action. **Fentanyl,** which is 50 to 100 times more potent than morphine, and related synthetic opioids sufentanil, alfentanil, and remifentanil are often used intravenously in anesthesia. Fentanyl is available as an oral lozenge, buccal tablets, sublingual solution, 72-hour transdermal patch, nasal spray, and IV solution. Meperidine is another synthetic opioid, which also affects serotonin and norepinephrine. It is less potent than morphine and is associated with significant drug interactions, especially with MAO inhibitors, selective serotonin reuptake inhibitor (SSRIs), and serotonin-norepinephrine reuptake inhibitors (SNRIs). Meperidine has a toxic metabolite, normeperidine, which can accumulate in patients with renal disease, and it can potentially cause CNS excitatory effects including seizures. Methadone potent μ-receptor agonist administered orally for opioid use disorder and chronic pain.

Mild to moderate mu agonists include codeine, hydrocodone, and the more potent oxycodone. Oxycodone is available orally in immediate-release or controlled-release forms for acute severe pain. Oxycodone is a commonly misused and abused oral opioid and has led to fatal overdoses.[46] Codeine is often used in combination with promethazine as a cough suppressant. Codeine is metabolized via phase I CYP2D6 to morphine (active). Hydrocodone is available in combination with acetaminophen or ibuprofen for acute moderate to severe pain, and with pseudoephedrine or guaifenesin as a cough suppressant.

Diphenoxylate and loperamide are used for the treatment of diarrhea. Diphenoxylate is a prescription schedule V drug combined with atropine to discourage abuse. Loperamide is available without a prescription, and it acts on peripheral mu receptors with limited access to the brain.

Mixed receptor agonists/antagonists include buprenorphine, which is a partial μ-receptor agonist and an antagonist at the δ and κ receptors. Buprenorphine was approved by the FDA for the management of opioid dependence, and it can be prescribed by clinicians with Drug Enforcement Administration waiver and training. Butorphanol is a kappa agonist with partial agonist activity at mu receptors; it is available intranasally and parenterally and can be used as an analgesic during labor in full-term pregnancy. Nalbuphine is an opioid with mixed agonist-antagonist properties used off-label for opioid-induced pruritus treatment.

Naloxone and naltrexone are pure opioid antagonists and are used for treatment of acute opioid overdose, opioid use disorder, and alcohol use disorders. **Acute opioid overdose** is treated specifically with IV naloxone or alternatively naloxone subcutaneously, or intramuscularly or via endotracheal tube at a dose to restore ventilation. Intramuscular and intranasal naloxone can be provided to bystanders to resuscitate opioid overdose patients in the community.[47] Naltrexone is longer acting than naloxone and is available orally or as a once-monthly injectable depot formulation.

Peripherally acting opioid antagonists (PAMORA) may be used for severe opioid-induced constipation. Methylnaltrexone may be given subcutaneously or orally for chronic treatment of constipation. Naloxegol, a pegylated form of naloxone, and naldemedine are other oral PAMORAs approved for refractory opioid-induced constipation. The PAMORAs do not induce opioid withdrawal, nor do they prevent analgesia.[48]

Miscellaneous opioid-like medications include tramadol and tapentadol. They are used for treatment of moderate to severe pain. Tramadol also blocks serotonin and norepinephrine reuptake, and tapentadol blocks norepinephrine reuptake. They both increase the risk of seizures, especially in patients with a history of epilepsy. Dextromethorphan is an antitussive (cough suppressant) available over-the-counter "cold/cough" medication. Dextromethorphan has been associated with increased accidental overdoses in young children and increased illicit use in young adults.[49,50]

Opioid addiction (Opioid use disorder [OUD]) is highly prevalent, and it is currently an epidemic in the United States. The basic definition of OUD is a "problematic pattern of opioid use leading to clinically significant impairment or distress" manifested by at least two specific criteria such as use of larger quantities than intended; persistent craving; excessive time spent on getting, using, or recovering from opioids; recurrent and continued use despite negative consequences and/or hazardous conditions; withdrawal; and tolerance over a 12-month period.[51]

Pharmacotherapy of OUD includes either methadone or buprenorphine alone or in combination with naloxone or naltrexone for maintenance treatment to prevent relapse in OUD. Methadone is a long-acting oral opioid agonist that reduces cravings, prevents withdrawal, and maintains tolerance. Methadone is only available at licensed opioid treatment programs and licensed inpatient hospital units. Adverse effects of methadone include constipation, mild drowsiness, sweating, peripheral edema, and decreased libido. Methadone can prolong the QT interval and may increase the risk of cardiac arrhythmias. Methadone can be used during pregnancy for women with OUD.

Buprenorphine is a partial mu-opioid agonist that can be prescribed in a clinician's office or clinic for medically supervised opioid withdrawal, e.g., detoxification and maintenance treatment.[52,53] Buprenorphine is combined with naloxone (an opioid antagonist) as a sublingual tablet, or a dissolvable sublingual or buccal film for induction and maintenance in the treatment of OUD. Naloxone, which is an opioid antagonist, is added to buprenorphine to prevent crushing or injecting the tablets or film. Buprenorphine (oral film, tablets) has been associated with dental problems, and patients should see a dentist before and during treatment.[54] There are also two long-acting buprenorphine formulations for maintenance of opioid abstinence: a buprenorphine 6-month subcutaneous implant, and long-acting monthly injectable (LAI) buprenorphine.

SECTION 8: Psychopharmacology

ANTIDEPRESSANTS (MIND MAP 8.7)

Unipolar major depression is a prevalent, often recurrent and disabling condition. There are several classes of antidepressant medications available, although the most widely prescribed class, and initial therapy, is SSRIs. **All antidepressants are associated with a boxed warning about an increased risk of suicidality in patients aged 18 to 24 years.** In general, antidepressants should be tapered to reduce discontinuation effects. Most antidepressants can begin to improve baseline symptoms by 2 weeks.[55] Antidepressant medications are illustrated in Mind Map 8.7.

The primary classes of antidepressants include:

Second-generation antidepressants:

- Selective serotonin reuptake inhibitors (SSRIs)

The medications in the SSRI class include fluoxetine, paroxetine, fluvoxamine, sertraline, citalopram, and escitalopram. In addition to unipolar major depression, most of the SSRIS are approved for anxiety disorders, panic disorder, posttraumatic stress disorder (PTSD), obsessive compulsive disorder (OCD), and premenstrual dysphoric disorder. The SSRIs act to increase serotonergic activity by blocking mechanism of action of the SSRIs.

The SSRIs are heavily metabolized by the liver, specifically CYP450. Some SSRIs, e.g., paroxetine, fluvoxamine, and fluoxetine, are moderate to potent inhibitors of hepatic cytochrome P450 and can cause drug interactions. Fluoxetine has the longest half-life and can be dosed once a day or once a week.

The primary adverse effects of the SSRIs are sexual dysfunction, specifically orgasm dysfunction and decreased libido, and a potential decrease in male fertility. Other adverse effects are drowsiness/sedation (paroxetine) or increased anxiety with fluoxetine, weight gain, nausea especially with fluvoxamine, and dizziness. Serotonin syndrome, which is a potentially fatal condition, can be caused by SSRIs especially in combination with MAO inhibitors, TCAs, and other drugs, which can increase serotonergic activity.

- Serotonin-norepinephrine reuptake inhibitors (SNRI)

The medications in the SNRI class include venlafaxine, its metabolite desvenlafaxine, duloxetine, and levomilnacipran. SNRIs are a first-line option for unipolar major depression, and they are also used for generalized anxiety, vasomotor symptoms of menopause, fibromyalgia, and neuropathic pain. The mechanism of action of the SNRIs is inhibition of serotonin and norepinephrine reuptake in the synaptic cleft. The primary adverse effects of the

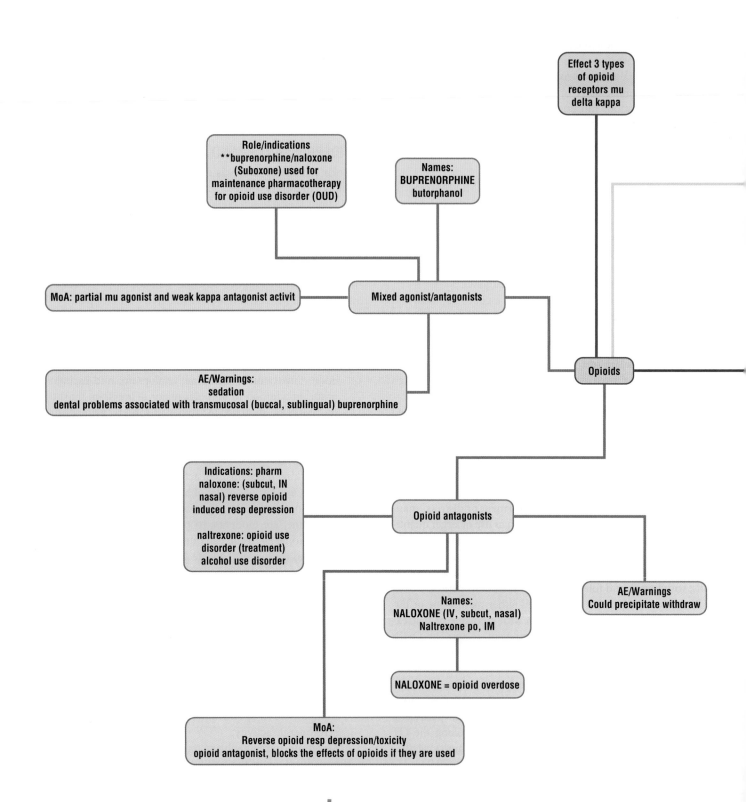

Effect 3 types of opioid receptors mu delta kappa

Role/indications
**buprenorphine/naloxone (Suboxone) used for maintenance pharmacotherapy for opioid use disorder (OUD)

Names:
BUPRENORPHINE
butorphanol

MoA: partial mu agonist and weak kappa antagonist activit

Mixed agonist/antagonists

Opioids

AE/Warnings:
sedation
dental problems associated with transmucosal (buccal, sublingual) buprenorphine

Indications: pharm
naloxone: (subcut, IN nasal) reverse opioid induced resp depression

naltrexone: opioid use disorder (treatment) alcohol use disorder

Opioid antagonists

AE/Warnings
Could precipitate withdraw

Names:
NALOXONE (IV, subcut, nasal)
Naltrexone po, IM

NALOXONE = opioid overdose

MoA:
Reverse opioid resp depression/toxicity
opioid antagonist, blocks the effects of opioids if they are used

MIND MAP 8.6

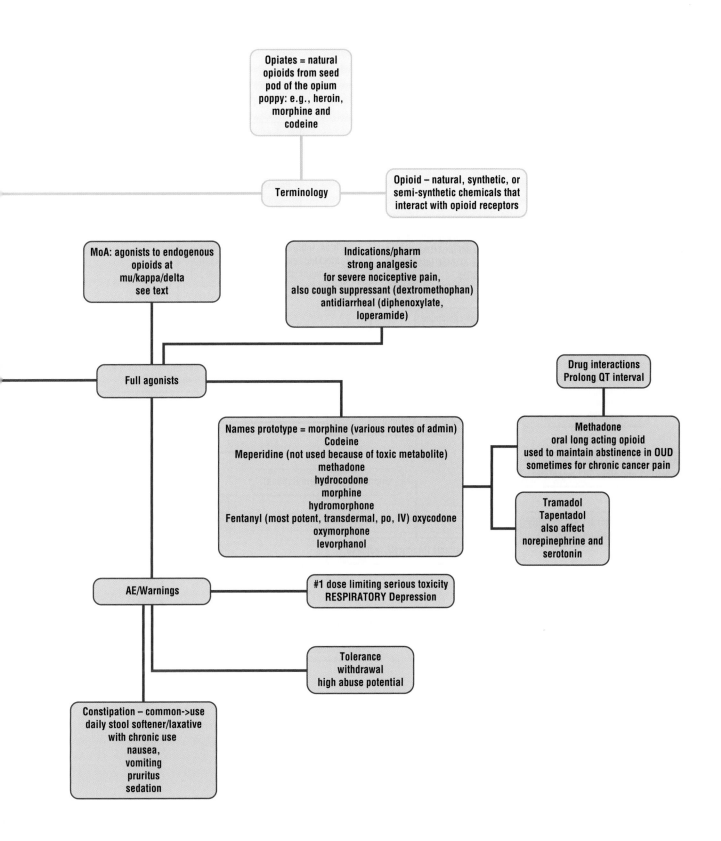

Opiates = natural opioids from seed pod of the opium poppy: e.g., heroin, morphine and codeine

Terminology

Opioid – natural, synthetic, or semi-synthetic chemicals that interact with opioid receptors

MoA: agonists to endogenous opioids at mu/kappa/delta see text

Indications/pharm
strong analgesic
for severe nociceptive pain,
also cough suppressant (dextromethophan)
antidiarrheal (diphenoxylate, loperamide)

Drug interactions
Prolong QT interval

Full agonists

Names prototype = morphine (various routes of admin)
Codeine
Meperidine (not used because of toxic metabolite)
methadone
hydrocodone
morphine
hydromorphone
Fentanyl (most potent, transdermal, po, IV) oxycodone
oxymorphone
levorphanol

Methadone
oral long acting opioid
used to maintain abstinence in OUD
sometimes for chronic cancer pain

Tramadol
Tapentadol
also affect
norepinephrine and serotonin

AE/Warnings

#1 dose limiting serious toxicity
RESPIRATORY Depression

Tolerance
withdrawal
high abuse potential

Constipation – common->use daily stool softener/laxative with chronic use
nausea,
vomiting
pruritus
sedation

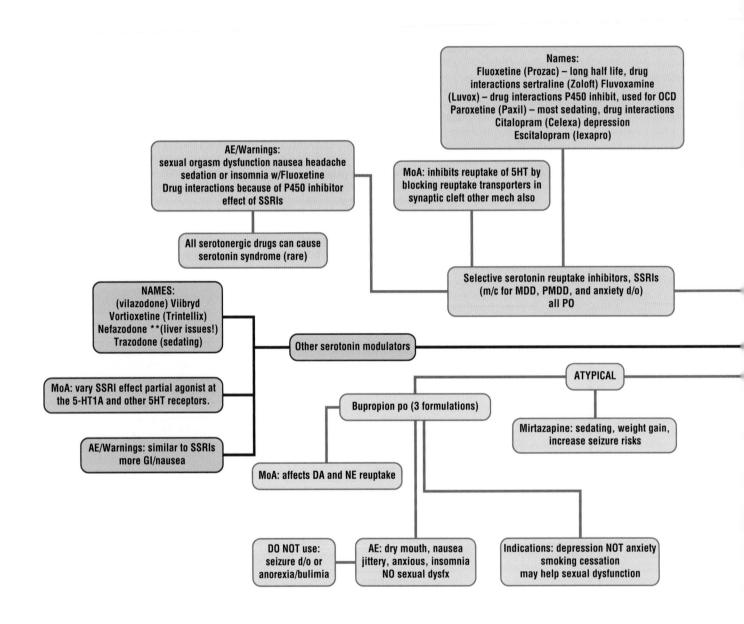

Names:
Fluoxetine (Prozac) – long half life, drug interactions sertraline (Zoloft) Fluvoxamine (Luvox) – drug interactions P450 inhibit, used for OCD Paroxetine (Paxil) – most sedating, drug interactions Citalopram (Celexa) depression Escitalopram (lexapro)

AE/Warnings:
sexual orgasm dysfunction nausea headache sedation or insomnia w/Fluoxetine Drug interactions because of P450 inhibitor effect of SSRIs

MoA: inhibits reuptake of 5HT by blocking reuptake transporters in synaptic cleft other mech also

All serotonergic drugs can cause serotonin syndrome (rare)

Selective serotonin reuptake inhibitors, SSRIs (m/c for MDD, PMDD, and anxiety d/o) all PO

NAMES:
(vilazodone) Viibryd
Vortioxetine (Trintellix)
Nefazodone **(liver issues!)
Trazodone (sedating)

Other serotonin modulators

MoA: vary SSRI effect partial agonist at the 5-HT1A and other 5HT receptors.

ATYPICAL

Bupropion po (3 formulations)

Mirtazapine: sedating, weight gain, increase seizure risks

AE/Warnings: similar to SSRIs more GI/nausea

MoA: affects DA and NE reuptake

DO NOT use: seizure d/o or anorexia/bulimia

AE: dry mouth, nausea jittery, anxious, insomnia NO sexual dysfx

Indications: depression NOT anxiety smoking cessation may help sexual dysfunction

|MIND MAP 8.7

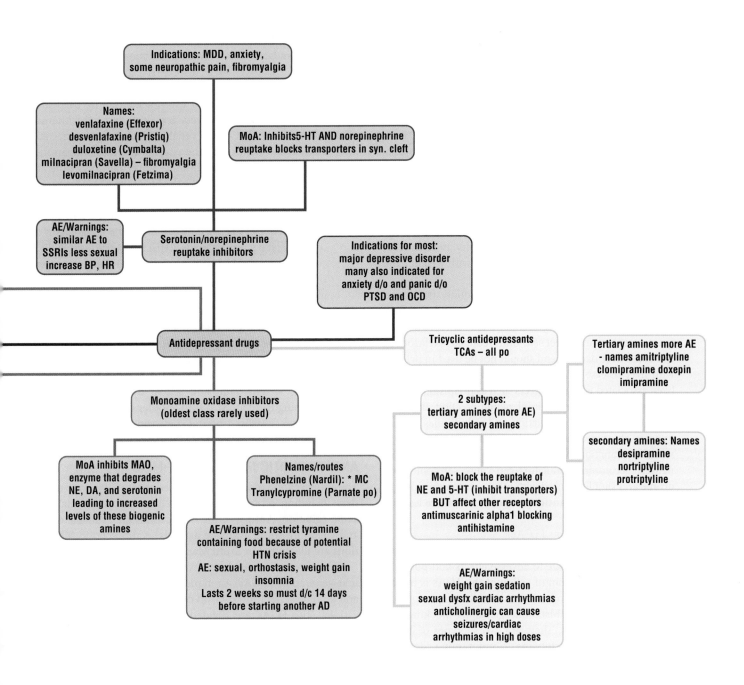

Indications: MDD, anxiety, some neuropathic pain, fibromyalgia

Names:
venlafaxine (Effexor)
desvenlafaxine (Pristiq)
duloxetine (Cymbalta)
milnacipran (Savella) – fibromyalgia
levomilnacipran (Fetzima)

MoA: Inhibits 5-HT AND norepinephrine reuptake blocks transporters in syn. cleft

AE/Warnings: similar AE to SSRIs less sexual increase BP, HR

Serotonin/norepinephrine reuptake inhibitors

Indications for most:
major depressive disorder
many also indicated for
anxiety d/o and panic d/o
PTSD and OCD

Antidepressant drugs

Tricyclic antidepressants
TCAs – all po

Tertiary amines more AE
- names amitriptyline
clomipramine doxepin
imipramine

Monoamine oxidase inhibitors
(oldest class rarely used)

2 subtypes:
tertiary amines (more AE)
secondary amines

secondary amines: Names
desipramine
nortriptyline
protriptyline

MoA inhibits MAO, enzyme that degrades NE, DA, and serotonin leading to increased levels of these biogenic amines

Names/routes
Phenelzine (Nardil): * MC
Tranylcypromine (Parnate po)

MoA: block the reuptake of NE and 5-HT (inhibit transporters) BUT affect other receptors antimuscarinic alpha1 blocking antihistamine

AE/Warnings: restrict tyramine containing food because of potential HTN crisis
AE: sexual, orthostasis, weight gain insomnia
Lasts 2 weeks so must d/c 14 days before starting another AD

AE/Warnings:
weight gain sedation
sexual dysfx cardiac arrhythmias
anticholinergic can cause
seizures/cardiac
arrhythmias in high doses

SNRIS are nausea, dizziness, diaphoresis, and sexual dysfunction, especially decreased libido, delayed ejaculation, and anorgasmia. SNRIs may elevate blood pressure but rarely cause sustained hypertension.[56] Duloxetine is an inhibitor of the hepatic cytochrome P450 enzyme CYP2D6 and can interact with several medications.

- Atypical antidepressants

The atypical antidepressants include bupropion and mirtazapine. Bupropion is a dopamine norepinephrine reuptake inhibitor. It is indicated for major depression, and is also used for seasonal affective disorder, attention-deficit hyperactivity disorder (ADHD), smoking cessation/tobacco dependence, hypoactive sexual disorder, and obesity. Bupropion is contraindicated in patients with **seizures disorder**s, bulimia nervosa, anorexia nervosa, and use of MAOIs in the past 2 weeks.[57] Adverse effects of bupropion are dry mouth, nausea, insomnia, tremor, anxiety, and weight loss.

Mirtazapine is used to treat major depression and generalized anxiety disorder. It has complex pharmacologic effects including alpha-2 antagonist, serotonergic, and antihistamine effects. Adverse effects of mirtazapine include sedation, dry mouth, and increased appetite with weight gain.

- Serotonin modulators

The serotonin modulators include nefazodone, trazodone, vilazodone, and vortioxetine. Serotonin modulators have antagonist and agonist effects at different subtypes of serotonin receptors and affect serotonin reuptake. Nefazodone can cause liver damage and should not be used in patients with liver disease. Trazodone is very sedating, and it has been associated with rare effects such as priapism, which is a persistent and often painful penile erection that lasts hours without sexual stimulation, and arrhythmias. Vilazodone is associated with diarrhea and nausea as well as sexual dysfunction. Vortioxetine is associated with more nausea. Serotonin modulators can cause serotonin syndrome and should be used with other serotonergic drugs.

Older, first-generation antidepressants, which are less frequently used, include:

- Tricyclic antidepressants (TCAs)

The TCAs are an older class of antidepressants, and they are less commonly used due to adverse effects and potential toxicity. The mechanism of action of the TCAs is inhibition of reuptake of both serotonin and norepinephrine, but they also have antihistaminergic, alpha-blocking, and antimuscarinic effects. There are two subtypes of TCAs: tertiary amines (amitriptyline, clomipramine, doxepin, imipramine, and trimipramine) and secondary amines (desipramine, nortriptyline, and protriptyline). The tertiary amines have more antihistaminergic and anticholinergic effects and are potent blockers of serotonin reuptake. The tetracyclic **maprotiline** is highly sedating and increases risk of seizures.

Amoxapine is a tricyclic that also blocks postsynaptic dopamine receptors and has antipsychotic effects.

The primary adverse effects of the TCAs include sedation, weight gain, sexual dysfunction, anticholinergic effects, and orthostasis; they also can prolong the QT interval and lower seizure threshold. The tertiary amine TCAs cause more adverse effects. Patients should undergo cardiac evaluation before initiating TCAs. Toxicity is more common with TCAs than with second-generation antidepressants. Overdosage of TCAs is mainly associated with **cardiotoxicity,** QT prolongation, cardiac conduction abnormalities with **widened and abnormal QRS,** anticholinergic clinical features (dry as a bone, mad as hatter, red as a beet, hot as a hare, blind as a bat), mental status changes, and **seizures**.

- MAOIs for psychiatric disorders, especially treatment-resistant major depression, include **phenelzine** and **tranylcypromine**. The MAOI are not commonly used and have several adverse effects and drug and food interactions. These MAOIs irreversibly block monoamine oxidase, and inhibition of the enzyme increases dopamine, norepinephrine, and serotonin. Since the drugs bind irreversibly, the effects last for the life of the MAO enzymes, usually 2 to 4 weeks.[58]

The most serious adverse effect of MAOI use is an **acute hypertensive crisis**. MAOIs can block the metabolism of certain dietary amino acids, especially **tyramine,** which can increase the levels of norepinephrine and epinephrine and lead to an acute hypertensive crisis. Patients must avoid food with tyramine including certain aged cheeses, cured meats, soy and yeast, beer, and fermented foods. MAOIs can cause **serotonin syndrome**, especially with other serotonergic medications including other antidepressants. Side effects of the MAOI include constipation, dry mouth, nausea, blurry vision, orthostasis, edema, weight gain, and sexual dysfunction. Patients switching from an MAOI to another antidepressant need a 2-week "washout period" between the last dose of the MAOI and the first dose of the new antidepressant.

ANTIPSYCHOTIC MEDICATIONS (MIND MAP 8.8)

The antipsychotic medications are used to treat psychotic disorders including schizophrenia as well as bipolar mania, and acute agitation. Antipsychotic medications are available orally, and there are some available as LAIs. Antipsychotic Medications are illustrated in Mind Map 8.8.

There are two general classes of antipsychotic medications: first-generation (FGAs) or typical, traditional antipsychotics; and second-generation (SGAs) or atypical antipsychotic medications. The FGAs are divided into high-potency and low-potency types. The high-potency FGAs (fluphenazine, haloperidol, loxapine, perphenazine, pimozide, thiothixene, and trifluoperazine) are highly potent postsynaptic brain **dopamine D2 receptors blockers**. The low-potency FGAs (chlorpromazine and thioridazine) are less potent D2 blockers with more antihistamine and anticholinergic effects. The high-potency FGAs have more **extrapyramidal effects,** e.g., akathisia (inner restlessness with compulsion to move), rigidity, bradykinesia, tremor, like clinical manifestations of PD, and acute dystonic reactions. **Acute dystonic reactions,** which are involuntary spasms of the face, mouth, eye muscles, and neck, usually occur rapidly within the first few doses. Acute dystonia is treated with either IV or IM diphenhydramine or benztropine. **Tardive dyskinesia (TD),** which is a movement disorder, is more common with chronic long-term use of FGAs, especially in older patients. TD is characterized by a range of involuntary and repetitive muscle movements of the mouth, tongue, face, extremities, or trunk, including lip smacking, tongue writhing or thrusting, grimacing, jaw movements, facial grimacing, twisting movements of the neck, trunk, or extremity writhing.

Other adverse effects of the FGAS antipsychotics include weight gain, increased diabetes mellitus, and metabolic syndrome (also with SGAs), **hyperprolactinemia** with potential galactorrhea and menstrual irregularities, sexual dysfunction, and sedation. Cardiovascular events, especially **QT prolongation**, and orthostatic hypotension, which can increase the risk for falls, are also associated with antipsychotic medications. Anticholinergic symptoms are more common with low-potency FGAs. **Neuroleptic malignant syndrome (NMS)**, which is rare but potentially fatal, is associated with FGAs; it can occur within 2 weeks of starting an antipsychotic medication. Features of NMS include mental status changes, extreme muscle rigidity, hyperthermia usually greater than 38°C, and autonomic lability with tachycardia, variations in blood pressure, and tachypnea. All antipsychotics are associated with a boxed warning about **increased mortality in older adult patients with dementia-related psychosis.**[59]

SGAs, or atypical antipsychotics, are more frequently used than FGAs and have less extrapyramidal effects. The pharmacology of this diverse group of medications is variable and involves D2 receptor agonist, D2 antagonist, and serotonin 5HT2 receptor antagonist actions. The SGAs are aripiprazole, asenapine, brexpiprazole, Cariprazine, Clozapine, Iloperidone, Lumateperone, Lurasidone, Olanzapine, Paliperidone, Pimavanserin, Quetiapine, Risperidone, and ziprasidone. Clozapine is reserved for schizophrenia resistant to treatment with other antipsychotic drugs.

Weight gain and metabolic effects such as diabetes and dyslipidemia are common effects of the SGAs, especially clozapine and olanzapine. Sedation is common with most SGAs, especially clozapine and quetiapine. Aripiprazole is less sedating and may cause insomnia. Sexual dysfunction is also common, especially with risperidone and paliperidone; elevated prolactin is also more common with risperidone and paliperidone. Several SGAs, especially ziprasidone, can prolong the QT interval, which can increase the risk for ventricular arrhythmias. **Clozapine** is associated with a potentially fatal **agranulocytosis,** which most often occurs in the first 3 months of treatment. **Clozapine** has a boxed warning about associated risks of **myocarditis** and **cardiomyopathy.** Patients taking clozapine require regular monitoring for neutropenia with absolute neutrophil counts. Seizures, increased risk for falls, and increased mortality of older adult patients with dementia-related psychosis are also associated with both FGA and SGA.

MEDICATIONS FOR BIPOLAR DISORDER

Bipolar disorder is a mood disorder characterized by alternating episodes of mania (abnormally elevated, irritable, and labile mood, increased energy, increased activity, decreased sleep, and associated behavioral, cognitive, speech, and interpersonal changes) and major depression. Medications for bipolar mania include **valproate,** an antiepileptic drug, or **lithium**, often in addition to an atypical antipsychotic such as aripiprazole, haloperidol, olanzapine, quetiapine, or risperidone. Valproate was discussed in the antiepileptic section of this chapter and is used for bipolar mania and maintenance treatment.

Lithium is used for acute bipolar mania and maintenance therapy. The mechanism of lithium may relate to its ability to affect neurotransmitters and second messenger systems. **Lithium has a narrow therapeutic index,** and it is associated with several acute and chronic adverse effects. **Weight gain** and cognitive impairment (memory, creativity, verbal learning, etc.) are common and often lead to poor adherence. **Renal effects of lithium** are common and include polyuria and polydipsia, nephrogenic diabetes insipidus, and chronic kidney disease with long-term use. Nausea and loose stools are also common. Lithium can also cause **thyroid dysfunction**, especially goiter and hypothyroidism, and cause hyperparathyroidism with hypercalcemia. Monitoring of lithium therapy includes serum lithium levels, renal, thyroid, and parathyroid function testing. Lithium toxicity presents with gastrointestinal symptoms, e.g., nausea, vomiting, and later neurologic features of course tremor, ataxia, confusion, myoclonic jerks, and severe toxicity seizures. Treatment of acute lithium intoxication includes supportive care, hydration, and possibly hemodialysis.

Other medications for bipolar disorder include lamotrigine, which was discussed in the antiepileptic section of this chapter, certain atypical antipsychotics, e.g., quetiapine, and the antiepileptic drug carbamazepine. Carbamazepine is an antiepileptic drug that is approved as monotherapy for bipolar disorder, but it has less evidence to support its use compared to first-line medications.[60,61] Newer atypical antipsychotics (SGA) asenapine, lurasidone, and paliperidone are also approved for bipolar disorder maintenance therapy.

ANXIOLYTICS

The anxiety disorders include generalized anxiety disorder, panic disorder, social anxiety disorder, PTSD, and OCD. Medications used to treat acute anxiety and panic attacks are usually BZs, e.g., alprazolam, clonazepam, or lorazepam. The BZs are described in the sedative/hypnotics section of this chapter. SSRIs and SNRIs are the first-line pharmacologic treatment for anxiety disorders. Buspirone is also indicated for generalized anxiety disorder. **Buspirone** is a serotonin partial agonist and blocks serotonin (5HT1A) auto-receptors; it is well tolerated, with dizziness as the primary adverse effect. Buspirone may be added to therapy for patients with a partial response to serotonergic reuptake inhibitor.[62,63]

ATTENTION-DEFICIT HYPERACTIVITY DISORDER

ADHD is a common neuropsychiatric condition that arises in children and can persist into adolescence and adulthood. The DSM-5 diagnostic criteria for ADHD centers around persistent symptoms of hyperactivity, impulsivity, and/or inattention, which lead to significant dysfunction and interference with social, academic, or occupational functioning.[51] **The most**

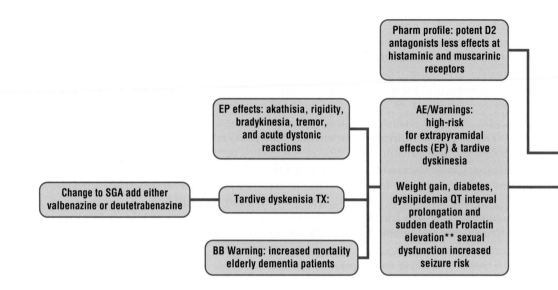

Pharm profile: potent D2 antagonists less effects at histaminic and muscarinic receptors

EP effects: akathisia, rigidity, bradykinesia, tremor, and acute dystonic reactions

AE/Warnings: high-risk for extrapyramidal effects (EP) & tardive dyskinesia

Weight gain, diabetes, dyslipidemia QT interval prolongation and sudden death Prolactin elevation** sexual dysfunction increased seizure risk

Change to SGA add either valbenazine or deutetrabenazine

Tardive dyskenisia TX:

BB Warning: increased mortality elderly dementia patients

MIND MAP 8.8

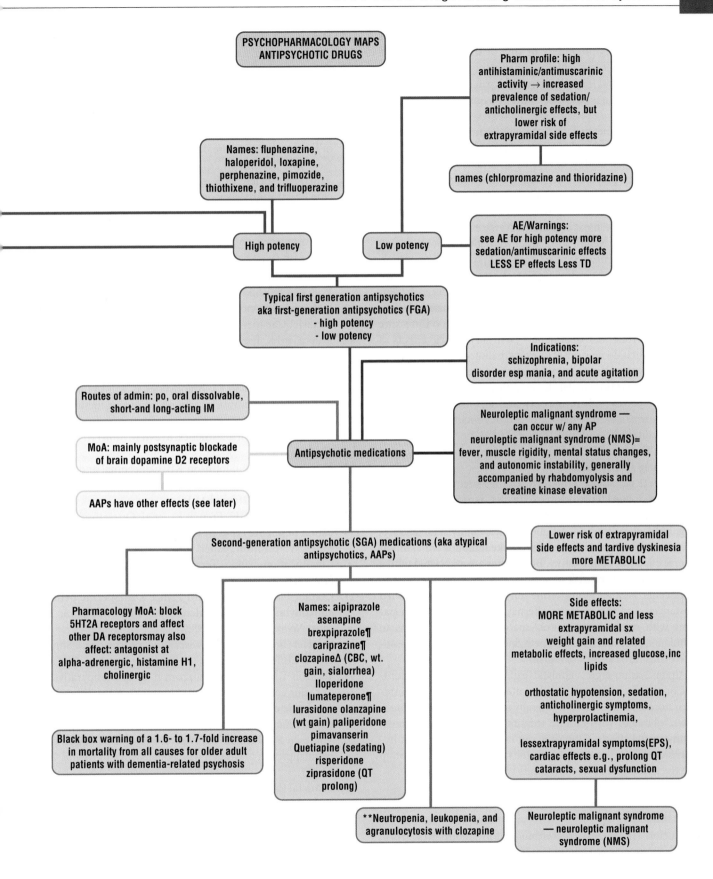

PSYCHOPHARMACOLOGY MAPS
ANTIPSYCHOTIC DRUGS

Pharm profile: high antihistaminic/antimuscarinic activity → increased prevalence of sedation/anticholinergic effects, but lower risk of extrapyramidal side effects

names (chlorpromazine and thioridazine)

Names: fluphenazine, haloperidol, loxapine, perphenazine, pimozide, thiothixene, and trifluoperazine

High potency

Low potency

AE/Warnings:
see AE for high potency more sedation/antimuscarinic effects LESS EP effects Less TD

Typical first generation antipsychotics aka first-generation antipsychotics (FGA)
- high potency
- low potency

Indications:
schizophrenia, bipolar disorder esp mania, and acute agitation

Routes of admin: po, oral dissolvable, short- and long-acting IM

Antipsychotic medications

Neuroleptic malignant syndrome — can occur w/ any AP neuroleptic malignant syndrome (NMS)= fever, muscle rigidity, mental status changes, and autonomic instability, generally accompanied by rhabdomyolysis and creatine kinase elevation

MoA: mainly postsynaptic blockade of brain dopamine D2 receptors

AAPs have other effects (see later)

Second-generation antipsychotic (SGA) medications (aka atypical antipsychotics, AAPs)

Lower risk of extrapyramidal side effects and tardive dyskinesia more METABOLIC

Pharmacology MoA: block 5HT2A receptors and affect other DA receptorsmay also affect: antagonist at alpha-adrenergic, histamine H1, cholinergic

Names: aipiprazole asenapine brexpiprazole¶ cariprazine¶ clozapineΔ (CBC, wt. gain, sialorrhea) Iloperidone lumateperone¶ lurasidone olanzapine (wt gain) paliperidone pimavanserin Quetiapine (sedating) risperidone ziprasidone (QT prolong)

Side effects:
MORE METABOLIC and less extrapyramidal sx weight gain and related metabolic effects, increased glucose,inc lipids

orthostatic hypotension, sedation, anticholinergic symptoms, hyperprolactinemia,

lessextrapyramidal symptoms(EPS), cardiac effects e.g., prolong QT cataracts, sexual dysfunction

Black box warning of a 1.6- to 1.7-fold increase in mortality from all causes for older adult patients with dementia-related psychosis

**Neutropenia, leukopenia, and agranulocytosis with clozapine

Neuroleptic malignant syndrome — neuroleptic malignant syndrome (NMS)

effective class of medications for ADHD is the stimulants class, either methylphenidate or one of the amphetamines. Methylphenidate is available in short-acting and long-acting, various types of oral formulations, and a patch. The mechanism of methylphenidate is blockade of the dopamine transporters in the synaptic cleft.

The amphetamines include dextroamphetamine-amphetamine, amphetamine, dextroamphetamine, and the prodrug lisdexamfetamine. The amphetamine stimulants are available in short- and long-acting oral preparations. Amphetamines work by blocking dopamine reuptake transporters and increasing dopamine release.

There are significant adverse effects and contraindications to the stimulants. The most common adverse effects of stimulants are **appetite loss,** weight loss, which can affect growth during childhood, insomnia, jitteriness, and emotional lability. Stimulants have potential **cardiovascular effects** including elevated heart rate and blood pressure. Patients should undergo a complete cardiovascular history and physical examination before stimulant treatment with regular monitoring of blood pressure and pulse throughout treatment.[64] Neuropsychiatric effects of stimulants include new onset or exacerbation of tics and, rarely, psychotic symptoms. Contraindications to stimulant medications include cardiovascular disease, moderate to severe hypertension, hyperthyroidism, anxiety and agitated states, motor tics or Tourette's, history of drug abuse, or concurrent use or use within 14 days of the administration of MAOIs.[65] Stimulants are **schedule II controlled substances** and have been associated with **misuse** and **diversion**.[66]

SNRIs (e.g., atomoxetine, viloxazine) are alternatives to stimulants for ADHD. Atomoxetine is associated with decreased appetite and weight loss, abdominal pain, nausea, vomiting, headache, dizziness, fatigue, and irritability. Viloxazine is a newer elective norepinephrine reuptake inhibitor with similar adverse effects as atomoxetine. Both drugs are associated with a boxed warning about risk of suicidal thinking in children and adolescents. Neither atomoxetine nor viloxazine are controlled substances, and they may be alternatives to stimulants in patients with substance use problems or severe side effects to stimulants. Atomoxetine and methylphenidate have been associated with rare cases of **priapism.**

Alpha-2-adrenergic agonists (e.g., extended-release clonidine or guanfacine) can be used as alternative therapy to stimulants/atomoxetine or add-on therapy for ADHD. Guanfacine is better tolerated, with fatigue/sedation and headache as most common side effects. Clonidine can cause bradycardia and hypotension. Clonidine and guanfacine have a delayed effect of up to 2 weeks compared to a few hours with stimulants.[67]

REFERENCES

1. Halcion (triazolam) [prescribing information]. New York, NY: Pharmacia & Upjohn Co; 2021.
2. Lunesta (eszopiclone) [prescribing information]. Marlborough, MA: Sunovion Pharmaceuticals Inc; 2019.
3. Ambien CR (zolpidem tartrate extended-release tablet) [prescribing information]. Bridgewater, NJ: Sanofi-Aventis US LLC; 2020.
4. Dayvigo (lemborexant) [prescribing information]. Woodcliff Lake, NJ: Eisai Inc; 2021.
5. Silenor (doxepin) [prescribing information]. Morristown, NJ: Currax Pharmaceuticals, LLC; 2020.
6. Rozerem (ramelteon) [prescribing information]. Lexington, MA: Takeda Pharmaceuticals America Inc; 2021.
7. Butterworth JF IV, Strichartz GR. Molecular mechanisms of local anesthesia: a review. *Anesthesiology*. 1990;72:711.
8. Neal JM, Barrington MJ, Fettiplace MR, et al. The Third American Society of Regional Anesthesia and Pain Medicine Practice Advisory on local anesthetic systemic toxicity: executive summary 2017. *Reg Anesth Pain Med*. 2018;43:113.
9. Hewer CL. The stages and signs of general anesthesia. *Br Med J*. 1937;2:274.
10. White PF, Eng MR. Intravenous anesthetics. In: Barash PG, ed. *Clinical Anesthesia*. 7th ed. Philadelphia: Lippincott Williams & Wilkins; 2013:478-500.
11. Diprivan (propofol) [product monograph]. Oakville, Ontario, Canada: Aspen Pharmacare Canada Inc; 2021.
12. Fruergaard K, Jenstrup M, Schierbeck J, Wiberg-Jørgensen F. Total intravenous anaesthesia with propofol or etomidate. *Eur J Anaesthesiol*. 1991;8:385.
13. Eger EI II, Saidman LJ, Brandstater B. Minimum alveolar anesthetic concentration: a standard of anesthetic potency. *Anesthesiology*. 1965;26:756.
14. Torri G. Inhalation anesthetics: a review. *Minerva Anestesiol*. 2010;76:215.
15. Naguib M, Brull SJ, Johnson KB. Conceptual and technical insights into the basis of neuromuscular monitoring. *Anaesthesia*. 2017;72(suppl 1):16.
16. Fisher RS, Cross JH, French JA, et al. Operational classification of seizure types by the International League Against Epilepsy: position paper of the ILAE Commission for Classification and Terminology. *Epilepsia*. 2017;58:522-530.
17. Coulter DA, Huguenard JR, Prince DA. Specific petit mal anticonvulsants reduce calcium currents in thalamic neurons. *Neurosci Lett*. 1989;98:74.
18. Briviact (brivaracetam) [prescribing information]. Smyrna, GA: UCB Inc; 2021.
19. Tomson T, Battino D, Bonizzoni E, et al. Comparative risk of major congenital malformations with eight different antiepileptic drugs: a prospective cohort study of the EURAP registry. *Lancet Neurol*. 2018;17:530.
20. Voinescu PE, Pennell PB. Delivery of a personalized treatment approach to women with epilepsy. *Semin Neurol*. 2017; 37:611.
21. Lamictal (lamotrigine) [prescribing information]. Research Triangle Park, NC: GlaxoSmithKline; 2021.
22. Depakote ER (divalproex sodium) [prescribing information]. North Chicago, IL: AbbVie Inc; 2021.
23. Zarontin capsule (ethosuximide) [prescribing information]. New York, NY: Pfizer; 2021.
24. Keppra (levetiracetam) tablets and oral solution [prescribing information]. Smyrna, GA: UCB Inc; 2019.
25. Drug Enforcement Administration, US Department of Justice. *Schedules of Controlled Substances: Placement of*

Perampanel into Schedule III. Available at: https://www.federalregister.gov/documents/2013/10/22/2013-24600/schedules-of-controlled-substances-placement-of-perampanel-into-schedule-iii.

26. Tfelt-Hansen P, De Vries P, Saxena PR. Triptans in migraine: a comparative review of pharmacology, pharmacokinetics, and efficacy. *Drugs.* 2000;60:1259.

27. Bartsch T, Knight YE, Goadsby PJ. Activation of the 5-HT(1B/1D) receptor in the periaqueductal gray inhibits nociception. *Ann Neurol.* 2004;56:371.

28. Jamieson DG. The safety of triptans in the treatment of patients with migraine. *Am J Med.* 2002;112:135.

29. Reyvow (lasmiditan) [prescribing information]. Indianapolis, IN: Lilly USA LLC; 2021.

30. Becker WJ. Acute migraine treatment in adults. *Headache.* 2015;55:778.

31. Silberstein SD, Holland S, Freitag F, et al. Evidence-based guideline update: pharmacologic treatment for episodic migraine prevention in adults: report of the Quality Standards Subcommittee of the American Academy of Neurology and the American Headache Society. *Neurology.* 2012;78:1337.

32. Pringsheim T, Davenport WJ, Becker WJ. Prophylaxis of migraine headache. *CMAJ.* 2010;182:E269.

33. US Food and Drug Administration. *Nurtec ODT [Package Insert].* Biohaven Pharmaceuticals Inc; 2023.

34. Qulipta (atogepant) [prescribing information]. North Chicago, IL: AbbVie Inc; 2021.

35. Ajovy (fremanezumab-vfrm) [prescribing information]. North Wales, PA: Teva Pharmaceuticals USA Inc; 2021.

36. Obermann M, Holle D, Naegel S, et al. Pharmacotherapy options for cluster headache. *Expert Opin Pharmacother.* 2015;16:1177.

37. Porritt M, Stanic D, Finkelstein D, et al. Dopaminergic innervation of the human striatum in Parkinson's disease. *Mov Disord.* 2005;20:810.

38. Connolly BS, Lang AE. Pharmacological treatment of Parkinson disease: a review. *JAMA.* 2014;311:1670.

39. Apokyn (apomorphine) [prescribing information]. Louisville, KY: US WorldMeds, LLC; 2020.

40. Mirapex (pramipexole dihydrochloride) [prescribing information]. Ridgefield, CT: Boehringer Ingelheim Pharmaceuticals Inc; 2021.

41. Nirenberg MJ. Dopamine agonist withdrawal syndrome: implications for patient care. *Drugs Aging.* 2013;30:587.

42. Amantadine hydrochloride tablets [prescribing information]. Yardley, PA: Vensun Pharmaceuticals Inc; 2019.

43. Chen R, Chan PT, Chu H, et al. Treatment effects between monotherapy of donepezil versus combination with memantine for Alzheimer disease: a meta-analysis. *PLoS One.* 2017;12:e0183586.

44. Cummings J, Aisen P, Apostolova LG, Atri A, Salloway S, Weiner M. Aducanumab: appropriate use recommendations. *J Prev Alzheimers Dis.* 2021;8(4):398-410.

45. Sano M, Ernesto C, Thomas RG, et al. A controlled trial of selegiline, alpha-tocopherol, or both as treatment for Alzheimer's disease. The Alzheimer's Disease Cooperative Study. *N Engl J Med.* 1997;336:1216.

46. Scholl L, Seth P, Kariisa M, et al. Drug and opioid-involved overdose deaths - United States, 2013-2017. *MMWR Morb Mortal Wkly Rep.* 2018;67:1419.

47. Doyon S, Aks SE, Schaeffer S. Expanding access to naloxone in the United States. *J Med Toxicol.* 2014;10:431.

48. Candy B, Jones L, Vickerstaff V, et al. Mu-opioid antagonists for opioid-induced bowel dysfunction in people with cancer and people receiving palliative care. *Cochrane Database Syst Rev.* 2018;6:CD006332.

49. Substance Abuse and Mental Health Services Administration. *Office of Applied Studies. The NSDUH Report: Misuse of Over-the-Counter Cough and Cold Medications Among Persons Aged 12 to 25.* Available at: http://www.oas.samhsa.gov/2k8/cough/cough.cfm.

50. LoVecchio F, Pizon A, Matesick L, O'Patry S. Accidental dextromethorphan ingestions in children less than 5 years old. *J Med Toxicol.* 2008;4:251.

51. American Psychiatric Association. *Diagnostic and Statistical Manual of Mental Disorders.* 5th ed. APA; 2013. https://doi.org/10.1176/appi.books.9780890425596.

52. Mattick RP, Breen C, Kimber J, Davoli M. Buprenorphine maintenance versus placebo or methadone maintenance for opioid dependence. *Cochrane Database Syst Rev.* 2014;CD002207.

53. Buprenorphine: an alternative to methadone. *Med Lett Drugs Ther.* 2003;45:13.

54. Suboxone (buprenorphine/naloxone) sublingual film [prescribing information]. North Chesterfield, VA: Indivior Inc; 2021.

55. Stassen HH, Angst J, Hell D, et al. Is there a common resilience mechanism underlying antidepressant drug response? Evidence from 2848 patients. *J Clin Psychiatry.* 2007;68:1195.

56. Thase ME. Effects of venlafaxine on blood pressure: a meta-analysis of original data from 3744 depressed patients. *J Clin Psychiatry.* 1998;59:502.

57. Hamilton DV, Clayton AH. Bupropion. In: Schatzberg AF, Nemeroff CB, eds. *The American Psychiatric Association Publishing Textbook of Psychopharmacology.* 5th ed. Arlington, VA: American Psychiatric Association Publishing; 2017;495.

58. Krishnan KRR. Monoamine oxidase inhibitors. In: Schatzberg AF, Nemeroff CB, eds. *The American Psychiatric Association Publishing Textbook of Psychopharmacology.* 5th ed. Arlington, VA: American Psychiatric Association Publishing; 2017:283.

59. US Food and Drug Administration. *Public Health Advisory: Deaths with Antipsychotics in Elderly Patients with Behavioral Disturbances.* Available at: http://www.fda.gov/drugs/drugsafety/postmarketdrugsafetyinformationforpatientsandproviders/ucm053171.

60. Equetro (carbamazepine) [prescribing information]. Parsippany, NJ: Validus Pharmaceuticals LLC; 2021.

61. Smith LA, Cornelius V, Warnock A, et al. Effectiveness of mood stabilizers and antipsychotics in the maintenance phase of bipolar disorder: a systematic review of randomized controlled trials. *Bipolar Disord.* 2007;9:394.

61a. Ceron-Litvoc D, Soares BG, Geddes J, et al. Comparison of carbamazepine and lithium in treatment of bipolar disorder: a systematic review of randomized controlled trials. *Hum Psychopharmacol.* 2009;24:19.

62. Chessick CA, Allen MH, Thase M, et al. Azapirones for generalized anxiety disorder. *Cochrane Database Syst Rev.* 2006:CD006115.

63. Slee A, Nazareth I, Bondaronek P, et al. Pharmacological treatments for generalized anxiety disorder: a systematic review and network meta-analysis. *Lancet.* 2019; 393:768.

64. Perrin JM, Friedman RA, Knilans TK, et al. Cardiovascular monitoring, and stimulant drugs for attention-deficit/hyperactivity disorder. *Pediatrics.* 2008;122:451.

65. Kaplan G, Newcorn JH. Pharmacotherapy for child and adolescent attention-deficit hyperactivity disorder. *Pediatr Clin North Am.* 2011;58:99.

66. Drugs for ADHD. *Med Lett Drugs Ther.* 2015;57:37.

67. Biederman J, Faraone SV. Attention-deficit hyperactivity disorder. *Lancet.* 2005;366:237.

CHAPTER 9

Drug Therapy for Infectious Diseases

Antiinfective agents are generally classified by chemical structure, mechanism of action, and the spectrum of organism they kill or inhibit. Antiinfective agents must effectively cover the type of infecting organism and penetrate the site of infection in a high enough concentration to kill or inhibit the infecting organism, and should be based on a dosing schedule that maximizes antimicrobial effects of the antiinfective drug. The microbiology laboratory is essential to identify the infecting organism from a patient's specimen and perform susceptibility testing to guide the appropriate antiinfective medications.

There are several goals of antiinfective therapy. Prophylaxis is the antiinfective treatment of uninfected or asymptomatic patients to prevent infection. Examples of antimicrobial prophylaxis include surgical prophylaxis to prevent wound infections, prophylaxis against bacterial endocarditis, and postexposure prophylaxis to protect patients after exposure to an infective agent. Empirical treatment treats a symptomatic patient based on the clinical presentation and basic laboratory techniques, and it is often a broad-spectrum antiinfective agent. Definitive therapy is a narrow-spectrum therapy based on pathogen identification and susceptibility testing. Suppressive therapy is a long-term lower dose treatment to suppress or prevent recurrence of an infection, eg, acquired immunodeficiency syndrome (AIDS) and prophylaxis for pneumocystis pneumonia.

ANTIBACTERIAL DRUGS

Antibacterial drugs or antibiotics are an essential class of medications used to inhibit the growth of (bacteriostatic) or kill bacteria (bactericidal) that cause infections. Some of the medically important bacteria that cause various infections, classified by Gram stain and morphology, include:

- Gram-positive cocci: *Staphylococcus, Streptococcus, Enterococcus*
- Gram-negative cocci: *Neisseria* (diplococcus, kidney shaped)
- Gram-positive rods: *Bacillus, Clostridium* (also anaerobic), *Listeria, Corynebacterium*
- Gram-negative rods (enteric): *Escherichia, Salmonella, Shigella, Vibrio, Campylobacter, Helicobacter, Klebsiella, Enterobacter, Proteus, Serratia, Pseudomonas* (requires specific antipseudomonal antibiotics), *Bacteroides* (common cause

of anaerobic infections), *Prevotella*, and *Fusobacteria* (mouth flora)
- Gram-negative respiratory pathogens: *Hemophilus, Bordetella, Legionella* (poor stains), *Acinetobacter*
- Gram negatives acquired from animal contact: *Pasteurella, Brucella, Yersinia, Bartonella.*

Mycobacteria are aerobic acid-fast bacteria not seen on Gram stain and can cause tuberculosis and leprosy. *Mycoplasma*, which has no cell wall, and *Chlamydia* are atypical bacteria that are not seen on Gram stain. Spirochetes are spiral shaped and include *Treponema, Borrelia*, and *Leptospira*.

Antibacterial drugs can be classified into major groups by mechanism of action and chemical structure. The spectrum of activity of antibiotics refers to the genera and species that it inhibits or kills. Refer to Mind Maps 9.1 and 9.2.

The antibacterial drugs can be classified as:
- The cell wall inhibitor group
  - Beta-lactam group
    - Penicillins
    - Cephalosporins
    - Carbapenems
    - Monobactam (aztreonam)
  - Non–beta-lactams
    - Vancomycin, teicoplanin, telavancin, dalbavancin, oritavancin
    - Bacitracin
- The protein synthesis inhibitors
  - Aminoglycosides
  - Tetracyclines
  - Chloramphenicol
  - Macrolides
  - Aminoglycosides
  - Clindamycin
  - Oxazolidinones
  - Streptogramins
  - Pleuromutilins
- The deoxyribonucleic acid (DNA)/nucleic acid synthesis inhibitors
  - Fluoroquinolones
  - Rifamycins

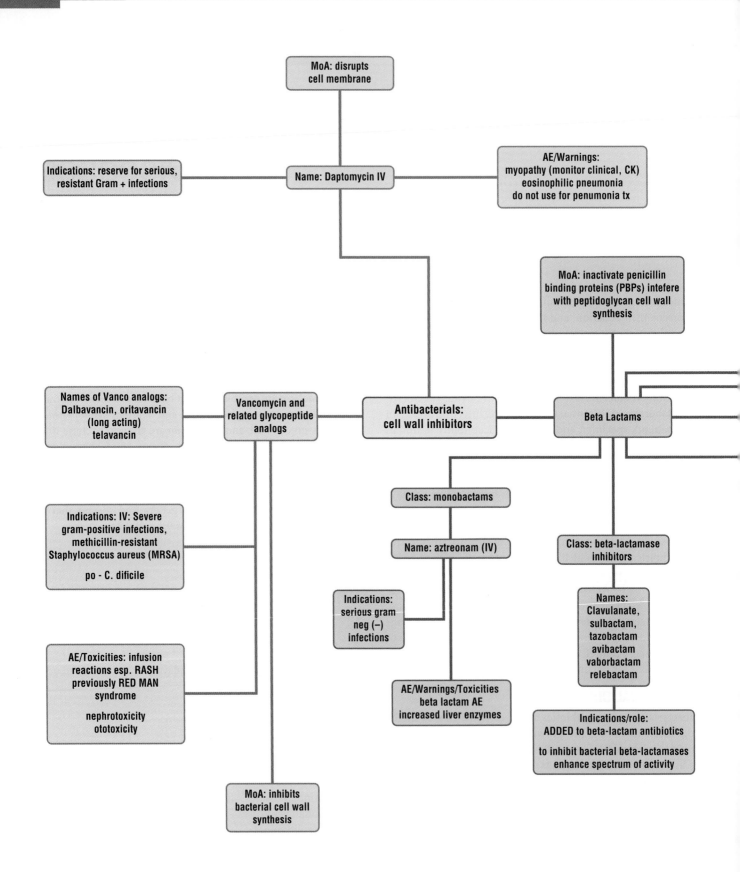

MIND MAP 9.1

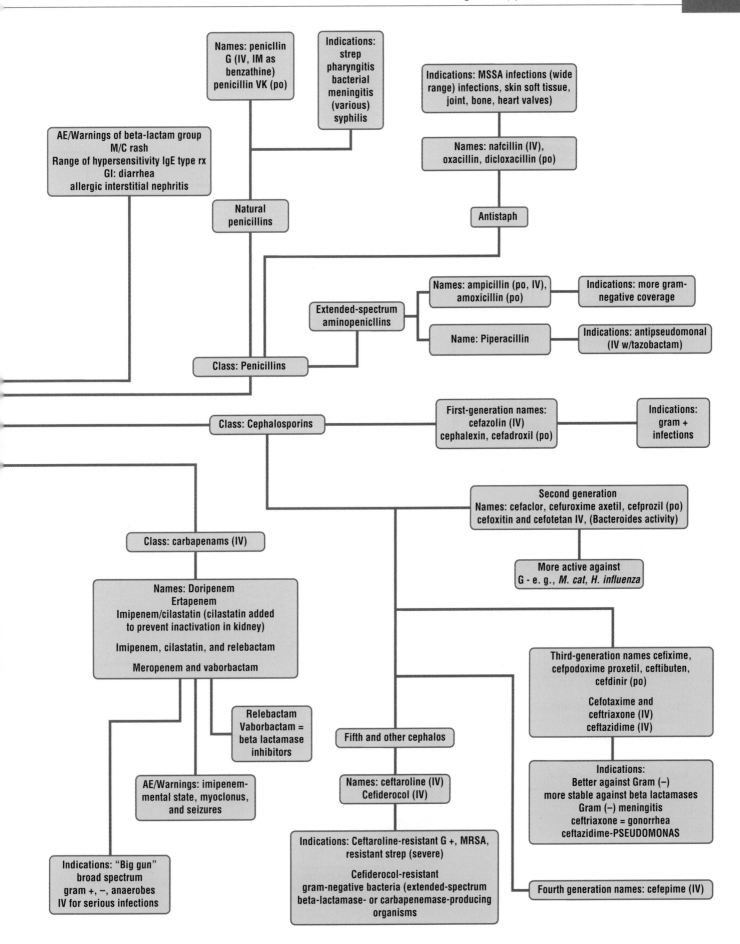

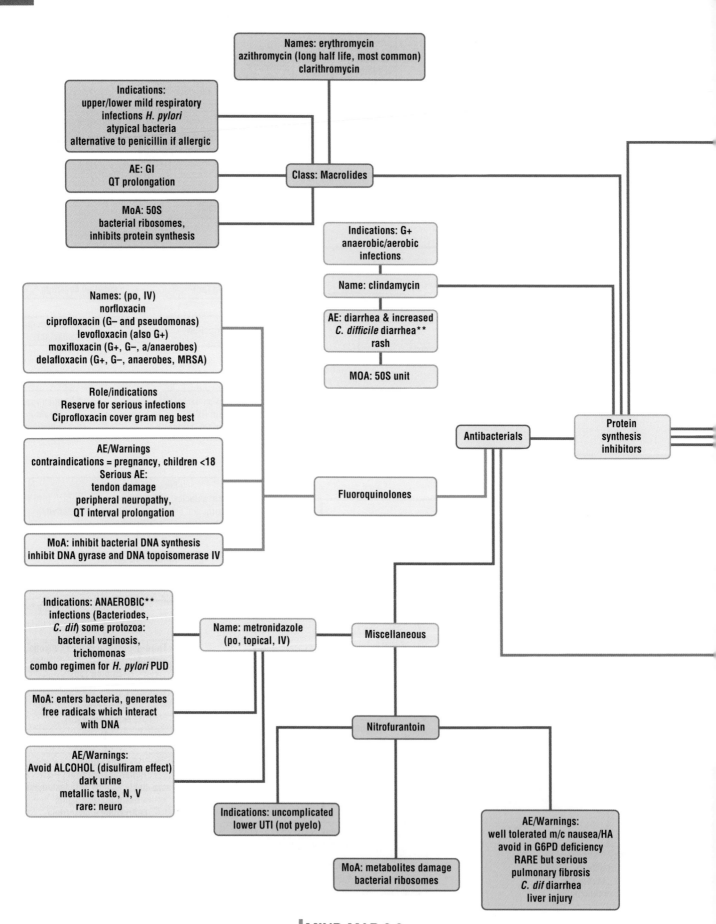

MIND MAP 9.2

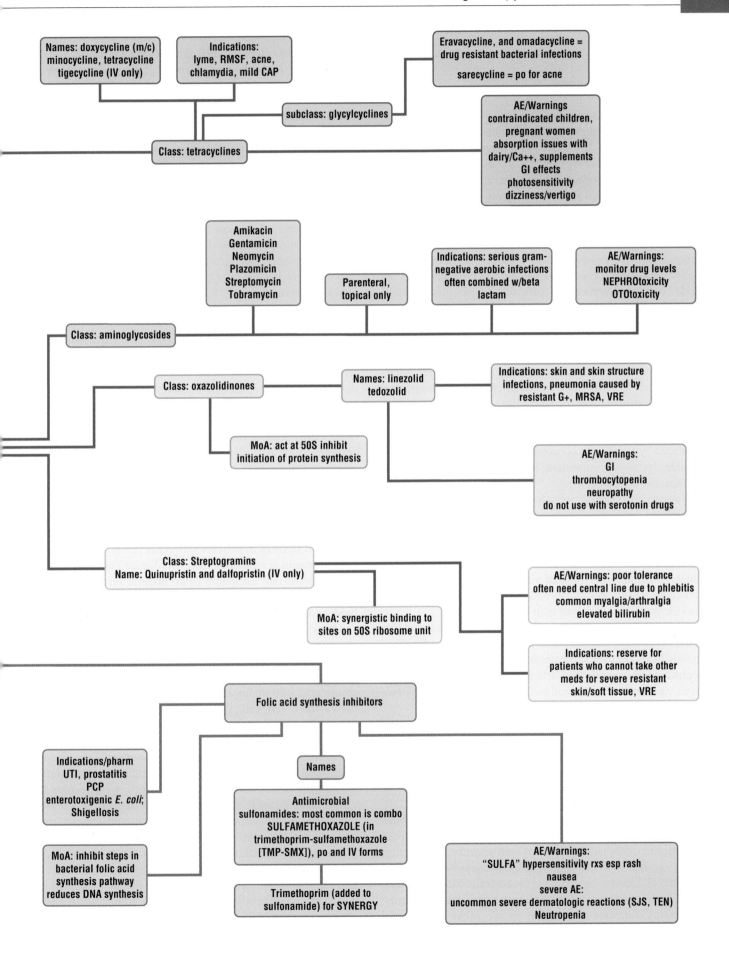

Names: doxycycline (m/c) minocycline, tetracycline tigecycline (IV only)

Indications: lyme, RMSF, acne, chlamydia, mild CAP

Eravacycline, and omadacycline = drug resistant bacterial infections

sarecycline = po for acne

subclass: glycylcyclines

Class: tetracyclines

AE/Warnings contraindicated children, pregnant women absorption issues with dairy/Ca++, supplements GI effects photosensitivity dizziness/vertigo

Amikacin
Gentamicin
Neomycin
Plazomicin
Streptomycin
Tobramycin

Parenteral, topical only

Indications: serious gram-negative aerobic infections often combined w/beta lactam

AE/Warnings: monitor drug levels NEPHROtoxicity OTOtoxicity

Class: aminoglycosides

Class: oxazolidinones

Names: linezolid tedozolid

Indications: skin and skin structure infections, pneumonia caused by resistant G+, MRSA, VRE

MoA: act at 50S inhibit initiation of protein synthesis

AE/Warnings:
GI
thrombocytopenia
neuropathy
do not use with serotonin drugs

Class: Streptogramins
Name: Quinupristin and dalfopristin (IV only)

MoA: synergistic binding to sites on 50S ribosome unit

AE/Warnings: poor tolerance often need central line due to phlebitis common myalgia/arthralgia elevated bilirubin

Indications: reserve for patients who cannot take other meds for severe resistant skin/soft tissue, VRE

Folic acid synthesis inhibitors

Indications/pharm
UTI, prostatitis
PCP
enterotoxigenic *E. coli*;
Shigellosis

Names

Antimicrobial sulfonamides: most common is combo SULFAMETHOXAZOLE (in trimethoprim-sulfamethoxazole [TMP-SMX]), po and IV forms

MoA: inhibit steps in bacterial folic acid synthesis pathway reduces DNA synthesis

Trimethoprim (added to sulfonamide) for SYNERGY

AE/Warnings:
"SULFA" hypersensitivity rxs esp rash
nausea
severe AE:
uncommon severe dermatologic reactions (SJS, TEN)
Neutropenia

- Folate inhibitors
  - Sulfonamides
  - Trimethoprim
- Cell membrane disruptors
  - Daptomycin
  - Polymyxin B colistin.

The **cell wall inhibitor** group of antibacterials include the **beta-lactam** antibiotics, which share a **beta-lactam** ring in their structure. There are four types of beta-lactam antibacterial agents: penicillins, cephalosporins, carbapenems, and the monobactam, aztreonam. Beta-lactam antibacterial agents inhibit transpeptidation in the formation of **peptidoglycan** in the bacterial cell wall. Beta-lactams target penicillin-binding proteins, which form cross-links in the peptidoglycan chains. Bacteria can produce **beta-lactamases** of various types that can inactivate beta-lactam antibiotics.

The **penicillin** class of beta-lactam cell wall inhibitors include (1) **natural penicillins** (penicillin G, parenteral; benzathine penicillin, intramuscular; and penicillin V, oral); (2) **semisynthetic penicillins, antistaphylococcal** penicillins (methicillin, which is no longer used; nafcillin, parenteral; oxacillin; dicloxacillin, oral); and (3) aminopenicillins, which have an extended spectrum, including more Gram-negative coverage, and include amoxicillin, ampicillin, and **antipseudomonal penicillins, piperacillin** and **ticarcillin**.

Beta-Lactamase inhibitors are often added to beta-lactam inhibitor antibiotics to inactivate the beta-lactamase enzymes produced by many types of bacteria. **Beta-lactamase inhibitors** include clavulanate, sulbactam, tazobactam, avibactam, vaborbactam, and relebactam.

The penicillin class is well tolerated, and most adverse effects are related to hypersensitivity reactions. Allergic reactions range from common skin rashes to serum sickness–delayed reactions, interstitial nephritis, and, rarely, anaphylaxis. Amoxicillin and ampicillin can cause skin rashes in patients with viral illness, especially Epstein–Barr virus. Large doses of penicillin can cause nausea and diarrhea. Superinfections with *Candida* and *Clostridioides* can occur with penicillins.

The **cephalosporins** are beta-lactam antibiotics classified into generations: first, second, third, fourth, fifth, or "unclassified," mainly based on their spectrum of activity. The first-generation cephalosporins are the most active against Gram-positive infections, e.g., staph and strep, and include cefazolin (IV), cephalexin (po), and cefadroxil (po).

The second-generation cephalosporins (oral cefaclor, oral cefuroxime, and oral cefprozil, and cefoxitin parenteral and cefotetan parenteral) have more Gram-negative activity, including Enterobacteriaceae, and are more stable against beta-lactamases. Cefoxitin and cefotetan are active against anaerobes such as *Bacteroides*.

Third-generation cephalosporins, (cefotaxime, ceftazidime, ceftriaxone, cefixime, cefpodoxime proxetil, cefdinir, cefditoren pivoxil, and ceftibuten) have more Gram-negative coverage, less activity against staph and Gram-positive bacteria, beta-lactamase stability, and many can cross the blood-brain barrier. **Ceftazidime** is also active against the highly resistant *Pseudomonas aeruginosa*. Cefotaxime and ceftriaxone are useful for bacterial meningitis.

Later-generation cephalosporins include **fourth-generation cephalosporin cefepime, fifth generation ceftaroline,** and the **unclassified siderophore, cefiderocol.** Cefepime is parenteral and more active against many types of beta-lactamases produced by Gram-negative bacteria, including pseudomonas. Ceftaroline is parenteral with a similar activity to third-generation cephalosporins but is active against resistant Gram-positive methicillin-resistant staphylococci and *Staphylococcus pneumoniae* (pneumococcus). Cefiderocol is a parenteral cephalosporin that is highly active against **multidrug-resistant Gram-negative infections** such as extended-spectrum beta-lactamase or carbapenemase-producing organisms.

The adverse effects and toxicity of the cephalosporins are similar to the penicillins: hypersensitivity reactions ranging from skin rashes and serum sickness to, rarely, anaphylaxis. There is a low frequency of cross-allergenicity between penicillins and cephalosporins. Superinfections including *Candida* and *Clostriodoides* can occur.

Carbapenems (doripenem, ertapenem, imipenem, and meropenem) are parenterally administered, broad-spectrum beta-lactams used for serious infections. **Imipenem is administered with cilistatin** to prevent its breakdown by renal dehydropeptidase enzymes. There is some variability in the spectrum of activity between the four carbapenems, but they are generally active against most Gram-negative rods, including *P. aeruginosa*, Gram-positive organisms, and anaerobes. Carbapenem-resistant Enterobacteriaceae, or CRE, produce carbapenemase enzymes that degrade carbapenems. **Vaborbactam** is a broad-spectrum beta-lactamase inhibitor combined with meropenem to stabilize against certain carbapenemases. The most common adverse effects of carbapenems are infusion site reactions, nausea, vomiting, diarrhea, and skin rashes. Imipenem can increase the risk of seizures in patients with renal failure.[1]

Aztreonam is a **monobactam** beta-lactam antibiotic administered parenterally for serious Gram-negative aerobic infections, including pseudomonas. It penetrates well into the cerebrospinal fluid, and it is well tolerated with occasional skin rashes.

Other **non–beta-lactam cell wall inhibitors** include the **glycopeptide vancomycin** and its **analogs dalbavancin, oritavancin,** and **telavancin.** Vancomycin and its analogs dalbavancin, oritavancin, and telavancin bind to peptidoglycan amino acid side chains and interrupt cross-linking, disrupting the bacterial cell wall. Vancomycin is active against resistant Gram-positive infections, including methicillin-resistant *Staphylococcus aureus* (MRSA) and highly resistant streptococcus. Vancomycin is usually administered parenterally for serious infections but can be used orally for *Clostridioides difficile* infections of the bowel. Adverse effects of vancomycin include the vancomycin infusion reaction previously termed as *red man syndrome*, which is a common idiopathic reaction characterized by acute flushing, erythema, pruritus of the face, neck, and upper body, and sometimes muscle spasms, dyspnea, and hypotension, which occurs during the infusion. Vancomycin can also cause local phlebitis at the injection site, and rarely nephrotoxicity. Telavancin is also parenterally administered and is effective against MRSA, vancomycin intermediate *S. aureus*, and vancomycin-resistant *S. aureus*, but it is associated with labeled warnings of nephrotoxicity and teratogenic effects. Dalbavancin and oritavancin are long-acting lipoglycopeptides parenterally administered as a single dose or once weekly for highly resistant Gram-positive infections.[2]

Bacitracin is a cell wall inhibitor that inhibits the transfer of peptidoglycan subunits. It is used topically for conjunctivitis and in an ointment for prevention of mild skin infections.

The protein synthesis inhibitor antibiotics inhibit bacterial protein synthesis at ribosomes. Bacterial ribosomes have a 30S and a 50S subunit, which assemble during protein synthesis.

Tetracyclines and aminoglycosides bind to the **30S** subunit.

The **tetracycline** class that binds to the 30S ribosomal subunit includes tetracycline, doxycycline, and minocycline and newer glycylcyclines, which are eravacycline, sarecycline, and omadacycline. Tetracyclines are broad spectrum and bacteriostatic against many common aerobic Gram-positive, some Gram-negative, and atypical pathogens such as *Rickettsia* spp., *Borrelia* spp., *Treponema* spp., *Chlamydia* spp., and *Mycoplasma pneumoniae*. Doxycycline is the most used and is available orally and intravenously. Oral absorption of the tetracyclines is decreased with dairy products and antacids containing divalent cations. Tetracyclines should be avoided in children less than 8 years old due to the risk of yellow discoloration of permanent teeth and possible accumulation in long bones. Tetracyclines should NOT be used by pregnant women due to hepatotoxicity risk and potential effects on fetal teeth and bone, and should not be used by breastfeeding women. The adverse effects of tetracyclines are mainly gastrointestinal (GI), especially epigastric pain, nausea, vomiting, and diarrhea. Photosensitivity skin reactions are possible, and dizziness and vertigo are more likely with minocycline. Tigecycline (intravenous [IV]) has a boxed warning of increased mortality compared to other antibacterial drugs.[3]

Newer tetracycline-like drugs include eravacycline, omadacycline, and sarecycline (oral agent for inflammatory acne vulgaris). Eravacycline (IV agent) and omadacycline (oral and IV) are used for certain drug-resistant bacterial infections. Eravacycline is approved for complicated intraabdominal infections and omadacycline is approved for community-acquired pneumonia and bacterial skin and soft tissue infections.

The **aminoglycosides** are **parenterally** administered, bactericidal protein synthesis inhibitors, which bind to 30S ribosomal subunits. Currently available aminoglycosides include gentamicin, tobramycin, amikacin, plazomicin, streptomycin, neomycin, and paromomycin; tobramycin, gentamicin, and amikacin are the most used. Aminoglycosides are active against **aerobic, mainly Gram-negative, bacteria** and they are NOT active against anaerobes. Aminoglycosides are mainly used synergistically with other antibiotics such as beta-lactams for serious infections such as complicated urinary tract infections or intraabdominal septicemia. Tobramycin is most active against the notorious *P. aeruginosa*, and amikacin may be effective against certain tobramycin/gentamicin-resistant organisms.

Aminoglycosides are associated with other pharmacologic characteristics. They exhibit postantibiotic effect for a short time after discontinuation, concentration-dependent killing, and synergy with cell-wall inhibitors. Aminoglycosides have a narrow therapeutic index and the primary adverse effects are

nephrotoxicity with increased creatinine and **ototoxicity** with tinnitus and high-frequency hearing loss especially when given in high cumulative doses. Aminoglycosides can cause a neuromuscular blockade, which is rare. Serum trough levels of aminoglycosides are often monitored during treatment.[4]

Macrolides, clindamycin, chloramphenicol, streptogramins (quinupristin-dalfopristin), oxazolidinones (linezolid, tedizolid), and pleuromutilin (levamulin) bind to the 50S subunit.

Macrolide antibiotics are protein synthesis inhibitors, which bind to the 50s ribosomal subunit. Macrolide antibiotics include the prototype erythromycin and derivatives clarithromycin and azithromycin. Fidaxomycin is a macrolide which is used to treat *Clostridioides difficile* infection. Macrolides are active against many Gram-positive bacteria, several atypical organisms, nontuberculous mycobacteria, and some Gram negatives such as *Haemophilus* spp., *Moraxella catarrhalis*, *Helicobacter pylori*, and *Bordetella pertussis*. Azithromycin is the most used macrolide, available orally in 1-, 3-, or 5-day regimens and intravenously and it has a long tissue half-life of 2 to 4 days. Adverse effects of macrolides are mainly GI especially nausea, vomiting, and diarrhea; these GI effects are more common with erythromycin. Macrolides can prolong the QT interval, which can increase the risk for certain ventricular arrhythmias including torsades de pointes.

Clindamycin inhibits protein synthesis by binding to the 50s ribosomal subunit of bacteria. It is available orally, intravenously, and topically for mainly Gram-positive anaerobic and aerobic bacterial infections. It is used alone or in combination for various infections including abscesses, bone, joint, skin, soft tissue, gynecologic, and intraabdominal infections. Clindamycin is commonly associated with **antibiotic-associated diarrhea,** including *C. difficile* **colitis.** Other adverse effects of clindamycin include nausea, vomiting, metallic taste, and maculopapular rash.

Chloramphenicol is a broad-spectrum antibiotic that inhibits protein synthesis by binding to the 50S ribosomal subunit. Chloramphenicol use is restricted due to toxicity, specifically bone marrow suppression and rarely **aplastic anemia.** Chloramphenicol resulted in cases of serious multisystem dysfunction termed "*gray baby syndrome*" in neonates due to immature liver metabolism and toxic accumulation.

Oxazolidinone class includes linezolid (oral and IV) and tedizolid (oral and IV), which block the initiation of protein synthesis at the 50S ribosome. These drugs are generally used for infections caused by drug-resistant Gram-positive organisms, especially MRSA and vancomycin-resistant enterococci (VRE). Important adverse effects of the oxazolidinones include GI effects, myelosuppression especially **thrombocytopenia**, and peripheral and optic neuropathies with sensory and visual disturbances. **Lactic acidosis** has occurred in patients taking a prolonged course of linezolid.[5] Linezolid has been associated with **serotonin syndrome** when taken with serotonergic drugs, eg, nonselective monoamide oxidase inhibitors, selective-serotonin reuptake inhibitors, serotonin and norepinephrine reuptake inhibitors.[6]

Streptogramins include the parenteral combination medications, quinupristin and dalfopristin, which synergistically block the sites on the 50S ribosomal subunit. Quinupristin-dalfopristin is reserved as an alternative for severe infection caused by multidrug-resistant Gram-positive strep, staph (MRSA), and *Enterococcus faecium*. Quinupristin-dalfopristin may need to be infused with a central line because of vein irritation. Adverse effects include infusion pain, phlebitis, myalgias, and arthralgias, which are very common, and elevated bilirubin.[7]

The **pleuromutilins** include **lefamulin** (oral and IV formulations), which bind to 50S and inhibits bacterial transfer RNA from binding to its site on ribosomes. Lefamulin is used as an alternative to other antibacterials for community-acquired pneumonia, because it is effective against lower respiratory tract pathogens including atypical pathogens. Nausea and diarrhea are the most common adverse effects.[8]

The DNA/Nucleic Acid Synthesis Inhibitors

The **fluoroquinolones** are broad-spectrum antibiotics that inhibit DNA synthesis by inhibiting one or both DNA gyrase and DNA topoisomerase IV enzymes. Ciprofloxacin (oral, IV, and topical eye and ear formulations) is most active against Gram-negative organisms, including *Pseudomonas*. Newer fluoroquinolones such as levofloxacin, moxifloxacin, and delafloxacin are more active against Gram positives, including some strep and staph. Moxifloxacin is also active against some anaerobes. While the fluoroquinolones are generally well tolerated, there are some serious adverse effects that have restricted their use. The most serious adverse effects of the fluoroquinolones are **tendinopathies, peripheral neuropathy** that can persist, altered mental status including delirium, and QT prolongation. The most common adverse effects are mild GI upset, headache, and dizziness. Fluoroquinolones are contraindicated in children less than 18 years of age, and pregnant or breastfeeding women.[9]

The rifamycins include rifampin, rifapentine, and rifabutin, of which rifampin is the most used. Rifamycins inhibit bacterial RNA synthesis and are the most used in combination regimens for treatment of active and latent tuberculosis (discussed at the end of this section with antimycobacterials).

Folate Inhibitors

Sulfonamides are a diverse class of antifolate drugs, which compete with para-amino benzoic acid and inhibit dihydropteroate synthase in the synthesis of bacterial folic acid. Sulfonamides are active against many Gram-negative bacteria, some Gram-positive bacteria, and some protozoa. **Sulfonamide antibiotics can be combined with either trimethoprim** or pyrimethamine to synergistically block another enzyme in folic acid synthesis. There are several sulfonamides, most commonly **sulfamethoxazole**, which is usually combined with **trimethoprim** (oral and IV formulations) for urinary tract infection, prostatitis, *Pneumocystis jirovecii* pneumonia, and certain skin and soft-tissue infections caused by staph. Pyrimethamine and **sulfadiazine** are used for toxoplasmosis.

The sulfonamides and trimethoprim are associated with adverse effects and hypersensitivity reactions. Adverse effects of sulfonamides include myelosuppression, anemia and leukopenia, rashes, fever, and crystalluria. **Hypersensitivity reactions**

to **sulfonamide antimicrobials are a common** cause of drug allergic reactions and most commonly present as a morbilliform, maculopapular rash, and fever within a week of therapy. **Sulfonamide** antibiotics are also associated with severe skin reactions, including **Stevens–Johnson syndrome and toxic epidermal necrolysis.**[10]

Cell Membrane Disruptors

Daptomycin is an intravenously administered antibacterial that binds to and disrupts bacterial cell membranes in mainly Gram-positive organisms. Its use is restricted to patients with serious infections caused by drug-resistant staph (MRSA), drug-resistant strep, and *Enterococcus spp.*, including VRE. Serious adverse effects include myopathy with elevated creatine phosphokinase levels, which can progress to rhabdomyolysis and drug-induced eosinophilic pneumonia. Daptomycin should not be used for pneumonia because it binds to surfactant, which reduces its effectiveness.[11]

Polymyxin B and colistin are narrow-spectrum bactericidal drugs that disrupt the outer cell membrane of Gram-negative bacteria. Polymyxin B is administered intravenously, and it is reserved for serious multidrug-resistant infections with Enterobacteriaceae, *P. aeruginosa*, and *Acinetobacter baumannii*. Nephrotoxicity (with a range of clinical manifestations) is a common adverse effect of polymyxin and colistin and renal function should be monitored during therapy. Polymyxins can cause a range of neurologic effects such as dizziness, paresthesia, confusion, and ataxia. Colistin is associated with a greater incidence of nephrotoxicity than polymyxin B.[12]

Antimycobacterials

Mycobacteria are slow growing, intracellular bacteria that are resistant to many antibiotics. They require longer duration combinations of two or more drugs for effective treatment. Isoniazid (INH), rifampin (or other rifamycin), pyrazinamide, and ethambutol are first-line drugs for treatment of active tuberculosis (TB) disease. TB disease treatment has two phases: an intensive phase with a four-drug regimen of "RIPE therapy" for 2 months followed by a continuation phase with two drugs for an additional 26 weeks. "RIPE therapy" consists of rifampin, INH, pyrazinamide, and ethambutol. **INH** is selective for mycobacteria as it inhibits mycolic acid necessary for cell wall synthesis. INH is used orally for latent and active tuberculosis treatment. The primary adverse effects of INH are most commonly **hepatotoxicity,** especially in older patients and during the first 2 months of therapy. INH can cause **peripheral neuropathy** by interfering with vitamin **B6 (pyridoxine)** utilization; concomitant B6 supplementation reduces INH neuropathy. **Rifampin** is a rifamycin used to treat tuberculosis and other mycobacterial infections. **Rifampin is a potent inducer of several drug-metabolizing enzymes (CYP450),** which leads to many drug interactions. Ribabutin is similar to rifampin but has less potential for drug interactions. Rifapentine is a rifamycin with a long half-life, permitting once-weekly oral dosing, but it is also associated with drug interactions. Rifampin causes a distinctive but harmless orange or orange reddish discoloration to body fluids. Rifampin can cause flu-like symptoms, GI effects, and less commonly hepatitis. **Ethambutol** is a first-line antimycobacterial used in the four-drug treatment of TB disease. Ethambutol may inhibit an enzyme in the formation of the mycobacterial cell wall. The most important toxicity of **ethambutol is optic neuropathy** causing changes in visual acuity and red-green color blindness; this is usually dose related and more common with longer durations of treatment. **Pyrazinamide** is a first-line antituberculous drug during the four-drug initiation phase of treatment, which disrupts the mycobacterial cell membrane functions. Adverse effects of pyrazinamide are **hepatotoxicity** and **hyperuricemia,** which can exacerbate gout, nausea, and arthralgias.[13]

ANTIVIRALS

Viruses are intracellular microorganisms that contain either a DNA or RNA genome covered with a protein coat, and, in some cases, a lipoprotein envelope. Antiviral medications target various components in the viral life cycle. Antiviral drugs are illustrated in Mind Map 9.3, antivirals for hepatitis C are shown in Mind Map 9.4, and antiretrovirals for treatment of human immunodeficiency virus (HIV) are given in Mind Map 9.5.

There are three classes of drugs for influenza prevention and treatment: (1) the neuraminidase inhibitors, zanamivir, oseltamivir, and peramivir; (2) selective inhibitor of influenza cap-dependent endonuclease, baloxavir; and (3) adamantanes, amantadine, and rimantadine, which are only active against influenza A. Neuraminidase inhibitors work by interfering with the release of influenza virions from infected host cells to prevent new cells from being infected. **Oseltamivir** is administered orally twice daily for 5 days. The main adverse effects of oseltamivir are nausea and vomiting. Zanamivir is an inhalation powder used twice daily for 5 to 10 days. Zanamivir is not recommended for patients with underlying pulmonary disease, eg, chronic obstructive pulmonary disease. Peramivir is administered as a single IV dose and the most common adverse effect is diarrhea. Neuraminidase inhibitors are effective against influenza A and B.

Amantadine and rimantadine are oral medications that target the M2 protein in the viral membrane, which is required for viral replication. These drugs are not commonly used because of resistance, and they are only effective against influenza A. Amantadine can cause neuropsychiatric effects such as anxiety, insomnia, confusion, and lightheadedness.

Baloxavir is a one-dose orally administered antiviral for treatment of acute uncomplicated influenza. It is an inhibitor of influenza cap-dependent endonuclease, which inhibits messenger RNA synthesis.[14] It is administered as a single weight-based dose in patients presenting with flu symptoms for less than 48 hours' duration. Diarrhea is the primary adverse effect, which occurs in a small number of patients.

Antiherpetic medications are available for the treatment of the following herpes viruses: herpes simplex virus types 1 and 2, varicella-zoster virus, and cytomegalovirus (CMV). **Acyclovir, valacyclovir**, and **famciclovir** are used to prevent and treat infections with herpes simplex viruses 1 and 2 and varicella-zoster virus. Acyclovir is a nucleoside analog that inhibits viral replication; **valacyclovir** is an oral prodrug of acyclovir with

better oral bioavailability and less frequent dosing. Acyclovir is available orally, intravenously, and as a topical cream or ointment for recurrent herpes labialis (cold sores) and as an ophthalmic ointment. Acyclovir is well tolerated but has been associated with two toxic reactions: acute renal failure with IV therapy and neurologic toxicity, especially in patients with preexisting renal disease. **Famciclovir** is an oral prodrug that inhibits viral herpes and varicella DNA polymerase and viral replication. Valacyclovir (two to three times daily) and famciclovir (two to three times daily) are dosed less frequently than acyclovir (five times daily).

CMV can cause congenital symptomatic infection in neonates and disseminated multisystem disease in immunocompromised patients, especially AIDS patients and transplant recipients on immunosuppressive therapies. CMV can also cause a mild, self-limited, infectious mononucleosis–type syndrome in children and adults. There are several antiviral agents for CMV infection specifically in immunocompromised patients: **ganciclovir** and **valganciclovir** are the most used. Foscarnet and cidofovir are also available for CMV in certain cases. Ganciclovir (IV) and its oral prodrug valganciclovir are used to prevent and treat CMV infections and they are analogs of the nucleoside guanosine, which inhibit viral DNA polymerases.[15] Ganciclovir and valganciclovir are both associated with a boxed warning of bone marrow suppression especially leukopenia. IV ganciclovir may be associated with increased creatinine. Ganciclovir and valganciclovir have GI adverse effects including nausea and loss of appetite, and diarrhea with ganciclovir.[16]

Foscarnet and cidofovir are also available for CMV in certain cases. Foscarnet (IV) may be used for CMV-resistant infection in immunocompromised patients. Foscarnet binds to and inhibits viral DNA polymerases and blocks DNA synthesis. The primary adverse effects of foscarnet are **renal insufficiency** and renal tubular damage, **hypocalcemia**, hypomagnesemia, nausea, and possibly increased seizures. IV cidofovir is mainly used to treat CMV retinitis in patients with AIDS. **Cidofovir** is a nucleoside analog that inhibits viral DNA polymerases. There is a boxed warning of **nephrotoxicity**, which requires IV prehydration before each cidofovir infusion and close monitoring of kidney function.[17]

Hepatitis B is a DNA virus that is transmitted mainly by blood and bodily fluids, and it can cause chronic hepatitis, cirrhosis, liver failure, and hepatocellular carcinoma. Antivirals used for the treatment of hepatitis B include interferon and more commonly nucleos(t)ide analogs, entecavir and tenofovir. Interferon alfa, which induces antiviral genes in multiple cells, is administered by once weekly subcutaneous injection for 48 weeks. Interferon is associated with several common adverse effects, especially an **initial flu-like syndrome** in most patients. Other adverse effects include neutropenia, thrombocytopenia, depressed mood, induction of autoimmune disease, eg, thyroid disease, and flares of hepatitis. Interferon should not be given to pregnant women or patients with suicidal tendencies or severe psychiatric disease.[18]

Tenofovir and entecavir are preferred for most patients with chronic hepatitis B infection. These orally administered antiviral agents are also used to treat HIV infection (see section on

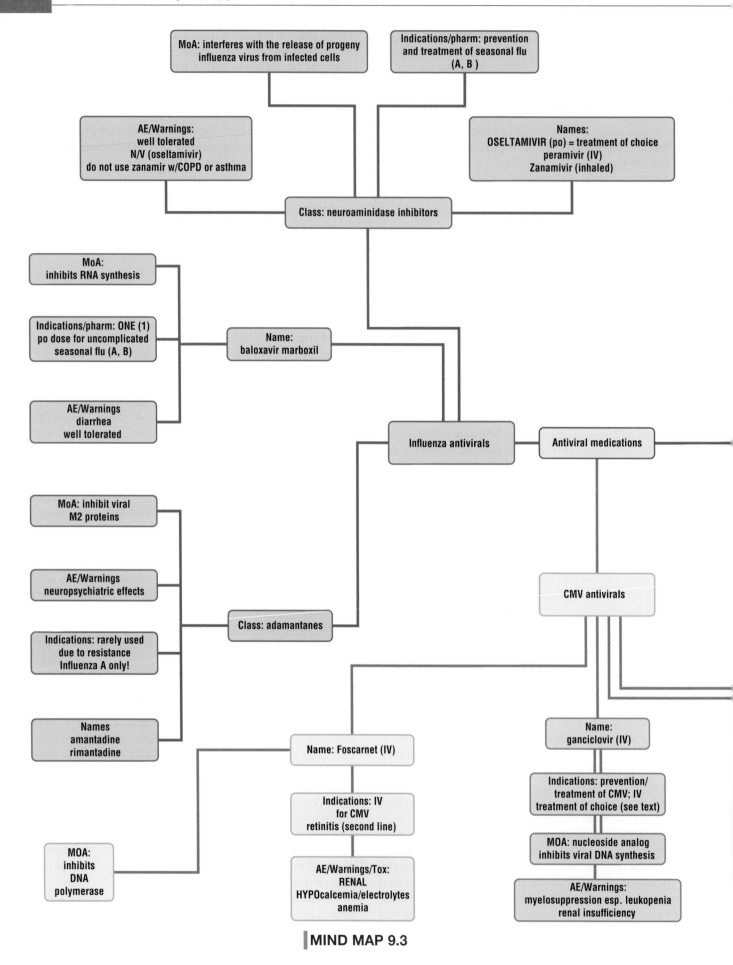

MoA: interferes with the release of progeny influenza virus from infected cells

Indications/pharm: prevention and treatment of seasonal flu (A, B)

AE/Warnings:
well tolerated
N/V (oseltamivir)
do not use zanamir w/COPD or asthma

Names:
OSELTAMIVIR (po) = treatment of choice
peramivir (IV)
Zanamivir (inhaled)

Class: neuroaminidase inhibitors

MoA:
inhibits RNA synthesis

Indications/pharm: ONE (1) po dose for uncomplicated seasonal flu (A, B)

Name:
baloxavir marboxil

AE/Warnings
diarrhea
well tolerated

Influenza antivirals

Antiviral medications

MoA: inhibit viral M2 proteins

AE/Warnings
neuropsychiatric effects

Indications: rarely used due to resistance Influenza A only!

Class: adamantanes

CMV antivirals

Names
amantadine
rimantadine

Name: Foscarnet (IV)

Name:
ganciclovir (IV)

Indications: IV for CMV retinitis (second line)

Indications: prevention/ treatment of CMV; IV treatment of choice (see text)

MOA:
inhibits DNA polymerase

AE/Warnings/Tox:
RENAL
HYPOcalcemia/electrolytes
anemia

MOA: nucleoside analog inhibits viral DNA synthesis

AE/Warnings:
myelosuppression esp. leukopenia
renal insufficiency

┃MIND MAP 9.3

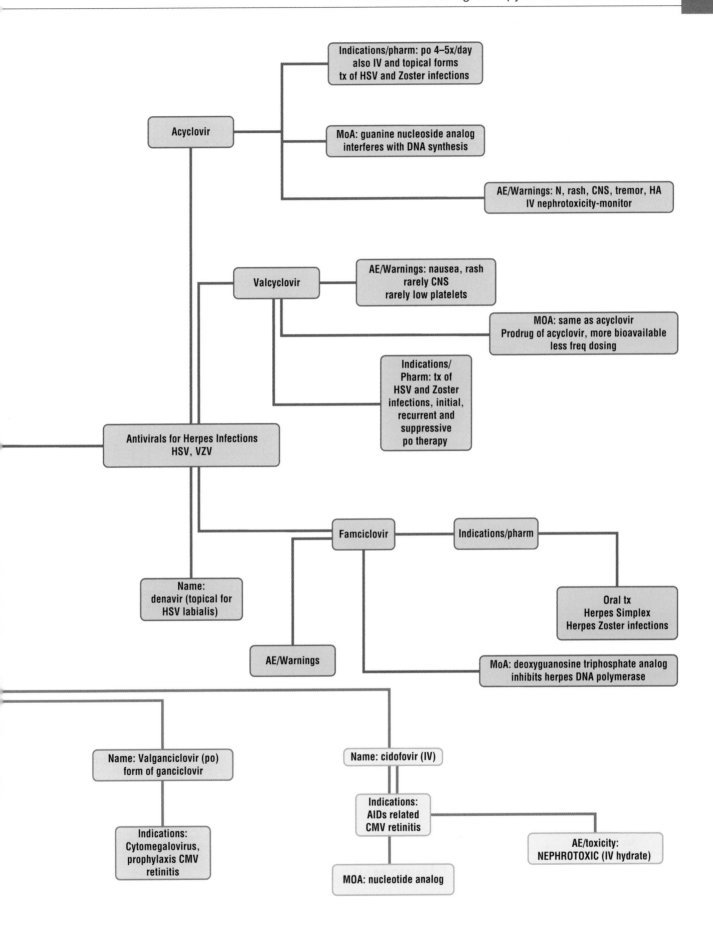

Acyclovir

Indications/pharm: po 4–5x/day
also IV and topical forms
tx of HSV and Zoster infections

MoA: guanine nucleoside analog
interferes with DNA synthesis

AE/Warnings: N, rash, CNS, tremor, HA
IV nephrotoxicity-monitor

Valcyclovir

AE/Warnings: nausea, rash
rarely CNS
rarely low platelets

MOA: same as acyclovir
Prodrug of acyclovir, more bioavailable
less freq dosing

Indications/
Pharm: tx of
HSV and Zoster
infections, initial,
recurrent and
suppressive
po therapy

**Antivirals for Herpes Infections
HSV, VZV**

Famciclovir   Indications/pharm

Name:
denavir (topical for
HSV labialis)

Oral tx
Herpes Simplex
Herpes Zoster infections

AE/Warnings

MoA: deoxyguanosine triphosphate analog
inhibits herpes DNA polymerase

Name: Valganciclovir (po)
form of ganciclovir

Name: cidofovir (IV)

Indications:
AIDs related
CMV retinitis

AE/toxicity:
NEPHROTOXIC (IV hydrate)

Indications:
Cytomegalovirus,
prophylaxis CMV
retinitis

MOA: nucleotide analog

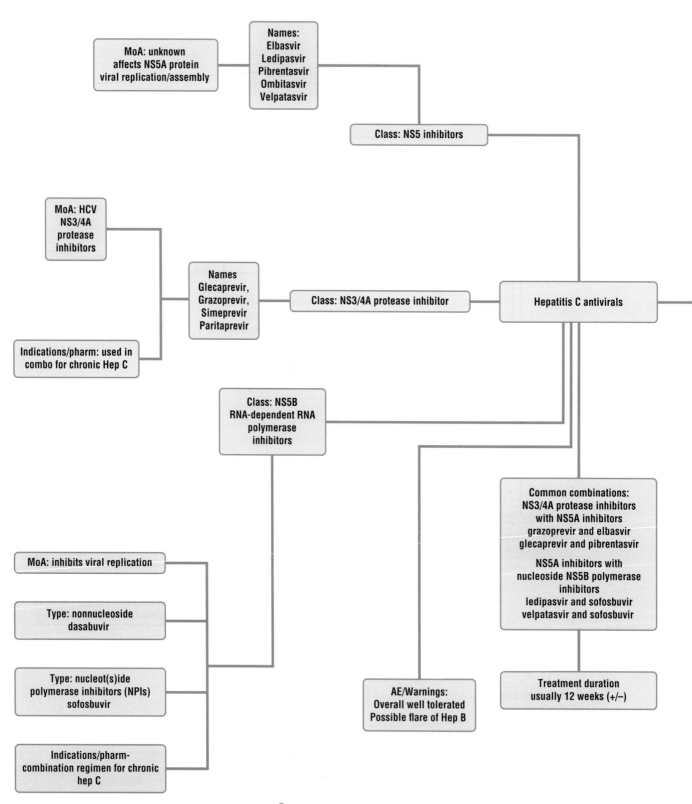

MIND MAP 9.4

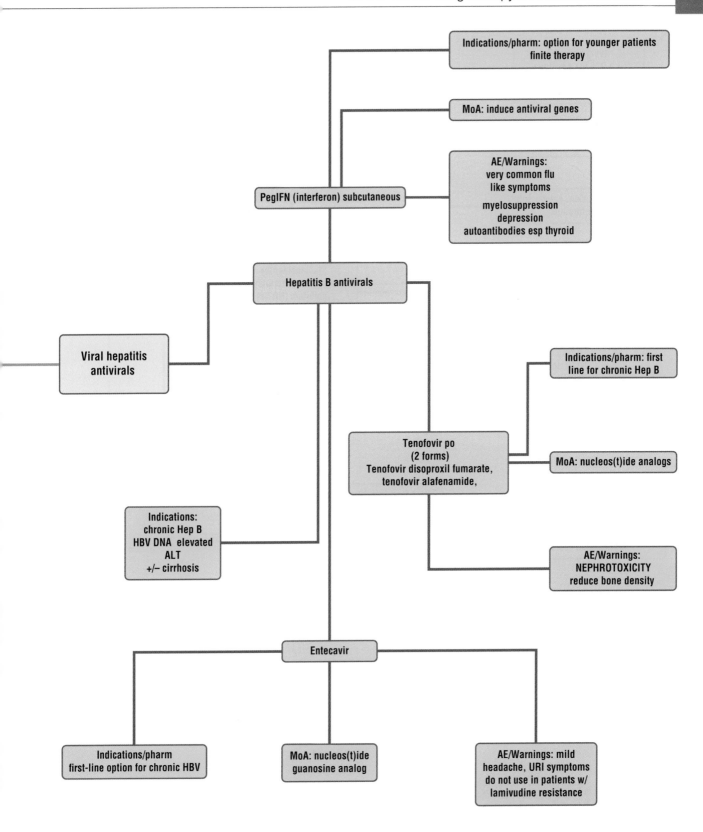

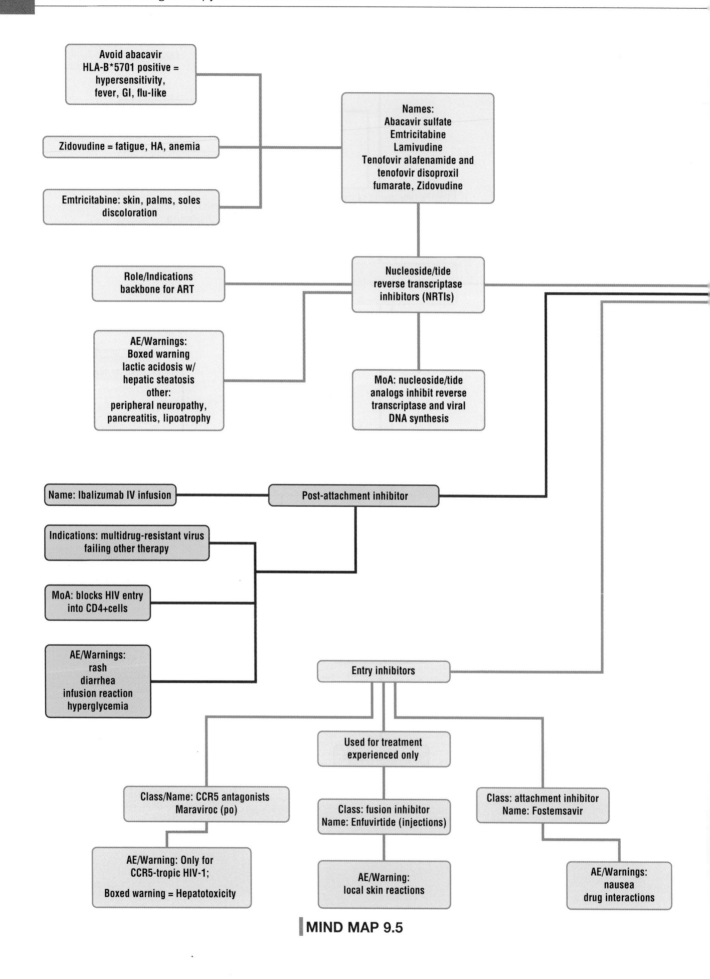

MIND MAP 9.5

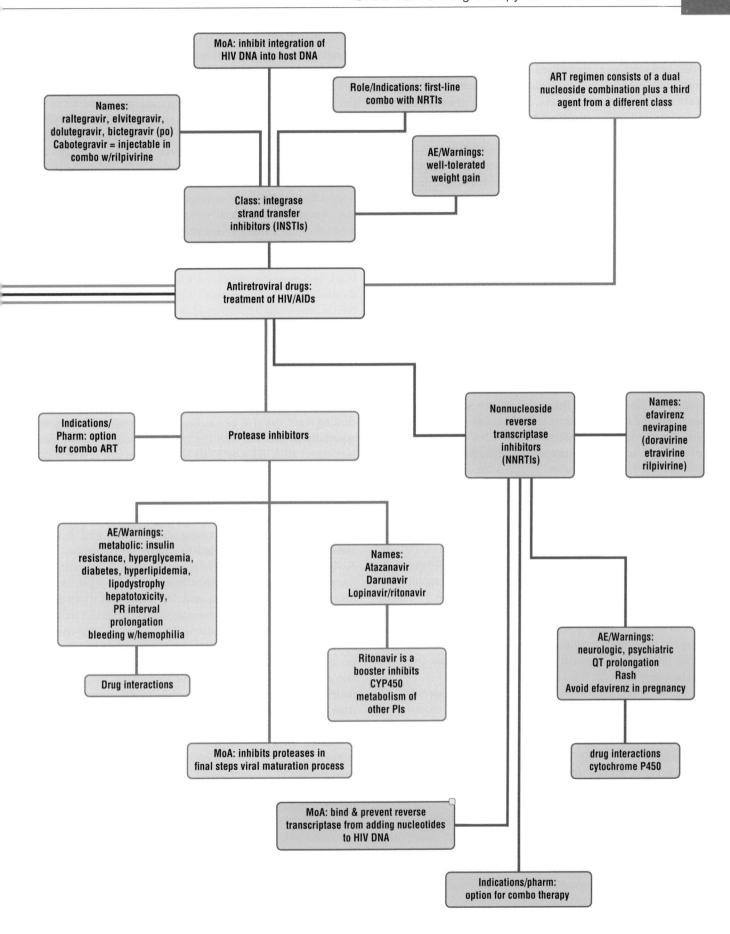

MoA: inhibit integration of HIV DNA into host DNA

Role/Indications: first-line combo with NRTIs

ART regimen consists of a dual nucleoside combination plus a third agent from a different class

Names: raltegravir, elvitegravir, dolutegravir, bictegravir (po) Cabotegravir = injectable in combo w/rilpivirine

AE/Warnings: well-tolerated weight gain

Class: integrase strand transfer inhibitors (INSTIs)

Antiretroviral drugs: treatment of HIV/AIDs

Indications/ Pharm: option for combo ART

Protease inhibitors

Nonnucleoside reverse transcriptase inhibitors (NNRTIs)

Names: efavirenz nevirapine (doravirine etravirine rilpivirine)

AE/Warnings: metabolic: insulin resistance, hyperglycemia, diabetes, hyperlipidemia, lipodystrophy hepatotoxicity, PR interval prolongation bleeding w/hemophilia

Names: Atazanavir Darunavir Lopinavir/ritonavir

AE/Warnings: neurologic, psychiatric QT prolongation Rash Avoid efavirenz in pregnancy

Drug interactions

Ritonavir is a booster inhibits CYP450 metabolism of other PIs

drug interactions cytochrome P450

MoA: inhibits proteases in final steps viral maturation process

MoA: bind & prevent reverse transcriptase from adding nucleotides to HIV DNA

Indications/pharm: option for combo therapy

antiretroviral therapy). Entecavir can be used in treatment-naïve patients without lamivudine-resistant hepatitis B infections, and tenofovir can be used in treatment naïve and those with prior exposure to lamivudine antiviral therapy. Antiviral treatment for chronic hepatitis C is long term, usually at least 4 to 5 years, and some patients with cirrhosis may require lifelong treatment.[19]

Hepatitis C virus is a leading cause of chronic hepatitis, which can cause cirrhosis and hepatocellular carcinoma. The **direct-acting antivirals (DAAs)** have changed the impact of chronic hepatitis C and most patients can be cured with a several-week course of oral therapy. DAAs target different steps in the life cycle of the hepatitis C virus. The four classes of DAAs are **nonstructural proteins 3/4A (NS3/4A) protease inhibitors (PIs), NS5B nucleoside polymerase inhibitors (NPIs), NS5B nonnucleoside polymerase inhibitors (NNPIs), and NS5A inhibitors.** The hepatitis C antiviral regimen depends on the genotype and patient factors such as the presence of cirrhosis and history of previous medication regimens.[20] **NS3/4A PIs** include glecaprevir, grazoprevir, simeprevir, paritaprevir, and voxilaprevir, which affect polypeptide processing and viral replication. The PIs are used in combination with NS5A inhibitors or NS5B RNA-dependent RNA polymerase inhibitors. **NS5A protein inhibitors** affect viral replication and assembly and include elbasvir, ledipasvir, ombitasvir, pibrentasvir, velpatasvir, and daclatasvir. **NS5B RNA-dependent RNA polymerase inhibitors** include sofosbuvir, which is a nucleotide inhibitor, and dasabuvir, which is an NNPI. DAAs are available in oral fixed dose combination regimens and are generally well tolerated. There have been reports of reactivation of hepatitis B virus infection in patients taking DAAs.

The virus that causes **COVID-19** is a coronavirus called *severe acute respiratory syndrome coronavirus 2 (SARS-CoV-2)*. Antiviral medications for SARS-CoV-2 (COVID-19) include nirmatrelvir-ritonavir (oral), remdesivir (IV), and molnupiravir (oral). Nirmatrelvir-ritonavir is a combination PI that is orally administered on an outpatient basis twice daily for 5 days in symptomatic patients who are at high risk for severe disease. Nirmatrelvir-ritonavir is well tolerated but does have drug interactions especially related to cytochrome P450 3A metabolism.[21]

Remdesivir is a nucleotide analog that is administered intravenously over 3 days in patients at high risk for progression to severe COVID-19. Bradycardia, which can be severe, is an associated adverse effect of remdesivir. Molnupiravir is a nucleoside analog that is orally administered twice daily for 5 days as an alternative therapy for COVID-19 high-risk patients. It is not authorized for children <18 years of age due to a potential risk of cartilage and bone toxicity.[22]

Anti–SARS-CoV-2 monoclonal antibodies include sotrovimab, casirivimab-imdevimab, and bamlanivimab-etesevimab, which are therapeutic options for high-risk symptomatic outpatients. They are administered as a single dose parenterally as soon as possible after symptom onset. Sotrovimab is also effective against the Omicron variant of SARS-CoV-2.[23] Infusion-related reactions can occur with monoclonal antibodies usually during or immediately after the infusion.

Antiretrovirals

Antiretroviral drugs or antiretroviral therapy (ART) are medications to prevent and treat HIV infection. HIV is an RNA retrovirus that infects and destroys $CD4^+$ T cells. HIV has distinctive life-cycle steps, which are therapeutic targets for six major classes of antiretroviral drugs. Treatment regimens for HIV combine antiretrovirals from more than one class. The nucleoside/nucleotide reverse transcriptase inhibitor (NRTI) class forms the backbone of ART and includes the following drugs: abacavir sulfate, a guanosine analog; emtricitabine and lamivudine, which are cytosine analogs; tenofovir alafenamide (TAF) and tenofovir disoproxil fumarate, which are adenosine-monophosphate analogs; and zidovudine, which is a thymidine analog. The NRTIs act by binding to reverse transcriptase and incorporating into DNA causing DNA chain termination. The **black box warning** associated with the NRTI class is **hepatic steatosis and lactic acidosis**, which is rare but can be fatal. NRTIs are usually administered in pairs and common regimens include emtricitabine, TAF, and tenofovir disoproxil fumarate. Emtricitabine can cause skin discoloration especially of the palms and soles. Tenofovir can cause nephrotoxicity and decrease bone density; TAF has less kidney and bone effects than tenofovir disoproxil fumarate but an increased risk of weight gain.[24,25]

Abacavir is associated with a **hypersensitivity reaction** including fever, malaise, headache, GI symptoms, and often rash especially in patients with the major histocompatibility complex class I allele **HLA-B*57:01** marker. Abacavir is contraindicated in persons who test positive for HLA-B*5701.

The **nonnucleoside reverse transcriptase inhibitors (NNRTIs)** include efavirenz and nevirapine and later-generation doravirine, etravirine, and rilpivirine. NNRTIs bind to a site on reverse transcriptase, decreasing its flexibility and reducing ability of nucleosides to bind to reverse transcriptase. Many NNRTIs are associated with drug interactions. Efavirenz commonly causes central nervous system effects such as vivid dreams, dizziness, insomnia, and depression and it can elevate liver enzymes. Efavirenz is associated with drug interactions as an inducer of certain cytochrome P450 enzymes. Etravirine can be used for drug-resistant HIV, and it is associated with a mild, usually self-limiting rash. Rilpivirine is available as a combination oral tablet and as an injectable formulation used in combination with the integrase strand inhibitor, cabotegravir. Rilpivirine can cause insomnia and depressive symptoms (like efavirenz) and it can prolong the QT interval.

The **PI class** includes the commonly used **atazanavir, darunavir**, the older, less commonly used lopinavir, and the rarely used indinavir, fosamprenavir, nelfinavir, saquinavir, and tipranavir. PIs interfere with the cleavage of polypeptides required for viral assembly leading to immature and noninfectious virions. The class-related adverse effects of the PIs include increased blood glucose and insulin resistance, dyslipidemia, lipodystrophy and maldistribution of fat, increased bleeding risk in hemophilia, elevated liver enzymes and bilirubin, and PR prolongation. Ritonavir is a PI that is added to other PIs as a pharmacologic "booster." Ritonavir is a potent inhibitor of the hepatic enzyme CYP (450) 3A4, which boosts the concentration by inhibiting the metabolism of coadministered drugs.

Ritonavir is associated with many drug interactions. **Cobicistat** is another cytochrome P-450 inhibitor administered with atazanavir or darunavir to **boost** the increase in systemic exposure. Atazanavir requires gastric acid for better absorption, and it has been associated with kidney stones. Darunavir is well tolerated, with nausea, diarrhea, and increased liver enzymes as the most common adverse effects.[26]

Integrase strand transfer inhibitors (INSTIs) include oral raltegravir, elvitegravir, dolutegravir, and bictegravir, and injectable long-acting INSTI (cabotegravir). Integrase inhibitors inhibit the integration of viral HIV DNA into the host cell genome, and they are considered a first-line component to ART regimens. INSTIs are well tolerated, and the most common adverse effects are weight gain and certain psychiatric effects, e.g., insomnia, dizziness, and depressed mood.[26] Cabotegravir is available orally and as an intramuscular monthly injection, and it is administered with the NNRTI rilpirivine. The most common adverse effect of injectable cabotegravir and rilpivirine is injection site discomfort.

ART entry and fusion inhibitors include the chemokine co-receptor 5 (CCR5) inhibitor maraviroc, the fusion inhibitor enfuvirtide, and fostemsavir, which is an attachment inhibitor. Maraviroc is an oral ART that blocks the entry of HIV into CD4$^+$ cells and it is only effective against CCR5-tropic R5-type HIV infections. Maraviroc is associated with hepatotoxicity, which may be related to a systemic allergic reaction. Enfuvirtide is an injectable fusion inhibitor that binds HIV glycoprotein 41 and prevents fusion to CD4$^+$ cells. Enfuvirtide is used for treatment-experienced patients, and it is commonly associated with injection site reactions, nausea, and diarrhea.[27] Fostemsavir is an oral attachment inhibitor that binds to HIV glycoprotein gp120 and prevents attachment to T cells. It is used for treating experienced patients only and can cause nausea, elevated liver enzymes, and prolonged QT interval.[28]

The ART fusion and attachment inhibitors and the **postattachment inhibitor, ibalizumab**, are used for treatment-experienced patients who are failing ART. Ibalizumab is a monoclonal antibody administered intravenously, which prevents HIV entry after it attaches to the T-cell membrane. Ibalizumab can cause infusion and hypersensitivity reactions, immune reconstitution inflammatory (IRIS) syndrome, nausea, diarrhea, leukopenia, and anemia. IRIS is a worsening of preexisting infections, especially an opportunistic infection, in patients with HIV and usually AIDS, which begins after initiating ART.[26]

ANTIFUNGALS

Antifungal medications are classified into four major categories: **azoles, allylamines, polyenes**, and **echinocandins.** Antifungal medications are illustrated in Mind Map 9.6. Ibrexafungerp is currently the only drug in a new class, the triterpenoids. Fungi are categorized morphologically as yeasts or molds. Superficial fungal infections affect the hair, nails, and mucous membranes and include dermatophytes (Epidermophyton, Microsporum, Trichophyton) and *Candida* species especially *Candida albicans.* Subcutaneous fungal infections may be caused by Sporothrix. Opportunistic fungi can cause serious systemic infections in immunocompromised patients; these include *Aspergillus, Mucor,*

Rhizopus, Pneumocystis, Cryptococcus, and *Candida.* **Endemic mycoses** that affect people who live in or travel to certain regions include Blastomyces (certain regions in midwestern, south-central, and southeastern states of the United States), Coccidioides or Valley Fever in the southwest, and certain parts of Mexico and Central America, and Histoplasma, which is found in soil with bird and bat droppings near Ohio and the Mississippi River valley regions of the Unites States.[29]

Certain characteristics of fungal morphology are therapeutic targets for antifungal drugs. The **polyenes nystatin** and **amphotericin B** bind to ergosterol in the fungal cell cytoplasmic membrane, which causes pore formation and leakage of cellular components. Nystatin is used for superficial mucocutaneous infections caused by *Candida* species only. Nystatin is available orally as a suspension for thrush and a tablet and topically as a powder or cream. Amphotericin B is an IV polyene antifungal agent used for serious systemic fungal infections caused by *Candida spp., Aspergillus spp.,* the Mucorales, all the endemic mycoses (blastomyces, coccidioides, *Histoplasma*), and most hyaline and brown-black molds.[30] Amphotericin is available for IV use in standard and in the more commonly used lipid-based formulations. Adverse effects of amphotericin are common and include acute infusion reactions with nausea, vomiting, chills, and rigors, thrombophlebitis, reversible **nephrotoxicity,** and electrolyte imbalances, especially hypokalemia and hypomagnesemia, which can require electrolyte repletion. Liposomal amphotericin has fewer adverse effects and less toxicity than other formulations.

Azole antifungals are commonly used antifungals that interrupt the fungal membrane by inhibiting the cytochrome P450-dependent enzyme lanosterol 14-alpha-demethylase and preventing the conversion of lanosterol to ergosterol. Lack of ergosterol causes fungal cell membrane damage, increased permeability, and fungal cell lysis. The azole antifungals are divided into the triazoles (fluconazole, itraconazole, voriconazole, posaconazole, and isavuconazole) and the imidazoles (ketoconazole). Indications for the systemic azole antifungals include systemic candidiasis, aspergillosis, and cryptococcal and endemic mycoses infections. Topical azole antifungals are used to treat dermatophyte infections (tinea), tinea versicolor caused by *Malassezia*, seborrheic dermatitis, and mucocutaneous candidiasis.

Azole antifungals are associated with adverse effects and drug interactions. GI side effects and hepatic function abnormalities are the most common adverse effects of azole antifungals. Voriconazole can cause abnormal vision, including photopsia or flashes of light, visual hallucinations, photosensitivity rash, and QT prolongation. Isavuconazole can also cause infusion reactions with chills, dyspnea, and hypotension. IV formulations of voriconazole and posaconazole contain cyclodextrin vehicle, sulphobutylether-beta-cyclodextrin, which can cause nephrotoxicity. Ketoconazole is associated with more GI and hepatic adverse effects, including potential severe liver injury (see ketoconazole product information).[31] **Most of the azoles are cytochrome P450 inhibitors and are associated with multiple drug interactions.**

The **allylamines** antifungals include terbinafine and naftidine. Allylamines inhibit ergosterol, which is the major sterol in the fungal cell membrane. Terbinafine is used orally and topically for

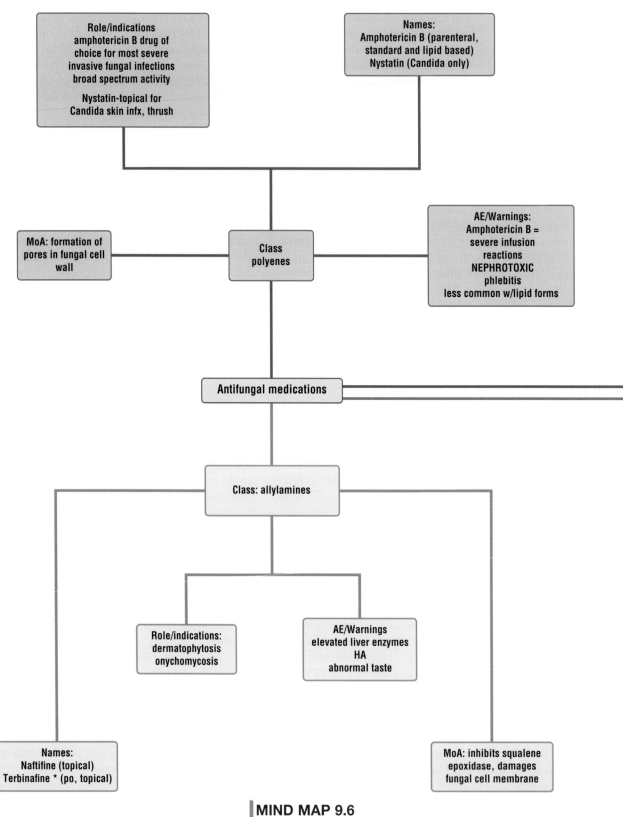

Role/indications
amphotericin B drug of choice for most severe invasive fungal infections broad spectrum activity

Nystatin-topical for Candida skin infx, thrush

Names:
Amphotericin B (parenteral, standard and lipid based) Nystatin (Candida only)

MoA: formation of pores in fungal cell wall

Class polyenes

AE/Warnings:
Amphotericin B = severe infusion reactions NEPHROTOXIC phlebitis less common w/lipid forms

Antifungal medications

Class: allylamines

Role/indications:
dermatophytosis onychomycosis

AE/Warnings
elevated liver enzymes HA abnormal taste

Names:
Naftifine (topical) Terbinafine * (po, topical)

MoA: inhibits squalene epoxidase, damages fungal cell membrane

MIND MAP 9.6

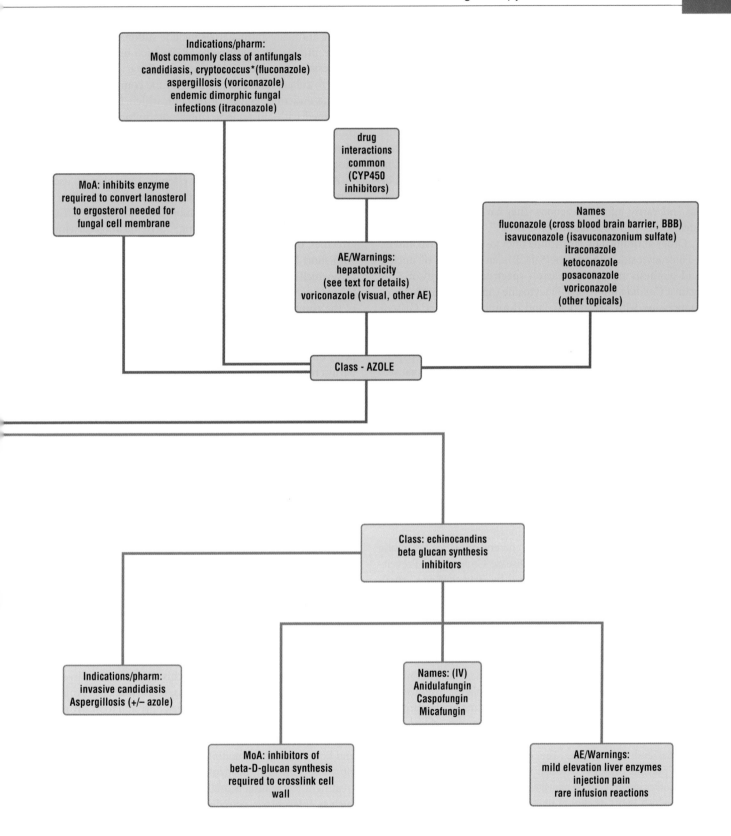

Indications/pharm:
Most commonly class of antifungals
candidiasis, cryptococcus*(fluconazole)
aspergillosis (voriconazole)
endemic dimorphic fungal
infections (itraconazole)

MoA: inhibits enzyme
required to convert lanosterol
to ergosterol needed for
fungal cell membrane

drug
interactions
common
(CYP450
inhibitors)

Names
fluconazole (cross blood brain barrier, BBB)
isavuconazole (isavuconazonium sulfate)
itraconazole
ketoconazole
posaconazole
voriconazole
(other topicals)

AE/Warnings:
hepatotoxicity
(see text for details)
voriconazole (visual, other AE)

Class - AZOLE

Class: echinocandins
beta glucan synthesis
inhibitors

Indications/pharm:
invasive candidiasis
Aspergillosis (+/− azole)

Names: (IV)
Anidulafungin
Caspofungin
Micafungin

MoA: inhibitors of
beta-D-glucan synthesis
required to crosslink cell
wall

AE/Warnings:
mild elevation liver enzymes
injection pain
rare infusion reactions

dermatophyte infections of the skin, hair, and nails. Naftidine is a topical cream or gel formulation. Terbinafine can cause headaches, dysgeusia, and increased hepatic transaminases.

The **echinocandin** class of antifungals include **caspofungin, micafungin,** and **anidulafungin**. Echinocandins inhibit beta-1,3-D-glucan synthase, which inhibits glucan synthesis, an essential component in the fungal cell wall. The echinocandins are administered intravenously and they are indicated for invasive candidiasis and in salvage regimens for invasive aspergillosis. Echinocandins are well tolerated, and the most common adverse effects include elevated hepatic transaminases, injection site pain, nausea, vomiting, and, rarely, infusion reactions. They have a lower risk of drug interactions than other antifungal classes.[32]

Other antifungal drugs include flucytosine and griseofulvin. 5-Fluorocytosine (flucytosine/5-FC) is an inhibitor of nucleic acid synthesis and it has a narrow spectrum of activity, mainly against *Candida* infections. Flucytosine can cause bone marrow suppression with neutropenia and thrombocytopenia. Griseofulvin affects microtubules and the formation of the mitotic spindle. It is used orally for dermatophyte infections, especially tinea capitis. Griseofulvin is available in different oral suspensions and tablet formulation; it is well tolerated with nausea, headache, and rashes as primary adverse effects.

ANTIPARASITIC DRUGS

Parasite infections are generally classified as protozoal or single-celled organisms or helminths multicellular parasites. Ectoparasites include blood-sucking arthropods mosquitoes and ticks, fleas, lice, and mites.

Malaria, a parasitic infection caused by *Plasmodium* protozoa, is a common cause of death globally and especially in sub-Saharan Africa.[33]

Parasitic infections classified as current priorities for public health action by the Centers for Disease Control and Prevention include Chagas disease (caused by *Trypanosoma cruzi*), cyclosporiasis (Cyclospora), cysticercosis (tapeworm *Taenia solium*), toxocariasis (*Toxocara* roundworms), toxoplasmosis (*Toxoplasma* parasite), and trichomoniasis (*Trichomonas vaginalis* sexually transmitted infection).[34]

Drugs for protozoal infections include several antimalarial drugs and other antiprotozoal medications. Antimalarials are grouped into quinoline derivatives, antifolates, artemisinins, and certain antimicrobials such as doxycycline or clindamycin.

The **antimalarial quinoline derivatives** are chloroquine, amodiaquine, quinine, quinidine, mefloquine, primaquine, lumefantrine, and halofantrine. The quinolines work by inhibiting heme polymerase activity, which increases cytotoxic hemoglobin metabolites in *Plasmodium* parasites. Chloroquine resistance is common, which limits its clinical utility. Quinine is the oldest antimalarial used for severe malaria and is available orally and parenterally. **Quinine and quinidine** have a narrow therapeutic index and they are associated with cardiotoxicity including QT prolongation, ventricular arrhythmias, and **cinchonism** (tinnitus, hearing loss, nausea, headaches, dizziness, and blurry vision). Primaquine and tafenoquine, which are used for prophylaxis and to prevent relapses, can cause hemolytic anemia in patients with glucose-6-phosphate dehydrogenase deficiency. Tafenaquine is used for primary malaria prophylaxis and prevention of relapse during travel to endemic areas.[35]

The antifolate antimalarials include sulfonamides, pyrimethamine, proguanil, and dapsone all of which interfere with folate synthesis required for DNA synthesis. There is significant resistance to sulfadoxine and pyrimethamine combinations in most malaria-endemic regions. Proguanil, which is an antifolate, is combined with atovaquone (interrupts mitochondrial electron transport), which is efficacious for the prevention and treatment of malaria. The most common adverse effects of atovaquone-proguanil are nausea, vomiting, diarrhea, and headache.[36]

Artemisinins are essential systemic antimalarials used in combination regimens; artemether-lumefantrine is the most widely adopted artemisinin combination therapy (ACT), followed by artesunate-amodiaquine.[37] Artemisinins (artemether, arteether, dihydroartemisinin, and artesunate) are rapid acting, with short half-lives, and they bind iron and generate free radicals, which damage and destroy malarial parasite proteins. Artemisimins are well tolerated and the most common adverse effects of the combination artemether and lumefantrine are headache, weakness, dizziness, nausea, anorexia, myalgia, and arthragia.[38]

Overall treatment and prophylaxis regimens for malaria depend on the type of *Plasmodium* and resistance patterns. Falciparum malaria is usually treated with ACT. Chemoprophylaxis in conjunction with mosquito avoidance measures should be used by travelers at risk of malarial infection. The chemoprophylaxis regimen should begin prior to travel and continue during the exposure period. Antimalarial prophylaxis regimens include atovaquone-proguanil, mefloquine, doxycycline, and tafenoquine and selection depends on patient factors and resistance patterns.[39]

Drugs for helminthic infections include drugs in the **benzimidazole** class, ivermectin, praziquantel, and pyrantel. The benzimidazoles, thiabendazole, mebendazole, albendazole, and triclabendazole inhibit polymerization of tubulin and affect microtubule formation. **Albendazole** is administered orally and is indicated for broad-spectrum helminthic infections including neurocysticercosis, echinococcosis, ascariasis, hookworm, and trichuriasis and is used for enterobiasis (pinworm) and giardiasis (*Giardia duodenalis*). Adverse effects of albendazole are mainly nausea, vomiting, and increased liver enzymes.[40] Mebendazole is orally available for intestinal nematode infections with abdominal pain and diarrhea as primary adverse effects. **Praziquantel** is orally available for schistosomiasis and liver fluke infections with headache, dizziness, and nausea as primary adverse effects. **Ivermectin** is available orally and topically and it is indicated for intestinal strongyloidiasis and onchocerciasis, as well as several intestinal nematodes and in some cases of scabies and lice (pediculosis capitis). Ivermectin is associated with pruritus and skin rash, particularly associated with onchocerciasis treatment.[41] **Pyrantel** is orally available for intestinal nematodes such as enterobiasis, roundworm, and hookworm.

REFERENCES

1. Asbel LE, Levison ME. Cephalosporins, carbapenems, and monobactams. *Infect Dis Clin North Am.* 2000;14:435.
2. Orbactiv (oritavancin) [prescribing information]. Lincolnshire, IL: Melinta Therapeutics LLC; 2022.
3. Tygacil (tigecycline) [prescribing information]. Philadelphia, PA: Wyeth Pharmaceuticals LLC, a subsidiary of Pfizer Inc; 2021.

4. Gilbert DN. Aminoglycosides. In: Mandell GL, Bennett JE, Dolin R, eds. *Principles and Practice of Infectious Diseases.* 6th ed. New York: Churchill Livingstone; 2005:328.

5. Wiener M, Guo Y, Patel G, Fries BC. Lactic acidosis after treatment with linezolid. *Infection.* 2007;35:278.

6. Zyvox (linezolid) [prescribing information]. New York, NY: Pharmacia and Upjohn; 2021.

7. Synercid (quinupristin dalfopristin) [prescribing information]. New York, NY: Pfizer Injectables; 2018.

8. Xenleta (lefamulin) [prescribing information]. Fort Washington, PA: Nabriva Therapeutics US Inc; 2021.

9. US Food and Drug Administration. *FDA Drug Safety Communication: FDA Updates Warnings for Oral and Injectable Fluoroquinolone Antibiotics Due to Disabling Side Effects.* Available at: https://www.fda.gov/drugs/drug-safety-and-availability/fda-drug-safety-communication-fda-updates-warnings-oral-and-injectable-fluoroquinolone-antibiotics.

10. Bactrim and Bactrim DS (sulfamethoxazole and trimethoprim) [prescribing information]. Cranbury, NJ: Sun Pharmaceutical Industries Inc; 2021.

11. Cubicin RF (daptomycin) [prescribing information]. Whitehouse Station, NJ: Merck Sharp & Dohme Corp; 2020.

12. Nation RL, Li J. Polymyxins. In: Grayson ML, Cosgrove SE, Crowe SM, et al., eds. *Kucers' The Use of Antibiotics: A Clinical Review of Antibacterial, Antifungal, Antiparasitic, and Antiviral Drugs.* 7th ed. Boca Raton: CRC Press; 2018:1420.

13. Nahid P, Dorman SE, Alipanah N, et al. Official American Thoracic Society/Centers for Disease Control and Prevention/Infectious Diseases Society of America clinical practice guidelines: treatment of drug-susceptible tuberculosis. *Clin Infect Dis.* 2016;63:e147.

14. Heo YA. Baloxavir: first global approval. *Drugs.* 2018;78:693.

15. Crumpacker CS. Ganciclovir. *N Engl J Med.* 1996;335:721.

16. Valcyte (valganciclovir) [prescribing information]. South San Francisco, CA: Genentech USA Inc; 2021.

17. Vistide (cidofovir) [prescribing information]. Foster City, CA: Gilead; 2010.

18. Pegasys (peginterferon alfa-2a) [prescribing information]. South San Francisco, CA: Genentech, Inc; 2021.

19. Terrault NA, Lok ASF, McMahon BJ, et al. Update on prevention, diagnosis, and treatment of chronic hepatitis B: AASLD 2018 hepatitis B guidance. *Hepatology.* 2018;67:1560.

20. AASLD-IDSA. *Recommendations for Testing, Managing, and Treating Hepatitis C.* Available at: http://www.hcvguidelines.org.

21. *Fact Sheet for Healthcare Providers: Emergency Use Authorization for Paxlovid (nirmatrelvir and ritonavir).* 2021. Available at: https://www.fda.gov/media/155050/download.

22. US Food and Drug Administration. *Fact Sheet for Healthcare Providers: Emergency Use Authorization for Molnupiravir.* 2021. Available at: https://www.merck.com/eua/molnupiravir-hcp-fact-sheet.pdf.

23. *Fact Sheet for Healthcare Providers Emergency Use Authorization (EUA) of Sotrovimab.* Available at: https://www.fda.gov/media/149534/download.

24. Tourret J, Deray G, Isnard-Bagnis C. Tenofovir effect on the kidneys of HIV-infected patients: a double-edged sword? *J Am Soc Nephrol.* 2013;24:1519.

25. Huang JS, Hughes MD, Riddler SA, et al. Bone mineral density effects of randomized regimen and nucleoside reverse transcriptase inhibitor selection from ACTG A5142. *HIV Clin Trials.* 2013;14:224.

26. Panel on Guidelines for the Prevention and Treatment of Opportunistic Infections in Adults and Adolescents with HIV. Guidelines for the Prevention and Treatment of Opportunistic Infections in Adults and Adolescents with HIV. National Institutes of Health, Centers for Disease Control and Prevention, HIV Medicine Association, and Infectious Diseases Society of America. Available at: https://clinicalinfo.hiv.gov/en/guidelines. Accessed August 2, 2022.

27. Fuzeon (enfuvirtide) [prescribing information]. South San Francisco, CA: Genentech USA, Inc; 2019.

28. Rukobia (fostemsavir) [prescribing information]. Research Triangle Park, NC: ViiV Healthcare; 2020.

29. Centers for Disease Control and Prevention, National Center for Emerging and Zoonotic Infectious Diseases (NCEZID), Division of Foodborne, Waterborne, and Environmental Diseases (DFWED). *Types of Fungal Diseases.* June 16, 2023. Available at:. https://www.cdc.gov/fungal/diseases/index.html.

30. McEvoy G, ed. *American Hospital Formulary Service — 1996.* Bethesda, MD: American Society of Health System Pharmacists; 1996.

31. Ketoconazole [product monograph]. Weston, Ontario, Canada: Apotex Inc; April 2021.

32. Cancidas (caspofungin acetate) for injection, for intravenous use, prescribing information. Available at: https://www.accessdata.fda.gov/drugsatfda_docs/label/2018/021227s038lbl.pdf.

33. World Health Organization. World malaria report. 2021. Available at:. https://www.who.int/teams/global-malaria-programme/reports/world-malaria-report-2021.

34. Global Health, Division of Parasitic Diseases and Malaria. *Parasites - Parasitic Infections in the United States.* August 22, 2023. Available at:. https://www.cdc.gov/parasites/npi/index.html.

35. Arakoda (tafenoquine) [prescribing information]. Washington, DC: Sixty Degrees Pharmaceuticals LLC; 2021.

36. Malarone (atovaquone and proguanil hydrochloride) tablets and pediatric tablets [prescribing information]. Research Triangle Park, NC: GlaxoSmithKline; April 2022.

37. Ramharter M, Kurth F, Schreier AC, et al. Fixed-dose pyronaridine-artesunate combination for treatment of uncomplicated falciparum malaria in pediatric patients in Gabon. *J Infect Dis.* 2008;198:911.

38. Coartem (artemether and lumefantrine) [prescribing information]. East Hanover, NJ: Novartis Pharmaceuticals Corp; 2019.

39. Chen LH, Keystone JS. New strategies for the prevention of malaria in travelers. *Infect Dis Clin North Am.* 2005; 19:185.

40. Albendazole tablets [prescribing information]. North Wales, PA: Teva Pharmaceuticals USA, Inc; 2020.

41. Ivermectin tablets [prescribing information]. Parsippany, NJ: Edenbridge Pharmaceuticals, LLC; 2014.

CHAPTER 10

Antineoplastic Drugs

DRUG THERAPY FOR CANCER (ANTINEOPLASTIC DRUGS)

Cancer is the leading cause of death in the United States. The most common types of cancer are breast, prostate, lung, and colorectal.[1] Cancer is defined as neoplastic transformation of human cells leading to abnormal differentiation, proliferation, and survival, and the ability to invade other tissues and spread or metastasize to distant sites. Anticancer or chemotherapy drugs are one of the modalities to treat cancer, and in most cases, drug combination regimens are used. Many cancer drugs kill actively dividing cells, which include both malignant cancer cells and rapidly dividing normal cells, especially in the gastrointestinal epithelium, mucous membranes, hair follicles, and bone marrow. Anticancer drugs kill a constant fraction of tumor cells, which is usually expressed in exponential log units.

Many classes of cancer chemotherapy drugs target different phases of the cell division cycle and are called *cell cycle–specific* (*CCS*) drugs. Cell cycle–nonspecific (CCNS) drugs can kill cancer cells in the resting (G_0) or cycling (G_1-M) phases. The cell division cycle or cell cycle is listed in Table 10.1.

Anticancer drugs are divided into broad classes: alkylating agents, platinum analogs, antimetabolites and antifolates, antimicrotubules/antimitotics such as vinca alkaloids and taxanes, camptothecins, antitumor antibiotics, and miscellaneous anticancer drugs such as antibodies, hormonal therapies, and targeted signal transduction inhibitors. See Mind Map 10.1 for a broad overview of classic cancer chemotherapy drugs.

Chemotherapeutic drugs are associated with a range of short- and long-term toxicities. The most common toxicities include myelosuppression, nausea and vomiting related to emetogenic drugs, gastrointestinal effects including mucositis, and skin and hair effects including rashes, hyperpigmentation, and alopecia. Drug-specific toxicities and, if relevant, management include:

- Hemorrhagic cystitis induced by cyclophosphamide managed with hydration and **mesna**, which neutralizes the toxic drug metabolites
- Neuropathy due to vinca alkaloids and taxanes

- Cardiotoxicity including heart failure from anthracyclines, especially doxorubicin, which can be prevented or treated with the iron-chelating agent **dexrazoxane**
- Nephrotoxicity and neurotoxicity with cisplatin; pre- and posttreatment hydration and replacement of electrolytes
- Pulmonary toxicity/fibrosis with bleomycin.

There are several management strategies for the common chemotherapy-associated toxicities. Myelosuppression can be treated with granulocyte colony-stimulating factor, e.g., filgrastim, to prevent or treat granulocytopenia. Neutropenia and other cancer-related conditions can increase the risk for serious infections including febrile neutropenia and systemic fungal infections. Prophylactic and empiric antimicrobials (and antifungals) can reduce and treat serious infectious complications of cancer. Anemia may be treated with erythropoiesis-stimulating agents, e.g., epoetin alfa or darbepoetin alfa for palliative treatment, or red cell transfusions. Chemotherapy-induced nausea and vomiting (CINV) is associated with highly emetogenic regimens such as cisplatin, cyclophosphamide, carmustine, and many other chemo drugs. CINV is prevented and treated with a combination of antiemetic drugs including 5HT3 antagonist, dexamethasone, neurokinin-1 receptor (NK-1) antagonist, and olanzapine.[2] Mucositis causing painful mouth sores can be treated with good oral hygiene, ice chips, and topical mouthwashes with lidocaine. Palifermin is an intravenous (IV) recombinant keratinocyte growth factor that can prevent oral mucositis in certain high-risk patients.[3] Diarrhea can be managed with loperamide and, if severe, IV hydration and electrolytes. **Leucovorin** is folinic acid that is used to "rescue" normal mucosal and bone marrow cells from damage by **methotrexate**.[4]

There is a long and growing list of miscellaneous cancer drugs that do not fit into the traditional classes. Some of these medications include tyrosine kinase inhibitors (TKIs), inhibitor of the 26S proteasome, epidermal growth factor receptor (EGFR) inhibitors, and vascular endothelial growth factor (VEGF) inhibitors. TKIs such as imatinib, dasatinib, nilotinib, and bosutinib are mainly useful for chronic myelogenous leukemia and

TABLE 10.1 Cell Cycle

State	Phase	Abbreviation	Description
Resting	Gap 0	G_0	The cell is quiescent has left the cycle and stopped dividing
Interphase	Gap 1	G_1	Cell growth and synthesis of requirements for deoxyribonucleic acid (DNA) synthesis
	Synthesis	S	DNA replication
	Gap 2	G_2	Growth and synthesis and elements needed for mitosis
Cell division	Mitosis	M	Cell division occurs

have various acute and chronic adverse effects and potential drug interactions related to CYP450 3A4 metabolism.

EGFRs are tyrosine kinase receptors that can be overexpressed in many solid tumors and can affect cellular growth and proliferation, invasion and metastasis, and angiogenesis.[5] Anti-EGFR monoclonal antibodies such as cetuximab and panitumumab inhibit the EGFR signaling pathway and are used for colorectal cancers. Erlotinib and afatinib are small molecule inhibitors of the tyrosine kinase domain of EGFR and are used for metastatic non-small cell lung cancer. Human epidermal growth factor receptor (HER2) or HER2/neu is a member of the EGFR, and it is overexpressed with certain types of breast cancer. Trastuzumab and pertuzumab are monoclonal antibodies that target HER2 and are used for HER2-positive breast cancer. Cardiotoxicity is associated with trastuzumab and pertuzumab.[6]

VEGF is a growth factor associated with angiogenesis. Tumors require blood vessels for growth, and drugs that inhibit VEGF binding to its VEGF tyrosine kinase receptors or interfere with VEGF signaling are useful for many solid tumors. Bevacizumab is a monoclonal antibody that targets VEGF and interferes with binding to its receptors. Sorafenib, sunitinib, and pazopanib are small molecules that inhibit multiple VEGF receptor tyrosine kinases. Hypertension is a common adverse effect of the anti-VEGF medications.

Hormonal therapies are useful for several types of cancers including prostate and breast cancers. Luteinizing hormone–releasing agonists (leuprolide, goserelin) and the luteinizing hormone–releasing hormone antagonist degarelix are used for metastatic prostate cancer. Enzalutamide and apalutamide bind to androgen receptor and function as androgen receptor inhibitors for certain metastatic prostate cancer. Aromatase inhibitors (anastrozole, letrozole, exemestane) are used for certain types of postmenopausal breast cancer. Tamoxifen is a selective estrogen receptor modulator used for premenopausal breast cancer risk reduction and breast cancer treatment. Fulvestrant is an estrogen receptor antagonist for hormone-receptor–positive advanced breast cancer.[7]

REFERENCES

1. *SEER*Explorer: An interactive website for SEER cancer statistics* [Internet]. Surveillance Research Program, National Cancer Institute; 2023 Apr 19. [updated: 2023 Jun 8; cited 2023 Sep 14]. Available at: https://seer.cancer.gov/statistics-network/explorer/.
2. Hesketh PJ, Bohlke K, Lyman GH, et al. Antiemetics: American Society of Clinical Oncology focused guideline update. *J Clin Oncol.* 2016;34:381.
3. Hong CHL, Gueiros LA, Fulton JS, et al. Systematic review of basic oral care for the management of oral mucositis in cancer patients and clinical practice guidelines. *Support Care Cancer.* 2019;27:3949.
4. Ackland SP, Schilsky RL. High-dose methotrexate: a critical reappraisal. *J Clin Oncol.* 1987;5:2017.
5. Hynes NE, Lane HA. ERBB receptors and cancer: the complexity of targeted inhibitors. *Nat Rev Cancer.* 2005;5:341-354.
6. *<800> Hazardous Drugs—Handling in Healthcare Settings.* United States Pharmacopeia and National Formulary (USP 43-NF 38). Rockville, MD: United States Pharmacopeia Convention; 2020:74-92.
7. NCCN Guidelines Treatment by Cancer Type. *NCCN Guidelines.* 2022. Available at: https://www.nccn.org/. Accessed April 6, 2022.

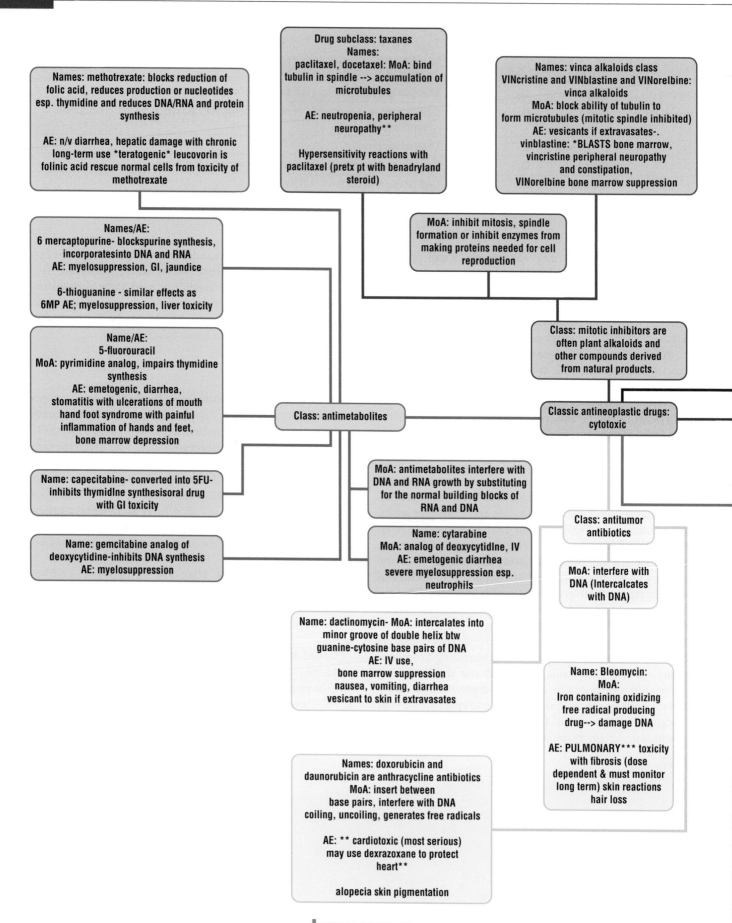

Names: methotrexate: blocks reduction of folic acid, reduces production or nucleotides esp. thymidine and reduces DNA/RNA and protein synthesis

AE: n/v diarrhea, hepatic damage with chronic long-term use *teratogenic* leucovorin is folinic acid rescue normal cells from toxicity of methotrexate

Drug subclass: taxanes
Names:
paclitaxel, docetaxel: MoA: bind tubulin in spindle --> accumulation of microtubules

AE: neutropenia, peripheral neuropathy**

Hypersensitivity reactions with paclitaxel (pretx pt with benadryland steroid)

Names: vinca alkaloids class
VINcristine and VINblastine and VINorelbine: vinca alkaloids
MoA: block ability of tubulin to form microtubules (mitotic spindle inhibited)
AE: vesicants if extravasates-.
vinblastine: *BLASTS bone marrow,
vincristine peripheral neuropathy and constipation,
VINorelbine bone marrow suppression

MoA: inhibit mitosis, spindle formation or inhibit enzymes from making proteins needed for cell reproduction

Names/AE:
6 mercaptopurine- blockspurine synthesis, incorporatesinto DNA and RNA
AE: myelosuppression, GI, jaundice

6-thioguanine - similar effects as 6MP AE; myelosuppression, liver toxicity

Class: mitotic inhibitors are often plant alkaloids and other compounds derived from natural products.

Name/AE:
5-fluorouracil
MoA: pyrimidine analog, impairs thymidine synthesis
AE: emetogenic, diarrhea, stomatitis with ulcerations of mouth hand foot syndrome with painful inflammation of hands and feet, bone marrow depression

Class: antimetabolites

Classic antineoplastic drugs: cytotoxic

Name: capecitabine- converted into 5FU-inhibits thymidIne synthesisoral drug with GI toxicity

MoA: antimetabolites interfere with DNA and RNA growth by substituting for the normal building blocks of RNA and DNA

Class: antitumor antibiotics

Name: gemcitabine analog of deoxycytidine-inhibits DNA synthesis
AE: myelosuppression

Name: cytarabine
MoA: analog of deoxycytidIne, IV
AE: emetogenic diarrhea severe myelosuppression esp. neutrophils

MoA: interfere with DNA (Intercalcates with DNA)

Name: dactinomycin- MoA: intercalates into minor groove of double helix btw guanine-cytosine base pairs of DNA
AE: IV use,
bone marrow suppression nausea, vomiting, diarrhea vesicant to skin if extravasates

Name: Bleomycin:
MoA:
Iron containing oxidizing free radical producing drug--> damage DNA

AE: PULMONARY*** toxicity with fibrosis (dose dependent & must monitor long term) skin reactions hair loss

Names: doxorubicin and daunorubicin are anthracycline antibiotics
MoA: insert between base pairs, interfere with DNA coiling, uncoiling, generates free radicals

AE: ** cardiotoxic (most serious) may use dexrazoxane to protect heart**

alopecia skin pigmentation

MIND MAP 10.1

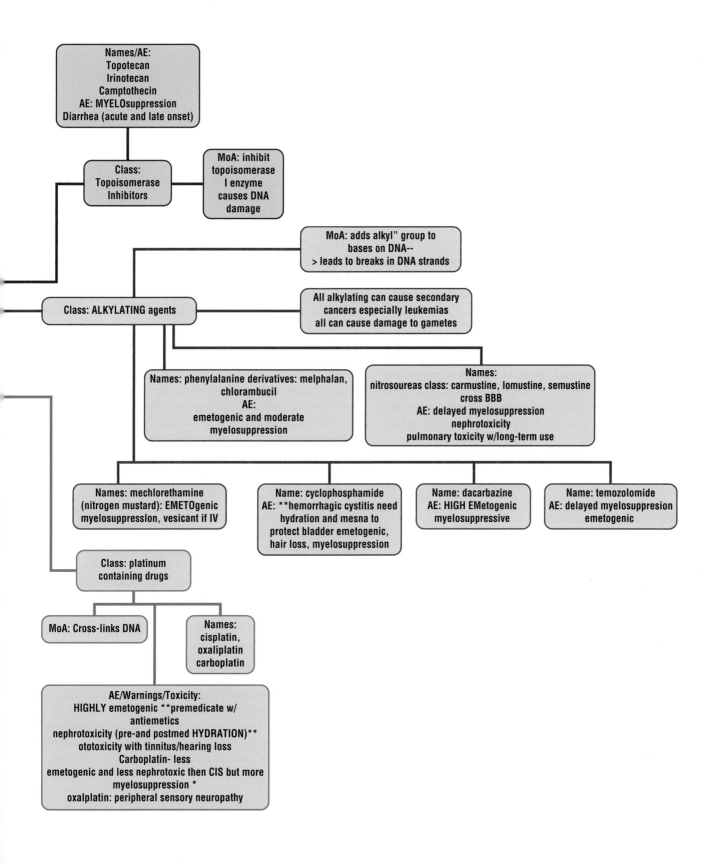

Names/AE:
Topotecan
Irinotecan
Camptothecin
AE: MYELOsuppression
Diarrhea (acute and late onset)

Class:
Topoisomerase
Inhibitors

MoA: inhibit
topoisomerase
I enzyme
causes DNA
damage

MoA: adds alkyl" group to
bases on DNA--
> leads to breaks in DNA strands

Class: ALKYLATING agents

All alkylating can cause secondary
cancers especially leukemias
all can cause damage to gametes

Names: phenylalanine derivatives: melphalan,
chlorambucil
AE:
emetogenic and moderate
myelosuppression

Names:
nitrosoureas class: carmustine, lomustine, semustine
cross BBB
AE: delayed myelosuppression
nephrotoxicity
pulmonary toxicity w/long-term use

Names: mechlorethamine
(nitrogen mustard): EMETOgenic
myelosuppresslon, vesicant if IV

Name: cyclophosphamide
AE: **hemorrhagic cystitis need
hydration and mesna to
protect bladder emetogenic,
hair loss, myelosuppression

Name: dacarbazine
AE: HIGH EMetogenic
myelosuppressive

Name: temozolomide
AE: delayed myelosuppresion
emetogenic

Class: platinum
containing drugs

MoA: Cross-links DNA

Names:
cisplatin,
oxaliplatin
carboplatin

AE/Warnings/Toxicity:
HIGHLY emetogenic **premedicate w/
antiemetics
nephrotoxicity (pre-and postmed HYDRATION)**
ototoxicity with tinnitus/hearing loss
Carboplatin- less
emetogenic and less nephrotoxic then CIS but more
myelosuppression *
oxalplatin: peripheral sensory neuropathy

CHAPTER 11

Drug Therapy for Select Eye Diseases

SECTION 1: Pharmacology of Ocular Therapeutics

This chapter reviews the basic pharmacology of ocular medications and therapeutics of select common eye diseases. Mind Map 11.1 illustrates the classes of commonly used eye medications.

GLAUCOMA

Glaucoma is a group of common chronic eye disorders associated with elevated intraocular pressure (IOP) and progressive damage to the optic nerve. Medications for glaucoma lower IOP, which reduces progressive damage to the optic nerve and visual field loss. Topical ocular medications for glaucoma are classified by the type and mechanism of action.

Medications that increase aqueous outflow include:
- prostaglandin analogs: Xalatan (latanoprost), Travatan Z (travoprost), Zioptan (tafluprost), and Lumigan (bimatoprost)
- alpha-adrenergic agonists
- cholinergic agonists
- rho kinase inhibitors.

Medications that decrease aqueous production include:
- alpha-adrenergic agonists
- beta-blockers
- carbonic anhydrase inhibitors.

Prostaglandin analogs include Xalatan (latanoprost), Travatan Z (travoprost), Zioptan (tafluprost), and Lumigan (bimatoprost), and they are generally the preferred initial therapy for open-angle glaucoma. The primary adverse effects of the topical ocular prostaglandin analogs are hyperemia, eye irritation, hyperpigmentation in iris and around eyelids, and increase in the number and length of eyelashes.[1]

Topical beta-blockers (betaxolol, carteolol, levobunolol, metipranolol, and timolol) are also alternative first-line options for open-angle glaucoma. They are well tolerated with ocular redness and burning sensation in the eyes in some patients.[2] Beta-blockers should not be used in patients with bradycardia, heart block, heart failure, asthma, or obstructive airway disease.

Other drugs for open-angle glaucoma include alpha-2 adrenergic agonists (apraclonidine, brimonidine), topical carbonic anhydrase inhibitors (dorzolamide, brinzolamide), cholinergic agonists (pilocarpine, carbachol), and netarsudil. Alpha-2 agonists have more ocular side effects such as allergic conjunctivitis, redness, and itching, and they may have some systemic effects such as reduced blood pressure and drowsiness. Topical carbonic anhydrase inhibitors may be less effective than other glaucoma medications, and their adverse effects are local eye irritation and redness.[2] Cholinergic agonists are not commonly used and are associated with significant ocular effects such as ciliary spasm with headache, myopia, fixed small pupils, and potential cataracts and iris-lens adhesions with long-term use. Netarsudil is a topical rho kinase inhibitor that increases aqueous humor outflow, and its role is unclear. Ocular adverse effects of netarsudil include eye redness, pain with application, and corneal deposits.

Age-related macular degeneration (AMD) is a common cause of severe visual loss and blindness. Exudative or wet AMD can be treated with intravitreous injections of a vascular endothelial growth factor (VEGF) inhibitor (e.g., bevacizumab, ranibizumab, and aflibercept). Dosing intervals for VEGF inhibitors vary from every month to less frequent intervals. Adverse effects include eye pain, floaters, punctate keratitis, endophthalmitis, and uveitis.[3]

Dry eye disease (DED) is associated with chronic eye irritation and dryness, which affects the tear film of the eye surface. First-line medical treatment includes artificial tears in liquid, gel, or ointment ocular formulations, which are available without a prescription. Prescription topical ocular medications for DED include the immunosuppressant cyclosporine in emulsion or solution, or the topical eye drop formulation lifitegrast, which is an integrin inhibitor. Topical cyclosporine emulsion or solution is well tolerated, and topical lifitegrast can cause a bad taste, eye irritation, and eye discomfort.[4]

CONJUNCTIVITIS

Conjunctivitis is a common condition causing a "red eye" and defined as inflammation of the conjunctivae. The conjunctiva is a mucous membrane that lines the inside surface of the eyelid and covers the front surface of the eye up to the limbus. Causes of conjunctivitis include infection (bacterial, viral, fungal, or parasitic), allergies, and toxins.

Allergic conjunctivitis is a common type of conjunctivitis caused by a type I immunoglobulin E-mediated hypersensitivity to airborne allergens that cause eye inflammation. Common causes include seasonal allergens, such as tree, grass, and weed pollens, and perennial allergens, e.g., dust mites, mold, or pet dander. Clinical manifestations include bilateral red, itchy eyes with watery discharge. Treatment of allergic conjunctivitis is avoidance and reduction of environmental exposure when possible and several classes of topical eye drops. The topical ophthalmic classes of medications for allergic conjunctivitis include **antihistamine/vasoconstrictor combination products, antihistamines with mast cell-stabilizing properties, mast cell stabilizers**, and, for severe cases, **topical glucocorticoids**.

Patients with seasonal or perennial allergic conjunctivitis often take topical antihistamine with mast cell–stabilizing properties such as olopatadine ([Patanol, Pataday, Pazeo]), alcaftadine ([Lastacaft]), bepotastine ([Bepreve]), azelastine hydrochloride ([Optivar]), cetirizine ([Zerviate]), epinastine ([Elestat]), and ketotifen fumarate ([Ketotifen]). Topical antihistamine/vasoconstrictor drugs include naphazoline and pheniramine and are useful for short-term treatment. Mast cell-stabilizing topical ophthalmic agents such as cromolyn sodium ([Opticrom]), nedocromil (Alocril [Alocril]), lodoxamide tromethamine (Alomide [brand name]), and pemirolast (Alamast [brand name]) have a delayed onset of effect of 5 to 14 days.[5] Topical ophthalmic glucocorticosteroids are reserved for short-term use in severe cases due to the risk of secondary infections, increased IOP, and cataracts. Some topical ophthalmic steroids include loteprednol ([Lotemax] and [Alrex]), rimexolone ([Vexol]), prednisolone ([Pred Mild]), fluorometholone (FML), and medrysone (HMS).

Infectious conjunctivitis is often caused by viruses, e.g., adenovirus, or bacteria, usually *Staphylococcus aureus, Streptococcus pneumoniae, Haemophilus influenzae*, and *Moraxella catarrhalis*.[6]

Bacterial conjunctivitis is treated with topical ophthalmic solutions or ointments applied for 5 to 7 days. Examples of topical ophthalmic antibiotics include erythromycin ophthalmic ointment or trimethoprim-polymyxin B drops. Patients who wear contact lenses are at a higher risk for Gram-negative infections including *Pseudomonas*. Topical fluoroquinolones such as ofloxacin or ciprofloxacin eye drops should be used in patients who wear contact lenses and develop bacterial conjunctivitis. Hyperacute bacterial conjunctivitis due to *Neisseria* is treated with systemic therapy, e.g., intramuscular ceftriaxone plus oral doxycycline or azithromycin for presumptive *Chlamydia trachomatis* infection.[7]

Serious viral infections of the eye can be caused by herpes simplex and varicella zoster virus. Herpes simplex keratitis (corneal infection and inflammation) is a serious condition requiring urgent treatment. Topical antiviral therapy and oral antiherpes antivirals are effective. Oral antiviral therapy with either acyclovir, valcyclovir, or famciclovir, or topical acyclovir 3% ophthalmic ointment are recommended. Herpes zoster ophthalmicus can cause acute keratitis and should be treated promptly with oral antiviral therapy (acyclovir, valacyclovir, or famciclovir).[8]

REFERENCES

1. Orme M, Collins S, Dakin H, et al. Mixed treatment comparison and meta-regression of the efficacy and safety of prostaglandin analogues and comparators for primary open-angle glaucoma and ocular hypertension. *Curr Med Res Opin.* 2010;26:511.
2. Vass C, Hirn C, Sycha T, et al. Medical interventions for primary open angle glaucoma and ocular hypertension. *Cochrane Database Syst Rev.* 2007:CD003167.
3. Holz FG, Tadayoni R, Beatty S, et al. Multi-country real-life experience of anti-vascular endothelial growth factor therapy for wet age-related macular degeneration. *Br J Ophthalmol.* 2015;99:220.
4. Donnenfeld ED, Karpecki PM, Majmudar PA, et al. Safety of Lifitegrast ophthalmic solution 5.0% in patients with dry eye disease: a 1-year, multicenter, randomized, placebo-controlled study. *Cornea.* 2016;35:741.
5. Nizami RM. Treatment of ragweed allergic conjunctivitis with 2% cromolyn solution in unit doses. *Ann Allergy.* 1981;47:5.
6. Friedlaender MH. A review of the causes and treatment of bacterial and allergic conjunctivitis. *Clin Ther.* 1995;17:800.
7. Haimovici R, Roussel TJ. Treatment of gonococcal conjunctivitis with single-dose intramuscular ceftriaxone. *Am J Ophthalmol.* 1989;107:511.
8. Pavan-Langston D. Herpes zoster ophthalmicus. *Neurology.* 1995;45:S50.

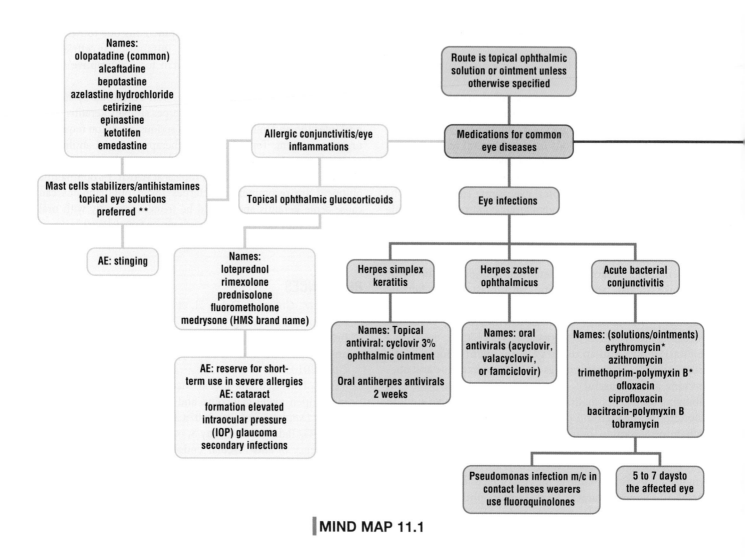

MIND MAP 11.1

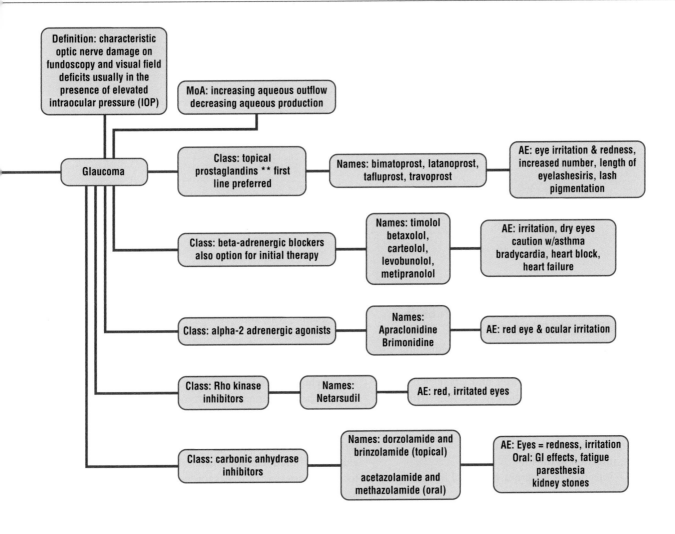

Definition: characteristic optic nerve damage on fundoscopy and visual field deficits usually in the presence of elevated intraocular pressure (IOP)

MoA: increasing aqueous outflow decreasing aqueous production

Glaucoma

Class: topical prostaglandins ** first line preferred

Names: bimatoprost, latanoprost, tafluprost, travoprost

AE: eye irritation & redness, increased number, length of eyelashesiris, lash pigmentation

Class: beta-adrenergic blockers also option for initial therapy

Names: timolol betaxolol, carteolol, levobunolol, metipranolol

AE: irritation, dry eyes caution w/asthma bradycardia, heart block, heart failure

Class: alpha-2 adrenergic agonists

Names: Apraclonidine Brimonidine

AE: red eye & ocular irritation

Class: Rho kinase inhibitors

Names: Netarsudil

AE: red, irritated eyes

Class: carbonic anhydrase inhibitors

Names: dorzolamide and brinzolamide (topical)

acetazolamide and methazolamide (oral)

AE: Eyes = redness, irritation
Oral: GI effects, fatigue paresthesia
kidney stones

CHAPTER 12

Dermatologic Pharmacology

PHARMACOLOGIC TREATMENT OF COMMON SKIN INFECTIONS AND INFESTATIONS (MIND MAP 12.1)

Fungal skin infections are common worldwide and include infections of the skin, hair, and nails. The dermatophyte fungi specifically *Trichophyton, Microsporum,* and *Epidermophyton* are the main causes of fungal infection of the skin, hair, and nails. Dermatophytes cause tinea infections of the skin, which are described as:

- Tinea corporis – infection of body surfaces
- Tinea pedis – infection of the foot
- Tinea cruris – infection of the groin, proximal inner thighs, or buttocks
- Tinea faciei – infection of the face
- Tinea manuum – infection of the hand.

Dermatophyte infections of the hair include tinea capitis (infection of scalp hair), tinea barbae (infection of beard hair), and tinea unguium (infections of the nails, also called dermatophyte onychomycosis). Most patients with dermatophyte infections of the skin can be treated with topical antifungal therapy. Systemic antifungal treatment is the treatment of choice for tinea capitis. Oral antifungal is the gold standard for onychomycosis because it results in high cure rates; however, topical antifungal therapy may be indicated for certain patients.

Topical antifungal therapy for dermatophyte infections of the skin is applied to affected areas once to twice daily for 1 to 3 weeks. Topical antifungals include the following antifungal classes: azoles, allylamines, butenafine, ciclopirox, and tolnaftate; these classes are summarized in Mind Map 12.1 and detailed in Chapter 9. Tinea pedis is treated with similar topical antifungal medications, which are generally applied once or twice daily and continued for 4 weeks.

Tinea capitis is more common in children and presents as patchy, scaling, pruritic areas of hair loss. Oral antifungal therapy is indicated for 6 to 12 weeks depending on the response to therapy. Oral griseofulvin is an antifungal available in two formulations: microsize (tablets or suspension) and ultramicrosize (tablets). Oral griseofulvin should be taken with fatty food to enhance absorption. It is well tolerated with some adverse effects such as nausea, headache, and skin rashes. Monitoring of liver function tests and a complete blood count may be required if griseofulvin therapy is prolonged for more than 8 weeks.[1] Oral terbinafine is an alternative antifungal for children over the age of 4 years.

Onychomycosis is a chronic fungal nail infection often involving the toenails and is most common in adults. Onychomycosis is most commonly treated with oral antifungals. Toenail infections generally require longer duration of treatment. Oral terbinafine is an allylamine antifungal and is the treatment of choice. Terbinafine is administered orally once daily for 6 weeks for fingernails and 12 weeks for toenail infections. Oral itraconazole, an azole derivative, is a second-line option for onychomycosis, which can be administered daily for 6 to 12 weeks or twice daily for 1 week per month for 2 to 3 months. Adverse effects and drug interactions of antifungals are discussed in Chapter 9. Topical antifungals and topical urea cream or ointment may be options for mild disease and in certain patients who cannot take oral antifungals. Topical antifungals for onychomycosis include efinaconazole, tavaborole, and ciclopirox, which are applied to the nail, nail bed, and undersurface of the nail plate once daily for up to 48 weeks. These topical antifungals are well tolerated with minor skin irritation and ingrown toenails as potential side effects.

Other superficial fungal skin infections include tinea versicolor caused by *Malassezia* species and cutaneous and mucosal candidiasis most caused by *Candida albicans.* Tinea versicolor (i.e., pityriasis versicolor) is a common superficial fungal infection caused by *Malassezia* yeasts. Lesions are typically hypo- or hyperpigmented macules and patches generally found on the upper trunk and proximal upper extremities. The first-line treatment options for tinea versicolor include topical antifungals, i.e., terbinafine, ciclopirox olamine, or ketoconazole for 1 to 2 weeks. Selenium sulfide shampoo as one 10-minute application daily for 1 week or zinc pyrithione shampoo as one 5-minute application daily for 2 weeks are also first-line treatment options. Pigmentation changes can persist for months after successful treatment. Oral antifungals such as itraconazole or fluconazole are reserved for severe and widespread or recalcitrant disease.[2]

CUTANEOUS AND MUCOSAL CANDIDIASIS

Oropharyngeal candidiasis, or thrush, is common in infants and in patients with predisposing factors, including use of antibiotics or certain chemotherapy drugs, certain immunodeficiencies including AIDS, radiation therapy to the head and neck, and in patients with other cellular immune deficiency states. Thrush is treated with topical antifungals for 7 to 14 days with either clotrimazole troches (one 10-mg troche dissolved in the mouth five times daily) or miconazole mucoadhesive buccal tablets (50 mg once daily applied to the mucosal surface over the canine fossa). Nystatin swish and swallow (400,000–600,000 units four times daily) is another option but may be less palatable and less effective.

Vulvovaginitis caused by *Candida* can be treated with topical antifungals or oral antifungals. Topical antifungals include clotrimazole, terconazole, miconazole, and tioconazole applied as creams with applicators or vaginal suppositories once daily for 1 to 7 days depending on the product. Adverse effects of topical therapy include local burning or irritation. Oral antifungals are generally preferred by patients and can be administered as one dose for uncomplicated infections. Single-dose fluconazole (150 mg) taken once orally is the preferred option and it is well tolerated. An alternative option for vulvovaginal candidiasis is ibrexafungerp, 150 mg two tablets orally twice in 1 day. It is available for patients with intolerance or allergies to azole antifungals. It is well tolerated with some nausea, diarrhea, and abdominal discomfort.

Cutaneous candidiasis often causes infections in moist areas of deeper skin folds referred to as intertrigo. It is more common with certain risk factors including obesity, immobility, poor hygiene, hyperhidrosis, and in patients with diabetes mellitus and human immunodeficiency virus (HIV)/AIDS infection. *Candida* can also exacerbate diaper dermatitis. Diaper dermatitis caused by *Candida* usually involves the skin folds, with red plaques and satellite papules and pustules; it is usually present for more than 3 days. It is treated with topical antifungal cream applied to the diaper area two to three times per day until the rash resolves. Intertrigo is managed by keeping the affected areas as clean, aerated, and dry as possible and applying drying powders and barrier creams with zinc oxide. Topical antifungal creams, e.g., clotrimazole, miconazole, and econazole, or allylamine antifungals naftifine and terbinafine are applied once to twice daily for 2 to 4 weeks.

BACTERIAL SKIN AND SOFT TISSUE INFECTIONS

Bacterial skin and soft tissue infections are variable and often caused by coagulase-positive *Staphylococcus aureus* or group A beta-hemolytic *Streptococci*. Impetigo is a common, contagious superficial skin infection usually caused by *S. aureus* and sometimes group A beta-hemolytic *Streptococci*. It is treated with a topical antibacterial agent usually either mupirocin ointment three times a day for 3 to 5 days or retapamulin ointment twice a day for 5 days. Folliculitis is an infection of the hair follicle often caused by *S. aureus* (methicillin-sensitive *S. aureus*, methicillin-resistant *S. aureus* [MRSA]) and sometimes *Pseudomonas aeruginosa* (hot tub) and certain fungi, e.g., *Candida*. Limited folliculitis can be managed with benzoyl peroxide cleansers

and topical mupirocin three times daily for 5 to 7 days. Extensive skin involvement or recurrence after topical therapy may require oral antibacterials (see Chapter 9), usually cephalexin or dicloxacillin for 7 to 10 days. MRSA skin infections require one of the following oral antibiotics: doxycycline (100 mg twice daily), trimethoprim-sulfamethoxazole (one to two double-strength tablets twice daily), or clindamycin (450 mg three times per day).

Deeper bacterial skin infections include furuncles, carbuncles, and abscesses. Furuncles are deep inflammatory nodules that arise from hair follicles, and carbuncles are interconnecting abscesses that coalesce into a mass that drains pus. An abscess is a collection of pus in the deeper dermis and subcutaneous tissues. Treatment of furuncles, carbuncles, and abscesses is incision and drainage with possible systemic antibiotics for large abscesses, immunocompromised patients, and systemic signs of serious infection.

Cellulitis, erysipelas, and skin abscesses are the most common skin and soft tissue infections. Cellulitis is a spreading infection of the deeper dermis and subcutaneous tissues often initiated by a portal of entry into the skin. Erysipelas is nonpurulent and involves the upper dermis and superficial lymphatics. The most common causes of cellulitis and erysipelas are beta-hemolytic *Streptococci* followed by *S. aureus*. Skin abscesses are mostly caused by *S. aureus* either methicillin-susceptible or MRSA. Patients with mild nonpurulent cellulitis or erysipelas can be treated with oral antibiotics as follows:

- No risk factors for MRSA
  - erysipelas: oral penicillin or amoxicillin
  - cellulitis: oral cephalexin.
- Risk factors for MRSA (including recent hospitalization, residence in a long-term care facility, recent surgery, hemodialysis, and HIV infection)
  - trimethoprim-sulfamethoxazole
  - clindamycin
  - doxycycline.

The duration of therapy is 5 to 14 days depending on clinical response. Patients should have symptomatic improvement within 24 to 48 hours of antibiotic treatment. Patients with mild purulent cellulitis can be treated with either clindamycin, trimethoprim-sulfamethoxazole, or doxycycline.[3]

Patients with cellulitis or erysipelas who have systemic signs of toxicity, rapid progression of clinical findings, or indwelling medical devices require parenteral antibiotics. Erysipelas is usually treated with either parenteral cefazolin or ceftriaxone. For patients with severe purulent cellulitis and patients with severe cellulitis and risk factors for MRSA, parenteral antibiotics options include either vancomycin or daptomycin.

SKIN INFESTATIONS: SCABIES AND PEDICULOSIS

Scabies is a highly contagious skin infestation caused by the mite *Sarcoptes scabiei* var. *hominis,* primarily transmitted through personal contact. Scabies infestation often causes intensely pruritic lesions, small papules with excoriations, and burrows typically in the interdigital web spaces, axillae and skin folds, genitalia, waist, posterior upper thighs, and areolae. Treatment is a topical scabicide applied to entire body left on for 8 to 14 hours, then washed off and repeated in 7 days. The most

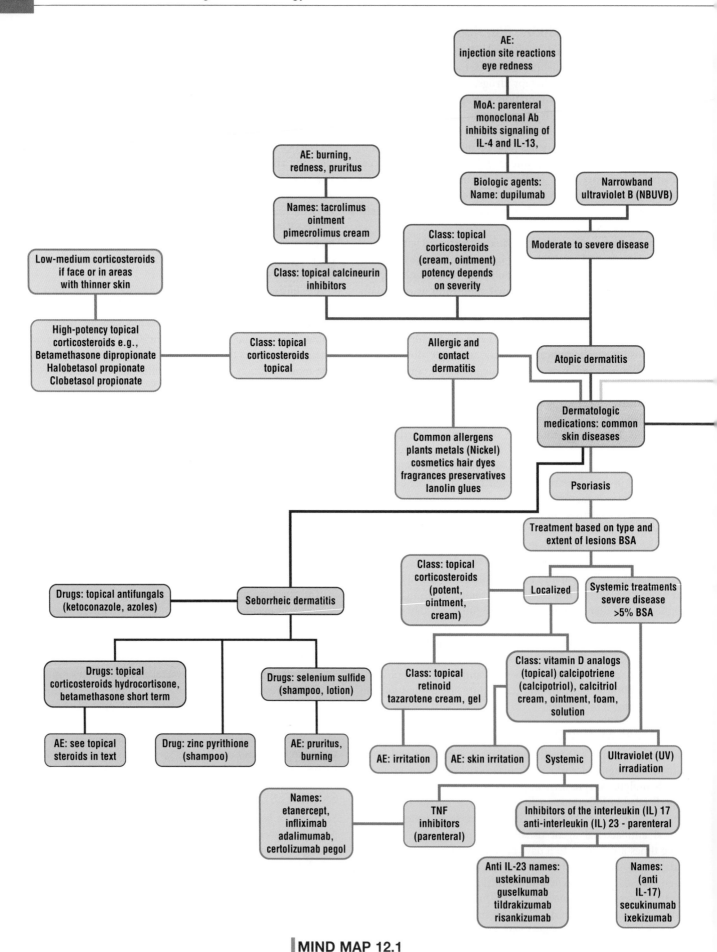

MIND MAP 12.1

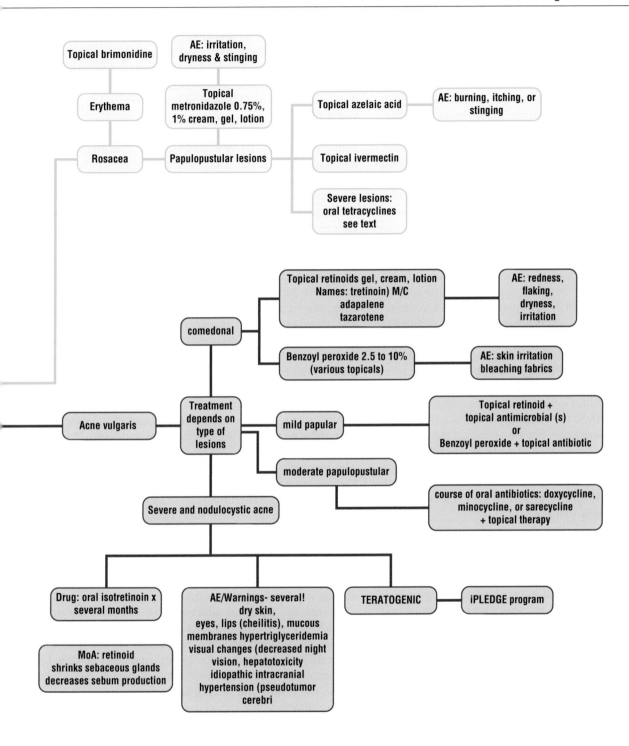

common treatment is permethrin 5% cream. Oral ivermectin 200 mcg/kg as a single dose followed by a repeat dose after 1 to 2 weeks is an alternative to topical therapy. Another topical option is spinosad 0.9% topical suspension for the treatment of scabies in children 4 years of age and older. Severe pruritus can be treated with oral antihistamines (nonsedating antihistamines [e.g., loratadine] during the day and sedating [e.g., diphenhydramine] at night). Close contacts should be treated, and items in contact should be placed in a plastic bag for at least 3 days or washed and dried on high heat settings.

Pediculosis is an infestation by lice, specifically (1) *Pediculus humanus capitis*, the head louse; (2) *Pediculus humanus humanus*, the body or clothing louse; and (3) *Phthirus pubis*, the pubic louse. Clinical manifestations of head lice are mainly scalp pruritus with visualization of live lice and nits, which are egg capsules stuck to hair shafts close to the scalp. Topical pediculicides are the treatment of choice for lice, and a second application should be repeated in approximately 1 week. A common first-line over-the-counter option is permethrin (1%) applied to saturate dry hair and left on for 10 minutes before rinsing, and repeated 9 days later. Other effective topical pediculicides include malathion, benzyl alcohol, spinosad, and topical ivermectin, which are available by prescription. Body lice can be managed by discarding or heat washing and drying infested clothing and bedding. Permethrin 5% cream applied to the entire body is also effective. Crab or pubic lice are sexually transmitted but can affect other hair-bearing areas of the body. The treatment of choice is permethrin 1% cream rinse or pyrethrins 0.33% with piperonyl butoxide 4% applied to all affected areas and left on for 10 minutes, then repeated in 9 to 10 days. The topical pediculicides are generally well tolerated.

Acne vulgaris is a common skin condition of the pilosebaceous unit that varies in types of lesions and severity. Mild acne has limited skin involvement, and the lesions are generally comedones or small scattered papules. Moderate to severe acne involves more surface area with an increased number of prominent papular and pustular lesions. Severe acne is extensive and involves face, chest, and back with diffuse inflammatory papules, pustules, nodules, and sometimes cysts, which can cause permanent scarring. Treatment of acne depends on the severity, clinical presentation, and patient preferences. Topical therapy includes topical retinoids, benzoyl peroxide, azelaic acid, salicylic acid, and topical antibiotics. Tretinoin, adapalene, tazarotene, and trifarotene are topical retinoids that decrease follicular plugging and prevent comedone formation. The topical retinoids (gels, creams, lotions) are very effective for comedonal acne and are applied once at night to dry skin. Skin irritation, dryness, and flaking of the skin are common and may be decreased by applying every other day. Topical retinoids, especially tazarotene, should not be used in pregnancy. Adapalene is available over the counter and may be a less irritating topical retinoid. Benzoyl peroxide is antibacterial and comedolytic, and it is available in a range of concentrations and in foams, cleansers, gels, lotions, creams, pads, masks, and washes. Benzoyl peroxide is also formulated in combination with topical antibiotics, which reduces antibiotic resistance. Skin irritation is the most common adverse effect of benzoyl peroxide. Salicylic acid in various concentra-

tions and vehicles is an over-the-counter keratolytic, which may be used as an alternative to benzoyl peroxide.[4] Topical clindamycin and, less commonly, topical erythromycin are antibiotics that are available alone or in combination with benzoyl peroxide for papulopustular acne. Azelaic acid is an alternative cream or gel that is also effective for rosacea.

Moderate to severe acne requires topical and systemic treatment, which includes oral antibiotics, oral isotretinoin, and hormonal agents. Oral antibiotics include one of the tetracyclines, preferably doxycycline, or alternatively minocycline or sarecycline, administered daily for 3 to 4 months. Antibiotics are discussed in Chapter 9. Tetracyclines are contraindicated in children 8 years of age and younger and in pregnant women. Postmenarchal females have the option of combined oral contraceptives or spironolactone hormonal therapies. US Food and Drug Administration–approved combined oral contraceptives for acne include ethinyl estradiol 20/30/35 mcg/norethindrone 1 mg, ethinyl estradiol 35 mcg/norgestimate 180/215/250 mcg, and ethinyl estradiol 20 mcg/drospirenone 3 mg.[5] The risks and benefits of the oral contraceptives are detailed in Chapter 6. Spironolactone is an antiandrogen oral medication that can be used in women who cannot tolerate or do not want combined oral contraceptive therapy. The pharmacology of spironolactone is detailed in Chapter 3.

Oral isotretinoin is a retinoid that is most effective for severe acne and acne resistant to other therapies in patients 12 years of age and older. It is typically dosed daily based on weight and administered for 20 to 24 weeks. Isotretinoin is teratogenic and has multiple adverse effects, which require monitoring. Patients who are taking isotretinoin are required to enroll in the iPLEDGE computer-based Risk Evaluation and Mitigation Strategy risk management program.[6] All patients must commit to using two forms of highly effective contraceptive 1 month before, during, and 1 month after treatment. Female patients using isotretinoin must have regular pregnancy testing before, during, and 1 month after treatment.

Isotretinoin has many adverse effects including mucocutaneous, eye, psychiatric, and other effects. Dry eyes, cheilitis, and xerosis are common, in addition to initial worsening of acne, epistaxis, and photosensitivity. Topical emollients on skin, lips, and intranasal saline can help with mucocutaneous adverse effects. Depression and suicidal behavior may be increased and require close monitoring and patient/caregiver education.[7,8]

Dyslipidemia, especially hypertriglyceridemia, can occur during isotretinoin therapy, and generally, it can be managed by lifestyle modification. Liver enzymes may increase during therapy but generally normalize within a few weeks of treatment.[9] Most patients have long-term improvement of acne lesions after one course of isotretinoin.[10]

ALLERGIC CONTACT DERMATITIS

Allergic contact dermatitis is common, and it is generally treated by identification of allergen, avoidance, and topical antiinflammatory medications. Plants, nickel from jewelry, coins, and zippers, and certain ingredients from cosmetics are common allergens. Topical corticosteroid creams are applied once to twice daily for 2 to 4 weeks or until symptoms resolve.[11]

Atopic dermatitis (AD) is a common chronic familial skin disease often presenting in childhood and associated with other allergic conditions such as asthma and allergic rhinitis. Skin lesions in AD are pruritic and vary in appearance and distribution. Acute AD is papulovesicular with weeping areas; chronic forms may have excoriated, lichenified, and scaly areas of dry skin. Infants often have AD on the face, scalp, and extensor surfaces of arms and legs; older children and adults have rashes in flexural folds of the extremities. Superficial viral and bacterial infections are more common in patients with AD.

AD management includes various classes of medications and general patient education about skin hydration, avoidance of aggravating factors, and controlling pruritus. Thick creams or ointments should be applied immediately to entire body after bathing every day. High heat, low humidity, stress, and excessive bathing can worsen AD. Pruritus can be managed with skin hydration, certain topical medications, and, if severe, oral antihistamines (see Chapter 5). Mild to moderate AD is managed with topical low- to medium-potency corticosteroid cream or ointment once to twice daily. Acute flares are treated with short-term super high- or high-potency topical corticosteroids for 2 weeks and tapered to lower potency until lesions resolve. Topical corticosteroid preparations are classified by potency group, according to the United States system, into groups 1 to 7; group 1 is the most potent, group 7 is the least potent. Table 12.1 illustrates some examples of topical corticosteroids in each potency group.

The adverse effects of topical corticosteroids are discussed in Chapter 6 and include skin thinning, striae, telangiectasias, folliculitis, hypertrichosis, and contact dermatitis. Facial, intertriginous, and genital areas are at higher risk for adverse effects and increased systemic absorption.

Alternative topical therapies for AD include nonsteroidal immunosuppressant calcineurin inhibitors and crisaborole 2%

ointment. The topical calcineurin inhibitors tacrolimus ointment and pimecrolimus cream are applied twice a day and are second-line therapeutic options in adults and children over the age of 2 years. There is a boxed warning on the prescribing information for these medications due to a small increase in the risk of lymphoma. Crisaborole is a topical phosphodiesterase 4 (PDE4) inhibitor ointment that is modestly effective and well tolerated for mild AD.[12]

Patients with moderate to severe AD may require narrow-band ultraviolet B phototherapy or systemic immunomodulatory therapy. Dupilumab is a subcutaneous interleukin-4 receptor antagonist approved for certain types of severe asthma and AD. It is administered by subcutaneous injection into the thigh or lower abdomen or upper arm every other week. The most common adverse events were injection site reaction, facial redness, and eye irritation. Severe refractory cases of AD may require systemic immunosuppressive therapy such as oral cyclosporine or oral methotrexate.

PSORIASIS

Psoriasis is a common chronic skin condition characterized by recurring papules and plaques with silvery scale, which can involve limited or extensive areas of the body. Chronic plaque psoriasis is the most common type, and other types include guttate, pustular, and erythrodermic psoriasis. Chronic plaque psoriasis most commonly affects the elbows, knees, sacral gluteal region, scalp, and palm/soles.

There are several topical and systemic medications for psoriasis. Patients with limited disease can be treated with topical therapies including topical corticosteroids, emollients, vitamin D analogs (e.g., calcipotriene and calcitriol), tar, and topical retinoids (tazarotene). Topical corticosteroid creams or ointments are generally first-line treatments for psoriasis on the skin. Potent steroid solutions or foams, shampoos, or sprays can be used on scalp and external ear lesions. A combination of topical corticosteroids and one of the vitamin D analogs, e.g., calcipotriene or calcitriol, is also used for localized psoriasis. Topical vitamin D analogs, calcipotriene or calcitriol, are applied twice daily to affected skin avoiding the face. Topical vitamin D analogs are well tolerated, and most common adverse effects are skin irritation, tingling, and burning; rarely hypercalcemia can occur in high doses.[13]

Tazarotene is a topical retinoid cream/gel that can be used as an adjunctive to topical corticosteroids once daily. It can be used on facial psoriatic lesions but can cause skin irritation, peeling, and burning. It is contraindicated in women who are or may become pregnant.

Other adjunctive topical therapies include topical tacrolimus 0.1% and pimecrolimus 1%, anthralin cream or shampoo, and topical tar preparations. Anthralin and tar preparations are older modalities with antiinflammatory effects. Both anthralin and coal tar preparations can stain clothing and skin; anthralin causes skin irritation, and coal tar has an unpleasant odor. Coal tar shampoo may be helpful for scalp lesions when applied and left on the scalp for 5 to 10 minutes.

Moderate to severe psoriasis involves more than 5% body surface area and requires treatment with either phototherapy

TABLE 12.1	Topical Corticosteroids	
Potency Group	**Names**
Super-high potency (group 1)	Betamethasone dipropionate, augmented Clobetasol propionate
High potency (group 2)	Betamethasone dipropionate Halcinonide
High potency (group 3)	Betamethasone valerate Diflorasone diacetate
Medium potency (group 4)	Fluticasone propionate Hydrocortisone valerate
Lower-mid potency (group 5)	Triamcinolone acetonide Hydrocortisone valerate
Low potency (group 6)	Desonide Triamcinolone acetonide (0.025%)
Least potent (group 7)	Hydrocortisone base (<2%)

(narrow ultraviolet B or psoralen plus ultraviolet A [PUVA]) or systemic therapies. PUVA is photochemotherapy that combines oral methoxsalen or direct application of psoralen to the skin prior to UVA treatment. Systemic therapies for moderate to severe psoriasis (Mind Map 12.2) include acitretin, methotrexate, cyclosporine, apremilast, or biologic immune-modifying agents. Methotrexate is a folic acid antagonist used for psoriasis, psoriatic arthritis, and nail disease for several decades. Methotrexate can be administered orally or subcutaneously (usually once weekly), and it is administered with folic acid 1 mg orally every day. Methotrexate is associated with significant adverse effects, which are reviewed in Chapter 5. Folic acid can protect against some of the adverse effects. Methotrexate is contraindicated in many conditions including pregnancy, breastfeeding, liver disease, immunodeficiency, and bone marrow cytopenias. Cyclosporine is an immunosuppressant drug that is administered orally and is rapidly effective for severe psoriasis. It is associated

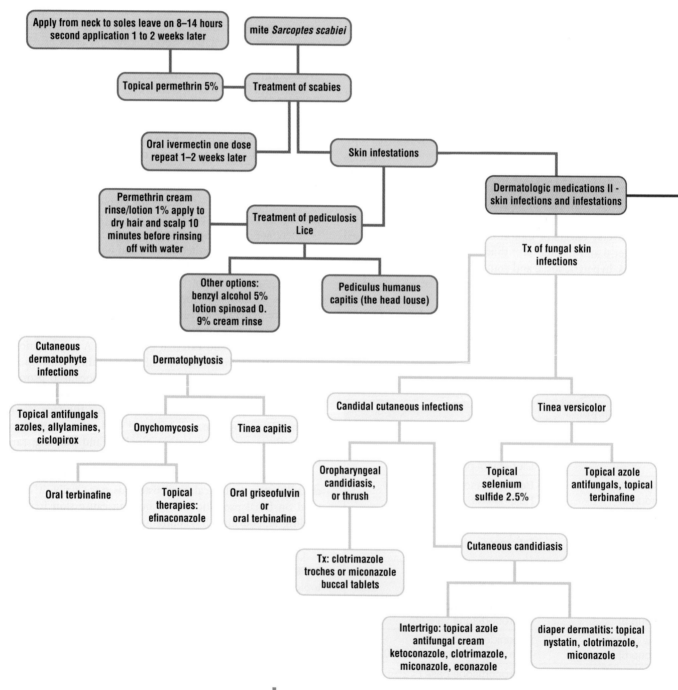

MIND MAP 12.2

with significant adverse effects including renal toxicity, hypertension, and increased risk for infections. Apremilast is an oral medication for moderate to severe psoriasis, or psoriatic arthritis that inhibits PDE4 and regulates inflammatory mediators. It may have lower efficacy than biologic agents and it is associated with short-term diarrhea and weight loss.[14]

Biologic agents for psoriasis are a highly effective treatment and include inhibitors of tumor necrosis factor (TNF)-alpha or inhibitors of various proinflammatory interleukins. The TNF-alpha inhibitors are long-term maintenance medications and include etanercept, adalimumab, and certolizumab pegol, which are administered by subcutaneous injection, and infliximab, which is administered as an intravenous infusion. TNF-alpha inhibitors are associated with multiple potential adverse events, including:

- Injection site reactions, which are common but usually minor inflammatory skin reactions that last a few days

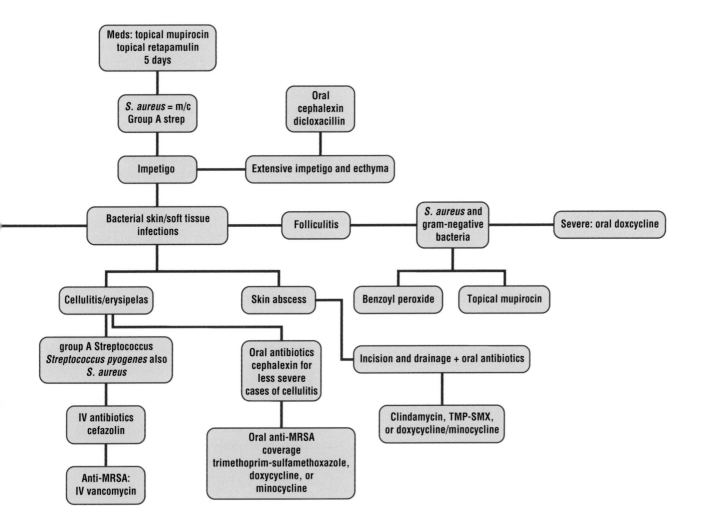

- Infusion reactions (with infliximab), which are most commonly acute, within 4 hours of infusion initiation, but sometimes delayed (several days after the infusion)
- Neutropenia is common and does not generally require discontinuation of therapy; monitoring of the complete blood count at baseline and periodically during treatment is required
- Infections, especially reactivation of latent tuberculosis, bacterial pneumonia, herpes zoster, and opportunistic infections are more common with TNF-alpha inhibitors
- Demyelinating disease such as multiple sclerosis MAY be exacerbated or initiated with TNF-alpha inhibitors
- Heart failure (HF) may be exacerbated and patients with psoriasis and symptomatic HF may need alternative therapy
- Cutaneous reactions, including psoriasis and eczema, may be increased with TNF-alpha inhibitors
- Malignancy risk may be increased especially nonmelanoma skin cancers, and a potential associated risk for lymphoma and solid organ cancers
- TNF inhibitors can increase autoimmune antibodies and formation of antidrug antibodies.

Monitoring for the associated adverse effects is important during treatment with TNF-alpha inhibitors.[15]

Biologic agents for moderate to severe psoriasis, which are inhibitors of the interleukin (IL)-17 pathway, include secukinumab, ixekizumab, and brodalumab. These agents are administered subcutaneously at specific intervals for induction and long-term maintenance therapy. There is a boxed warning in patients treated with brodalumab about risk for suicidal ideation and behavior. The major adverse effects of these medications include local injection site reactions, neutropenia with ixekizumab, upper respiratory infection, and increased overall infections.

Biologic antipsoriatic agents with anti-IL-23 activity include ustekinumab, guselkumab, tildrakizumab, and risankizumab. Ustekinumab blocks the proinflammatory cytokines IL-12 and IL-23. It is administered subcutaneously, and it is well tolerated with nasopharyngitis and production of anti-ustekinumab antibodies. Guselkumab, tildrakizumab, and risankizumab are subcutaneously injected anti–IL-23 biologics that are well tolerated, and the most reported adverse effects are upper respiratory tract infections, other infections, and antibody development. The anti-IL-23 antipsoriatics are costly but efficacious and generally well tolerated.

REFERENCES

1. Gupta AK, Cooper EA. Update in antifungal therapy of dermatophytosis. *Mycopathologia.* 2008;166:353.
2. Hu SW, Bigby M. Pityriasis versicolor: a systematic review of interventions. *Arch Dermatol.* 2010;146:1132.
3. Duong M, Markwell S, Peter J, Barenkamp S. Randomized, controlled trial of antibiotics in the management of community-acquired skin abscesses in the pediatric patient. *Ann Emerg Med.* 2010;55:401.
4. Bowe WP, Shalita AR. Effective over-the-counter acne treatments. *Semin Cutan Med Surg.* 2008;27:170.
5. Huber J, Walch K. Treating acne with oral contraceptives: use of lower doses. *Contraception.* 2006;73:23.
6. iPLEDGE. Prescriber isotretinoin educational kit. https://www.ipledgeprogram.com/iPledgeUI/rems/pdf/resources/Prescriber%20Isotretinoin%20Educational%20Kit.pdf.
7. Marqueling AL, Zane LT. Depression and suicidal behavior in acne patients treated with isotretinoin: a systematic review. *Semin Cutan Med Surg.* 2005;24:92.
8. Magin P, Pond D, Smith W. Isotretinoin, depression, and suicide: a review of the evidence. *Br J Gen Pract.* 2005;55:134.
9. Brelsford M, Beute TC. Preventing and managing the side effects of isotretinoin. *Semin Cutan Med Surg.* 2008;27:197.
10. Layton AM, Knaggs H, Taylor J, Cunliffe WJ. Isotretinoin for acne vulgaris—10 years later: a safe and successful treatment. *Br J Dermatol.* 1993;129:292.
11. American Academy of Allergy, Asthma and Immunology, American College of Allergy, Asthma and Immunology. Contact dermatitis: a practice parameter. *Ann Allergy Asthma Immunol.* 2006;97:S1.
12. Eucrisa Ointment 2% (crisaborole) [prescribing information]. New York, NY: Pfizer Labs; April 2023. Available at: https://www.accessdata.fda.gov/drugsatfda_docs/label/2020/207695s007s009s010lbl.pdf.
13. Silkis (calcitriol) [product monograph]. Thornhill, Ontario, Canada: Galderma Canada Inc; 2017.
14. Schmitt J, Rosumeck S, Thomaschewski G, et al. Efficacy and safety of systemic treatments for moderate-to-severe psoriasis: meta-analysis of randomized controlled trials. *Br J Dermatol.* 2014;170:274.
15. Dogra S, Khullar G. Tumor necrosis factor-α antagonists: side effects and their management. *Indian J Dermatol Venereol Leprol.* 2013;79(7):S35-S46.

CHAPTER 13

Pregnancy: Pharmacology of Select Conditions During Pregnancy

PHARMACOLOGIC CONSIDERATIONS DURING PREGNANCY AND LACTATION

Many women use prescription and over-the-counter medications during pregnancy and lactation despite limited data about drug disposition and potential maternal or fetal adverse reactions for most medications. Drug efficacy and safety during pregnancy and lactation affect the mother, fetus, and breastfeeding infant. Certain physiologic changes during pregnancy can affect the pharmacokinetic and pharmacodynamic characteristics of drugs. Maternal blood volume and cardiac output increase dramatically, and serum albumin decreases, which can affect the apparent volume of distribution of drugs. Hepatic and renal blood flow increases, and glomerular filtration rate increases, which can affect drug metabolism and excretion.

Many drugs can transfer to some degree from the mother to the fetus or the breastfeeding infant. During pregnancy, drugs transfer from maternal to fetal circulation transplacentally, mainly by passive diffusion. The ability of drugs to cross the placenta into fetal circulation depends on the drug's molecular weight, lipid solubility, and polarity. During lactation, passage of drugs across the alveolar apparatus of the breast into the breast milk is more likely with drugs that are lipid soluble, low in molecular weight, and relatively nonpolar. There is also a direct relationship between maternal plasma drug concentrations and concentrations in milk. Drug safety during lactation can be quantified by **relative infant dose** that is calculated by dividing the infant's dose (in milk) in mg/kg/day by the maternal dose in mg/kg/day. Although medications can transfer into breast milk, most medications are compatible with breastfeeding.[1]

Drugs can cause harmful effects on a developing embryo or fetus. A **teratogen** is a drug to which exposure during intrauterine development can impact growth, development, normal formation of anatomy and physiology, and postnatal development.[2,3] The most critical period for teratogen exposure is during organogenesis early in the first trimester of pregnancy.[4] Many drugs are known teratogens, including but not limited to ethanol, lithium, isotretinoin, warfarin derivatives, valproic acid and several other anticonvulsant agents, thalidomide, angiotensin-converting enzyme inhibitors, several antineoplastic agents, and folate antagonists (methotrexate).

In 2015, the US Food and Drug Administration (FDA) Pregnancy and Lactation Labeling Final Rule replaced the former pregnancy risk letter categories on prescription drug labels. The updated FDA drug labeling requirements include sections addressing risk and benefits of medication use during pregnancy, breastfeeding, and in males and females of reproductive potential including pregnancy testing and contraceptive requirements. Each section contains a detailed risk summary, clinical considerations, and data to guide patient counseling and clinical decision making about medication use during pregnancy, lactation, and potential reproductive effects of medications.[5]

Safety of Select Commonly Used Medications During Pregnancy

In general, fetal exposure to medications should be minimal, especially during the first trimester, as sufficient information to determine fetal risks of birth defects is limited. Certain antibiotics that may be safe during pregnancy include penicillins and cephalosporins as well as clindamycin and metronidazole. Acetaminophen can be used short term as an antipyretic and pain reliever during pregnancy.[6] For allergic conditions, second-generation antihistamines, loratadine (10 mg once daily), or cetirizine (10 mg once daily), or intranasal glucocorticoids such as budesonide, mometasone, or fluticasone seem to be safe during pregnancy.[7,8] Asthma during pregnancy can be managed with short-acting inhaled albuterol as needed, with long-term control therapy using one of the inhaled corticosteroids: budesonide, beclomethasone, or fluticasone.[9] Initial treatment of nausea associated with pregnancy is with pyridoxine-doxylamine succinate combination therapy.[10]

PHARMACOTHERAPY OF COMMON PREGNANCY-ASSOCIATED CONDITIONS

Gestational diabetes mellitus (GDM), which is defined as a diagnosis of diabetes at 24 to 28 weeks of gestation, is increasingly prevalent. GDM is associated with adverse maternal and fetal outcomes: preeclampsia, gestational hypertension, macrosomia, birth trauma to mother or newborn, operative delivery, perinatal mortality, and neonatal metabolic and respiratory problems.[11] Medical nutritional therapy and frequent daily self-blood glucose monitoring are the initial management strategies, although pharmacotherapy is needed for patients who do not adequately meet glycemic goals.

There are two options for pharmacotherapy for women with GDM that is inadequately controlled with medical nutritional therapy. Insulin therapy, which was discussed in Chapter 6, is a first-line option for GDM. Intermediate-acting basal insulin (neutral protamine Hagedorn) is often initiated once daily, with rapid-acting insulin (lispro or aspart) added before one or more meals based on blood glucose levels.[12] Blood glucose must be monitored frequently throughout the day to detect hypoglycemia and assess glycemic control. Oral hypoglycemic agents for GDM include the biguanide metformin and the sulfonylurea glyburide, which were discussed in Chapter 6. Metformin has primarily dose-related gastrointestinal adverse effects, i.e., mild anorexia, nausea, abdominal discomfort, and soft bowel movements. Glyburide can cause hypoglycemia. Insulin may be required if oral hypoglycemics are not effective.

Gestational hypertension is defined as the onset of hypertension (systolic blood pressure ≥140 mmHg and/or diastolic blood pressure ≥90 mmHg) at ≥20 weeks of gestation without evidence of preeclampsia or target organ damage.[13] Antihypertensive therapy of acute severe hypertension (blood pressure ≥160/110 mmHg) during pregnancy may include labetalol or hydralazine administered intravenously (IV) or oral nifedipine. Maintenance antihypertensive medications for gestational hypertension include either oral labetalol (alpha-1/beta antagonist) or intermediate-acting or extended-release nifedipine (dihydropyridine calcium channel blocker) or methyldopa. The details of antihypertensive medications are found in Chapter 3.

Preeclampsia and eclampsia are also hypertensive disorders caused by pregnancy. Preeclampsia is defined as the new onset of hypertension and proteinuria or the new onset of hypertension and significant end-organ dysfunction with or without proteinuria after 20 weeks of gestation or postpartum in a previously normotensive woman.[14,15] Preeclampsia with severe features may include severe hypertension with one or more organ/system disorders: central nervous system dysfunction; hepatic, renal, or platelet abnormalities; and/or pulmonary edema. Delivery at or close to term is the most effective management of preeclampsia. Pharmacotherapy of preeclampsia may include management of severe hypertension and a course of antenatal steroids to promote fetal maturity when preterm delivery is expected. All patients with preeclampsia with severe features are administered IV **magnesium sulfate** intrapartum and immediately postpartum for seizure prophylaxis. Adverse effects of magnesium sulfate are diaphoresis, flushing, and warmth. Patients should be monitored frequently for signs of magnesium sulfate toxicity. Magnesium sulfate is contraindicated in patients with myasthenia gravis. These include **loss of deep tendon reflexes** (patellar), which is the first sign of toxicity and occurs at 7 to 10 mEq/L (8.5–12.0 mg/dL or 3.5–5.0 mmol/L). More serious signs of magnesium toxicity, which occur as the serum levels increase, are respiratory paralysis at 10 to 13 mEq/L (12–16 mg/dL

or 5.0–6.5 mmol/L), cardiac conduction abnormalities at >15 mEq/L (>18 mg/dL or >7.5 mmol/L), and cardiac arrest at >25 mEq/L (>30 mg/dL or >12.5 mmol/L). **Calcium gluconate** administered IV over 2 to 5 minutes is the antidote for severe magnesium toxicity.[13]

Eclampsia is the onset of generalized, usually tonic-clonic type seizures in patients with preeclampsia. Patients should be treated with oxygen, blood pressure reduction for severe hypertension, magnesium sulfate to prevent seizure recurrence, and prompt delivery. **Magnesium sulfate** is administered IV as a loading dose followed by maintenance infusion for a short duration. Adverse effects, therapeutic range, signs of toxicity, and antidotes for magnesium sulfate have been discussed earlier.

Preterm labor is defined as the onset of labor (regular contractions and cervical changes) before the completion of 37 weeks of gestation. Preterm birth is a leading cause of infant morbidity and mortality. Tocolytic drugs can be administered to women with preterm labor <34 weeks of gestation, primarily to delay delivery for 48 hours to allow for administration of antenatal steroids. The most common tocolytic drugs include indomethacin, a nonspecific cyclooxygenase inhibitor, calcium channel blockers (e.g., nifedipine), beta-agonists (eg, terbutaline), and magnesium sulfate. Indomethacin is administered orally or per rectum as a first-line tocolytic for women at 24 to 32 weeks of gestation; it should not be used after 32 weeks due to potential ductal constriction. Indomethacin is contraindicated in women with bleeding disorders, liver or kidney disease, gastrointestinal ulcers, and asthma (in women with hypersensitivity to aspirin). Adverse effects of indomethacin include maternal gastrointestinal upset as well as constriction of the ductus arteriosus and oligohydramnios in the fetus.[16,17]

Nifedipine is a calcium channel blocker that is a first-line tocolytic agent in women at 32 to 34 weeks of gestation. It is well tolerated orally, with vasodilatory effects such as nausea, flushing, headache, dizziness, and palpitations. Nifedipine or any other calcium channel blocker **should not** be used with magnesium sulfate, and nifedipine is contraindicated in women with hypotension, severe heart failure, and cardiogenic shock.

Terbutaline is a beta-2 agonist that causes relaxation of the myometrium. Terbutaline is administered by intermittent subcutaneous injection for short-term tocolysis only, due to potential risk for maternal heart problems and increased mortality.[18] Terbutaline is associated with significant maternal adverse effects, specifically tachycardia, palpitations, and reduced blood pressure; fetal effects include tachycardia and hypoglycemia. Contraindications to terbutaline include maternal tachycardia-sensitive cardiac disease, poorly controlled hyperthyroidism, or diabetes mellitus.[16]

An important component to management of women at risk for preterm delivery is administration of antenatal corticosteroid therapy (ACS). Women who are at 23 to 33+6 weeks of gestation and at increased risk of preterm delivery are candidates for ACS. ACS accelerates neonatal lung maturity and pulmonary function and reduces the incidence of respiratory distress syndrome, intraventricular hemorrhage, necrotizing enterocolitis, sepsis, and neonatal mortality. ACS consists of either betamethasone suspension 12 mg intramuscularly every 24 hours for two doses or four doses of 6 mg dexamethasone intramuscularly 12 hours apart, ideally 2 to 7 days before delivery.[19]

INDUCTION OF LABOR

Induction of labor is defined as the stimulation of uterine contractions during pregnancy before the onset of spontaneous labor to accomplish delivery. Indications for induction may include certain high-risk pregnancy conditions such as postdate pregnancy, hypertensive disorders, prelabor rupture of membranes, and diabetes mellitus. Elective induction is defined as the induction of labor in low-risk women without other medical indications at 39 weeks of gestation.[20,21] Cervical ripening before induction of labor with oxytocin is preferrable in patients with an unfavorable cervix, e.g., low Bishop scores of cervical dilation, effacement, consistency, and position.[22] Pharmacologic cervical ripening is accomplished by the use of prostaglandin analogs, specifically prostaglandin E2 (PGE2) or prostaglandin E1 (misoprostol).

Prepidil (endocervical gel) and cervidil (vaginal insert controlled release; dinoprostone) are two PGE2, dinoprostone preparations commercially available for cervical ripening in the United States. Misoprostol is used off label for cervical ripening in the United States. Side effects of prostaglandins include tachysystole, fever, chills, vomiting, and diarrhea. Cervical ripening with prostaglandins is contraindicated in term pregnancies with a prior cesarean birth or other prior major uterine surgery.[20,21]

Synthetic oxytocin is the primary pharmacologic method of labor induction. Oxytocin normally stimulates uterine contractions, primarily by elevating intracellular calcium levels at or near term. Oxytocin is administered IV by an infusion pump with continuous monitoring of uterine activity and fetal heart rate (FHR) during labor induction. The most common side effects are tachysystole, which is >5 contractions in 10 minutes, averaged over a 30-minute window, pain, and sometimes lowered blood pressure and hyponatremia.[23,24] Contraindications to labor induction include prior uterine rupture, high-risk uterine surgery, placenta previa or vasa previa, abnormal (category III) intrapartum FHR tracings, cord prolapse, active genital herpes, and invasive cervical cancer.[23]

REFERENCES

1. Sachs HC, Committee on Drugs. The transfer of drugs and therapeutics into human breast milk: an update on selected topics. *Pediatrics*. 2013;132:e796.
2. Haas DM, Marsh DJ, Dang DT, et al. Prescription and other medication use in pregnancy. *Obstet Gynecol*. 2018;131:789.
3. Adam MP, Polifka JE, Friedman JM. Evolving knowledge of the teratogenicity of medications in human pregnancy. *Am J Med Genet C Semin Med Genet*. 2011;157C:175.
4. Sadler TW. *Langman's Medical Embryology*. 13th ed. Philadelphia: Wolters Kluwer; 2015.
5. FDA Pregnancy and Lactation Labeling Rule. Available at: https://www.federalregister.gov/documents/2014/12/04/2014-28241/content-and-format-of-labeling-for-human-prescription-drug-and-biological-products-requirements-for.
6. Black RA, Hill DA. Over-the-counter medications in pregnancy. *Am Fam Physician*. 2003;67:2517.
7. Källén B. Use of antihistamine drugs in early pregnancy and delivery outcome. *J Matern Fetal Neonatal Med*. 2002;11:146.
8. Namazy JA, Schatz M. The safety of intranasal steroids during pregnancy: a good start. *J Allergy Clin Immunol*. 2016;138:105.
9. Namazy J, Schatz M. The treatment of allergic respiratory disease during pregnancy. *J Investig Allergol Clin Immunol*. 2016;26:1.
10. Committee on Practice Bulletins-Obstetrics. ACOG Practice Bulletin No. 189: nausea and vomiting of pregnancy. *Obstet Gynecol*. 2018;131:e15. Reaffirmed 2020.
11. HAPO Study Cooperative Research Group, Metzger BE, Lowe LP, et al. Hyperglycemia and adverse pregnancy outcomes. *N Engl J Med*. 2008;358:1991.
12. Jovanovic L, Pettitt DJ. Treatment with insulin and its analogs in pregnancies complicated by diabetes. *Diabetes Care*. 2007;30(suppl 2):S220.
13. Gestational hypertension and preeclampsia: ACOG Practice Bulletin, Number 222. *Obstet Gynecol*. 2020;135:e237.
14. Magee LA, Pels A, Helewa M, et al. Diagnosis, evaluation, and management of the hypertensive disorders of pregnancy: executive summary. *J Obstet Gynaecol Can*. 2014;36:416.
15. Tranquilli AL, Dekker G, Magee L, et al. The classification, diagnosis and management of the hypertensive disorders of pregnancy: a revised statement from the ISSHP. *Pregnancy Hypertens*. 2014;4:97.
16. American College of Obstetricians and Gynecologists. Practice bulletin No. 130: prediction and prevention of preterm birth. *Obstet Gynecol*. 2012;120:964-973.
17. Vermillion ST, Scardo JA, Lashus AG, Wiles HB. The effect of indomethacin tocolysis on fetal ductus arteriosus constriction with advancing gestational age. *Am J Obstet Gynecol*. 1997;177:256.
18. US Food and Drug Administration. *FDA Drug Safety Communication: New Warnings Against Use of Terbutaline to Treat Preterm Labor*. Available at: http://www.fda.gov/Drugs/DrugSafety/ucm243539.htm#ds.
19. Committee on Obstetric Practice. Committee Opinion No. 713: antenatal corticosteroid therapy for fetal maturation. *Obstet Gynecol*. 2017;130:e102. Reaffirmed 2018 (interim update).
20. ACOG Committee on Practice Bulletins – Obstetrics. ACOG Practice Bulletin No. 107: Induction of labor. *Obstet Gynecol*. 2009;114:386. Reaffirmed 2019.
21. Voutsos L. Prophylactic induction. *Am J Obstet Gynecol*. 2020;222:290.
22. Bishop EH. Pelvic scoring for elective induction. *Obstet Gynecol*. 1964;24:266.
23. Smith JG, Merrill DC. Oxytocin for induction of labor. *Clin Obstet Gynecol*. 2006;49:594.
24. American College of Obstetricians and Gynecologists. ACOG Practice Bulletin No. 106: intrapartum fetal heart rate monitoring: nomenclature, interpretation, and general management principles. *Obstet Gynecol*. 2009;114:192. Reaffirmed 2021.

CHAPTER 14

Pediatric Pharmacology

There are important pharmacologic differences in pediatric patients, specifically in the preterm neonate and neonate, compared to children and adults. Pharmacokinetic parameters vary based on the age of the pediatric patient. Age definitions for pediatric patients are as follows[1]:

- A preterm neonate is born at <37 weeks' gestation
- A neonate is <1 month old
- An infant is between about 1 month and 1 year old
- A child is 1 to 11 years old
- An adolescent is 12 to 18 years old.

Drug absorption for medications can be affected by gastrointestinal functions such as gastric acid production, gastric emptying time, and gastrointestinal enzyme activity, especially in the preterm neonate. Drug distribution can vary in preterm neonates due to changes in body composition, e.g., less fat and more water, and reduced plasma protein binding of drugs. The neonatal blood-brain barrier is more permeable, which can cause bilirubin and certain medications to enter the central nervous system more readily. Drug-metabolizing enzyme activity is reduced in early neonatal life and matures gradually in the first few years of life. Drug excretion is also affected by a reduced glomerular filtration rate (GFR), especially in preterm neonates and newborns. The GFR reaches adult values by approximately 6 to 12 months, and in toddlers the GFR exceeds adult values.

DRUG DOSAGE

Drugs approved for pediatric patients generally have pediatric doses that are indicated in milligrams per kilogram or per pound. Some appropriate pediatric drug references include NeoFax and Pediatric & Neonatal Dosage Handbook.[2] If a pediatric dosage is not indicated, dosage calculations can be estimated based on age (Young's rule), weight (Clark's rule), or body surface area (BSA).

$$\text{Young's rule} = Dose = \text{Adult dose} \times \frac{\text{Age (years)}}{\text{Age} + 12}$$

$$\text{Clark's rule} = Dose = \text{Adult dose} \times \frac{\text{Weight (kg)}}{70}$$

The BSA, which is expressed in m², square meter, is a calculation that uses the infant's or child's weight (kg), height, and BSA to determine the percentage of adult dosage used to calculate the pediatric dosage:

$$\text{Pediatric dose} = (\text{Child's BSA in m}^2/1.73\text{m}^2) \times \text{Adult Dosage}$$

The child's BSA can be calculated from a nomogram as shown in Fig. 14.1.

Pediatric drug administration and adherence have certain unique differences from adult pharmacotherapeutics. Medication errors are more common in infants and children than in adults. Pediatric dosage forms for oral medications are often liquid forms such as elixirs or suspensions, and suspensions require shaking before each dose to distribute the medication. Dosing of liquid medications requires weight-based dosing (kg) in metric units dispensed, e.g., mL instead of teaspoons. Liquid medications should be dispensed with oral syringes to ensure accurate and standardized dosage volumes.[3] The unpalatable taste of many oral medications may interfere with appropriate dosing and affect therapy. Flavoring options can mask the taste of bitter medications, and providing sweet or chocolate-flavored foods can improve palatability.[4]

Administration of parenteral medications in pediatric and especially neonatal patients has important considerations. Some common concerns include limited vascular access, calculating small dose volumes, intravenous polypharmacy due to the need for multiple infusions of different medications, and potential incompatibilities of drug delivery devices, e.g., neonatal catheters and cannulas and medications.[5] Low flow rates and dead space in intravenous lines can further complicate intravenous drug delivery. Intramuscular injections are limited by the volume of the administered drug and small muscle mass of neonates. Vaccines are often delivered intramuscularly in the anterolateral thigh of infants.

Commonly used pediatric medications vary, but current trends indicate the following classes are most frequently used. Antibiotics, specifically amoxicillin, amoxicillin/clavulanic acid, azithromycin, and cephalosporins such as cefidinir and

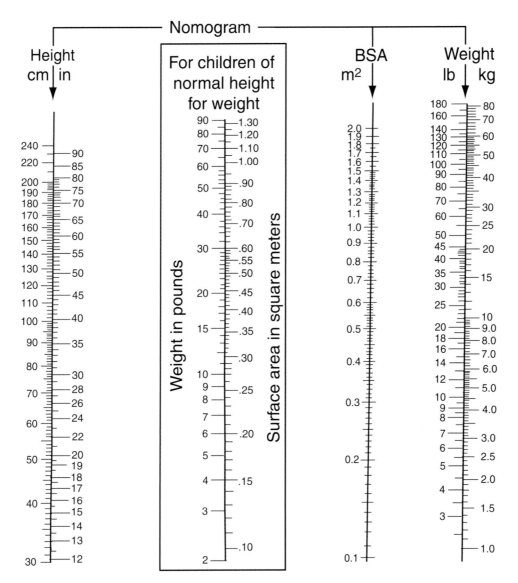

Nomogram

| Height cm \| in | For children of normal height for weight | BSA m² | Weight lb \| kg |

FIG. 14.1 West Nomogram (for estimation of body surface area [BSA]). The BSA is indicated where a straight line connecting the height and weight intersects the BSA column or, if the patient is roughly of normal proportion, from the weight alone (enclosed area). (Nomogram modified from data of Boyd E by West CCD; from Vaughan VC and McKay RJ, eds. *Nelson Textbook of Pediatrics*. 12th ed. Philadelphia: Saunders;1983.)

cephalexin, are most prescribed.[6] Topical mupirocin for bacterial infections and topical nystatin for candida fungal rashes are also commonly used. Other common medications include various drugs for allergic conditions and asthma, specifically inhaled albuterol and inhaled and nasal glucocorticosteroids, e.g., fluticasone, mometasone, triamcinolone, hydrocortisone (topical), and budesonide. Oral prednisone and prednisolone antiinflammatory glucocorticosteroids and oral montelukast (Singulair) for asthma are among the top prescribed medications. Attention-deficit hyperactivity disorder medications commonly prescribed include methylphenidate, amphetamine/dextroamphetamine, and lisdexamfetamine.[6] Cough and cold medications that are over the counter and commonly used include dextromethorphan/phenylephrine/chlorpheniramine. Generally, cold and

cold combination medications should not be used in children younger than 6 years of age.[7] Antipyretics commonly used were acetaminophen and ibuprofen; aspirin should be avoided in children due to the risk of Reye syndrome.[8]

REFERENCES

1. Eiland LS, Meyers RS. Caring for and assessing pediatric patients: aspects to consider as a pharmacy practitioner. *Am J Health Syst Pharm*. 2019;76:1463-1471.
2. Clinical Resource, Keeping Pediatric Patients Safe. *Pharmacist's Letter/Pharmacy Technician's Letter/Prescriber's Letter*. 2023.
3. Benavides S, Huynh D, Morgan J, Briars L. Approach to the pediatric prescription in a community pharmacy. *J Pediatr Pharmacol Ther*. 2011;16(4):298-307.

4. Eiland LS and Meyers RS. Caring for and assessing pediatric patients: aspects to consider as a pharmacy practitioner. *Am J Health Syst Pharm.* 2019;76(19):1463-1471.

5. O'Brien F, Clapham D, Krysiak K, et al. Making medicines baby size: the challenges in bridging the formulation gap in neonatal medicine. *Int J Mol Sci.* 2019;20(11):2688.

6. Chai G, Governale L, Mcmahon AW, Trinidad JP, Staffa J, Murphy D. Trends of outpatient prescription drug utilization in US children, 2002-2010. *Pediatrics.* 2012; 130(1):23-31.

7. Lowry J, Leeder J. Over-the-counter medications: update on cough and cold preparations. *Pediatr Rev.* 2015;36(7):286-298.

8. Rose E. Pediatric fever. *Emerg Med Clin North Am.* 2021; 39:627-639.

CHAPTER 15

Geriatric Pharmacology

BACKGROUND

The population aged 65 years and older is growing, and it is expected there will be 84 million persons aged 65 years and older in the United States in 2050. Globally, population aging is also increasing, especially in Europe and Japan. Appropriate pharmacotherapy is a fundamental component to caring for older adults. Older adults are more likely to have multiple chronic medical conditions and use multiple prescribed and over-the-counter medications. Polypharmacy, which is the use of multiple medications, is more common in older adults. Older adults are also using herbal and dietary supplements more frequently, many of which have adverse effects and drug interactions. Adverse drug events (ADE), drug interactions, inappropriate prescribing, and underutilization of certain medications are more common in older adults.[1,2]

ADEs are problems that result from use of medications. ADEs are a common cause of hospitalization and iatrogenic illness in older adults. Common classes of medications most likely to cause ADEs include: psychotropic drugs especially antipsychotics; sedative-hypnotics including benzodiazepines and nonbenzodiazepine; benzodiazepine-receptor agonist hypnotics (Z drugs); all drugs with anticholinergic activity such as first-generation antihistamines, tricyclic antidepressants, and bladder antimuscarinics; hypoglycemic agents, especially sliding-scale insulin; and sulfonylureas, anticoagulants, and cardiovascular medications especially alpha-1 antagonists, centrally acting alpha-2 agonists, and digoxin.[3] Cyclooxygenase (COX) nonselective nonsteroidal antiinflammatory drugs (NSAIDs) are associated with increased risk for gastrointestinal bleeding, elevated blood pressure, and kidney injury. Patient-specific risk factors for ADEs include renal impairment and long-term care residents.[4,5]

Certain medications are generally considered potentially inappropriate for use in older patients due to high risk for ADEs. The Beers criteria (website Beers, https://agsjournals.onlinelibrary.wiley.com/doi/full/10.1111/jgs.18372), which are applicable to drug therapy in the United States, include lists of drugs based on five categories: drugs that are potentially inappropriate in most older adults, drugs that should typically be avoided in older adults with certain conditions, drugs to use with caution, drug-drug interactions, and drug-dose adjustment based on kidney function. Drugs that are potentially inappropriate were discussed earlier and should generally be avoided in older adults. Certain drug classes can exacerbate underlying medical conditions. Examples of drug-disease interactions include NSAIDs or COX-2 inhibitors with heart failure, gastric or duodenal ulcers, and chronic kidney disease. Anticholinergic medications, antipsychotics, benzodiazepines, and sedative Z drugs should be avoided in patients with dementia or delirium. Patients with a history of falls or fractures should avoid medications that can cause balance disturbances or psychomotor impairment, including antiepileptics, antipsychotics, benzodiazepines, Z drugs, and certain antidepressants.[3]

Underutilization of medications is another issue in older adults.[6] Drugs most frequently associated with underuse included angiotensin-converting enzyme inhibitors for heart failure, antiplatelet therapy for cardiovascular diseases, statin therapy, regular inhaled β2-agonists, or antimuscarinic bronchodilators for asthma and chronic obstructive pulmonary disease, and vitamin D and calcium supplements for patients with osteoporosis and fractures. Underutilization of medications has been associated with increased hospitalization and mortality in elderly patients.[7] Some of the reasons for underprescribing in older adults are drug affordability, benefits of treatment or disease prevention not recognized by clinicians, or lack of dose availability.

There are some age-related changes in pharmacokinetic and pharmacodynamics in the geriatric population. Pharmacologically, the most significant age-related change is a decline in renal function, with a reduction in creatinine clearance, which is the measure of estimated glomerular filtration rate (eGFR). The Cockcroft-Gault formula estimates GFR as follows:

$$\text{Estimated creatinine clearance (mL/min)} = \frac{(140 - \text{Age}) \times (\text{Weight in kg})}{72 \times \text{Serum creatinine in mg/dL}}$$

For women, the result is multiplied by 0.85.[8] Significant reduction in renal function affects drug clearance, which can prolong the half-life of many drugs and lead to toxic accumulation. Dosage size or dosing frequency adjustments may be required in patients with significant renal insufficiency. Some important age-related pharmacodynamic changes include reduced responsiveness to beta-agonists such as albuterol, increased risk of orthostatic hypotension, and increased sensitivity to sedative-hypnotics and opioids.

There are methods that can improve pharmacotherapy in older adults. In addition to Beers, the screening tool of older people's prescriptions (STOPP) and screening tool to alert to right treatment (START) criteria provide guidance about which medication(s) to consider stopping in patients over 65 years and which medication to consider starting in patients over 65 years.[9] A systematic approach to managing medications in older adults requires regular follow-up and assessment to review a patient's drug regimen and evaluate the need for discontinuing or changing a medication is important.[10] Each medication should be evaluated to determine if current evidence supports the indication (reason) for which it is being used/prescribed. Changes in a patient's acute and chronic illnesses or overall functional status require medication reconciliation and potential adjustment. It is important to consider ADEs as a potential cause of new medical symptoms or problems. Dosing schedules of all medications should be reviewed to determine if a medication regimen can be simplified to reduce confusion, reduce cost, and improve medication adherence. Older adults may require lower dosages, especially if they have liver or kidney impairment, which can provide clinical benefit with less risk of dose-related ADEs.[10] Patients should be educated about reasons for stopping, starting, or adjusting medications, and to report the onset of new medical concerns as they may be related to ADEs. Patients should be counseled about nonpharmacologic options such as lifestyle modifications, e.g., dietary modification and increased physical activity, and other modalities such as physical and occupational therapy.

REFERENCES

1. Beijer HJ, de Blaey CJ. Hospitalisations caused by adverse drug reactions (ADR): a meta-analysis of observational studies. *Pharm World Sci.* 2002;24:46.
2. Steinman MA, Landefeld CS, Rosenthal GE, et al. Polypharmacy and prescribing quality in older people. *J Am Geriatr Soc.* 2006;54:1516.
3. 2019 American Geriatrics Society Beers Criteria® Update Expert Panel. American Geriatrics Society 2019 Updated AGS Beers Criteria® for potentially inappropriate medication use in older adults. *J Am Geriatr Soc.* 2019;67:674.
4. Breton G, Froissart M, Janus N, et al. Inappropriate drug use and mortality in community-dwelling elderly with impaired kidney function: the Three-City population-based study. *Nephrol Dial Transplant.* 2011;26:2852.
5. Gurwitz JH, Field TS, Judge J, et al. The incidence of adverse drug events in two large academic long-term care facilities. *Am J Med.* 2005;118:251.
6. Higashi T, Shekelle PG, Solomon DH, et al. The quality of pharmacologic care for vulnerable older patients. *Ann Intern Med.* 2004;140:714.
7. Wauters M, Elseviers M, Vaes B, et al. Too many, too few, or too unsafe? Impact of inappropriate prescribing on mortality, and hospitalisation in a cohort of community-dwelling oldest old. *Br J Clin Pharmacol.* 2016;82(5):1382-1392.
8. Cockcroft DW, Gault MH. Prediction of creatinine clearance from serum creatinine. *Nephron.* 1976;16:31.
9. O'Mahony D, O'Sullivan D, Byrne S, O'Connor MN, Ryan C, Gallagher P. STOPP/START criteria for potentially inappropriate prescribing in older people: version 2. *Age Ageing.* 2015;44(2):213-218.
10. Scott IA, Gray LC, Martin JH, Mitchell CA. Minimizing inappropriate medications in older populations: a 10-step conceptual framework. *Am J Med.* 2012;125:529.

Index

Note: page numbers followed by "b" indicate boxes, by "f" indicate figures, by "t" indicate tables.

A

Abacavir, hypersensitivity reaction, 136
Abaloparatide, 78
Abatacept, 59
Abciximab, 37
  for acute coronary syndrome, 25–30
Abscesses, pharmacologic treatment of, 151
Absorption, 6
Acetaminophen, 52, 55f
  during pregnancy, 159
Acetylcholine, 10
Acetylcholinesterase inhibitors, 11
Acne vulgaris, pharmacologic treatment of, 154
ACS. *see* Antenatal corticosteroid therapy
Active transport, 6
Acute coronary syndrome (ACS), treatment of, 17–30, 29f
Acute dystonic reactions, 114–115
Acute hypertensive crisis, 114
Acute opioid overdose, 109
Acyclovir, 129
Adapalene, for acne vulgaris, 154
Additivity, 8
ADE. *see* Adverse drug events
Adenosine, 31
Adrenal hormones, 74
Adrenergic blockers, 12–13, 14f
Aducanumab, for Alzheimer disease, 108
Adverse drug events (ADE), in older adults, 165
Afatinib, 143
Affinity, 4
Age-related macular degeneration (AMD), 146
Agonist, 4
Albendazole, 140
Albuterol, 12
Alcaftadine (Lastacaft), for allergic conjunctivitis, 147
Aldosterone antagonists, for hypertension, 20–22t
Alfuzosin, 13
Allergic conjunctivitis, 147
Allergic contact dermatitis, pharmacologic treatment of, 154–155
Allergic disease, 51
Allopurinol, for gout, 53
Allylamines antifungals, 137–140
Almotriptan, for migraines, 104
Alpha antagonist, 13
Alpha receptor agonists, 12
Alpha receptors, 11
5-Alpha reductase inhibitors (5-ARIs), for BPH, 71
Alpha-1 antagonists, for hypertension, 20–22t
Alpha-1 receptors, 11

Alpha-2 agonists, 13
  for hypertension, 20–22t
Alpha-2 receptors, 11
Alpha-2-adrenergic agonists, 118
Alprostadil, for erectile dysfunction, 71
Alteplase, 42
Alzheimer disease, 105–108
Amantadine, for Parkinson disease, 105
Amides, 97
Amiloride, for hypertension, 20–22t
Aminoglycosides, 127
Amiodarone, 30–31
Amlodipine
  for angina, 17, 25t
  for hypertension, 20–22t
Amoxapine, 114
Amphetamine stimulants, 118
Amphotericin B, 137
Analgesia state, 97
Anastrozole, 143
Andexanet alfa, 37
Androgen, 70–71, 72f
Anemia, drugs for, 59–62
Anesthetics, 96–100, 96f, 98f
Angina pectoris, treatment of, 17
Angiotensin II receptor blockers (ARBs), for heart failure, 23–24t
Angiotensin receptor blockers, for hypertension, 20–22t
Angiotensin-converting enzyme (ACE) inhibitors
  for heart failure, 17, 23–24t
  for hypertension, 16, 20–22t
Anidulafungin, 140
ANS. *see* Autonomic nervous system
Antacids, 80
Antagonist, 4
Antenatal corticosteroid therapy (ACS), for preterm labor, 160–161
Anthralin, for psoriasis, 155
Antiarrhythmic drugs, 30–31, 32f
Antibacterial drugs, 121–129, 122f, 124f
  antimycobacterials, 128–129
  cell membrane disruptors, 128
  DNA/nucleic acid synthesis inhibitors, 128
  folate inhibitors, 128
Antibiotics, for acne vulgaris, 154
Anticancer drug, 142
Anticholinergic toxicity, 12
Anticoagulants, 37–42, 40f, 42f
Anticonvulsants, 100

Antidepressant drugs, 109–114, 113f
Antidiarrheal medications, 81
Antiemetic drugs, 81, 85f, 86t
  for migraines, 104
Antiepileptics, 100–104, 103f
Antifungals, 137–140, 138f
  topical, for skin infections, 150
Antiherpetic medications, 129
Antihistamines, 51
  for allergic conjunctivitis, 147
Anti-IgE receptor therapy, for asthma, 48
Antiinfective agents, 121
Antiinflammatory drugs, for asthma, 45–48
Anti-interleukin (IL)-4 receptor alpha subunit antibody, for asthma, 48
Anti-interleukin (IL)-5 therapy, for asthma, 48
Antileukotrienes, for asthma, 45–48
Antimalarial quinoline derivatives, 140
Antimuscarinic agents, 12, 45
Antimycobacterials, 128–129
Antineoplastic drugs, 142–145
Antiparasitic drugs, 140
Antiplatelets, 36–37, 38f
Antiproliferative/antimetabolic agents, 53–58
Antipseudomonal penicillins, 126
Antipsychotic medications, 114–115, 117f
Antipyretics, for pediatric patients, 162–163
Antiretroviral drugs, 136–137
Anti-SARS-CoV-2 monoclonal antibodies, 136
Antistaphylococcal penicillins, 126
Antithyroid medications, 64–65, 67f
Antivirals, 129–137, 130f, 132f, 134f
  antifungals, 137–140, 138f
  antiretrovirals, 136–137
Anxiolytics, 115
Apalutamide, 143
Aplastic anemia, 127
Apraclonidine, for glaucoma, 146
Apremilast, for psoriasis, 155–157
Aprepitant, 86t
Argatroban, 42
Aromatase inhibitors, 143
Artemisinins, 140
Aspirin, 36, 52
  for acute coronary syndrome, 25–30
  toxicity, 52
Asthma
  drugs for, 44
  types of devices for, 44
  types of medications for, 44–49, 46f
Atazanavir, 136–137

Atenolol, 12
  for angina, 25t
  for hypertension, 20–22t
  for hyperthyroidism, 64
Atogepant, for migraines, 104–105
Atopic dermatitis (AD), pharmacologic treatment
    of, 155
ATP-binding cassettes, 6
Atropine, 12
Attention-deficit hyperactivity disorder, 115–118
Atypical antidepressants, 114
Autonomic ganglia, 11
Autonomic nervous system (ANS), pharmacology,
    10–15
  parasympathomimetic and parasympatholytic
     drugs, 11–12
  review of autonomic physiology, 10–11
  sympathomimetics and adrenergic blockers,
    12–13, 14f
Azathioprine, 58
Azelaic acid, for acne vulgaris, 154
Azelastine hydrochloride (Optivar), for allergic
    conjunctivitis, 147
Azilsartan, for hypertension, 20–22t
Azole antifungals, 137
Aztreonam, 126

B

Bacitracin, 127
Bacterial conjunctivitis, 147
Bacterial skin and soft tissue infections,
    pharmacologic treatment of, 151
Balsalazide, for ulcerative colitis, 81–87
Bamlanivimab-etesevimab, 136
Barbiturates, 96
Baricitinib, 59
Beclomethasone (Qvar), 45
Bempedoic acid, for dyslipidemia, 36
Benazepril, for hypertension, 20–22t
Benign prostatic hyperplasia (BPH), 71
Benralizumab, 48
Benzathine penicillin, 126
Benzimidazole, 140
Benzodiazepine (BZ) receptor agonists (BZRAs), 93
Benzoyl peroxide, for acne vulgaris, 154
Benztropine, 12
Benzylisoquinolinium compounds, 100
Bepotastine (Bepreve), for allergic conjunctivitis, 147
Beta agonists, 12
Beta antagonists, 12
  for angina, 25t
  for glaucoma, 146
  for heart failure, 23–24t, 30
  for hypertension, 20–22t
Beta receptors, 10–11
Beta-1 receptors, 10
Beta-2 adrenergic agonists, 44–45
Beta-2 agonists, 12
Beta-2 receptors, 10
Beta-3 receptor, 11
Beta-blockers. *see* Beta antagonists
Beta-lactamase inhibitors, 126
Betamethasone dipropionate, 155t
Betaxolol, for glaucoma, 146
Bethanechol, 11
Bile acid resins, 36
Bioavailability, 6
Biologic agents, 59

Biologics, for asthma, 48
Biotransformation, 7
Bipolar disorder, medications for, 115
Bisacodyl, for constipation, 90–91t
Bisoprolol, 12
  for heart failure, 23–24t
  for hypertension, 20–22t
Bisphosphonates, for osteoporosis, 78
Bivalirudin, 42
Blood disorder, drugs for, 59–62
Blood-brain barrier, 7
Body surface area (BSA), 162, 163f
Bosutinib, 142–143
Breast milk, 7
Brexafungerp, for vulvovaginitis, 151
Brimonidine, for glaucoma, 146
Brinzolamide, for glaucoma, 146
Brivaracetam, 101
Bronchodilators, for asthma, 44–45
BSA. *see* Body surface area
Budesonide (Pulmicort), 45
Bulk-forming laxatives, for constipation, 90–91t
Bumetanide, for hypertension, 20–22t
Bupivacaine, 97
Buprenorphine, 109
Buspirone, 115

C

Calcineurin inhibitors, 53
Calcitonin gene-related peptide (CGRP) antagonists,
    for migraines, 104
Calcium channel blockers (CCBs), 100
  for angina, 25t
  dihydropyridine type, for hypertension,
    16, 20–22t
  non-dihydropyridine type, for hypertension,
    20–22t
Calcium gluconate, for magnesium toxicity, 160
Canagliflozin, for heart failure, 23–24t
Cancer
  defined, 142
  drug therapy for, 142–143, 144f
Candesartan
  for heart failure, 23–24t
  for hypertension, 20–22t
Cangrelor, 37
  for acute coronary syndrome, 25–30
Captopril
  for heart failure, 23–24t
  for hypertension, 20–22t
Carbachol, for glaucoma, 146
Carbamazepine, 100–101
Carbapenems, 126
Carbidopa, for Parkinson disease, 105
Carbuncles, pharmacologic treatment of, 151
Cardiomyopathy, 115
Cardiotoxicity, 97
Cardiovascular function, drugs affecting, 16–43
  antiarrhythmic drugs, 30–31, 32f
  anticoagulants, 37–42, 40f, 42f
  antiplatelets, 36–37, 38f
  fibrinolytic drugs, 42
  for treatment of acute coronary syndrome,
    17–30, 29f
  for treatment of angina pectoris, 17
  for treatment of dyslipidemia, 31–36, 34f
  for treatment of heart failure, 16–17, 23–24t, 26f
  for treatment of hypertension, 16, 18f, 20–22t

Carteolol, for glaucoma, 146
Carvedilol, 12
  for hypertension, 20–22t
Casirivimab-imdevimab, 136
Caspofungin, 140
Catecholamine, 10
Catechol-O-methyltransferase (COMT)
    inhibitors, 105
Cefdinir, 126
Cefditoren, 126
Cefiderocol, 126
Cefixime, 126
Cefotaxime, 126
Cefotetan, 126
Cefoxitin, 126
Cefpodoxime proxetil, 126
Cefprozil, 126
Ceftazidime, 126
Ceftibuten, 126
Ceftriaxone, 126
Cefuroxime, 126
Cell cycle, drug therapy of cancer, 143t
Cell membrane disruptors, 128
Cell wall inhibitor group, 121
Cellulitis, pharmacologic treatment of, 151
Central nervous system, drugs affecting, 93–120
  Alzheimer disease, 105–108
  anesthetics, 96–100, 96f, 98f
  antiepileptics, 100–104, 103f
  for migraines and cluster headaches, 104–105
  opioids, 108–109, 111f
  for Parkinson disease, 105, 107f
  psychopharmacology, 109–118
  sedative hypnotics, 93–96, 95f
Cephalosporins, 126
  second-generation, 126
  third-generation, 126
Cerebral vasodilation, with increased intracranial
    pressure, 100
Cetirizine (Zerviate), for allergic
    conjunctivitis, 147
Cevimeline, 11
Chemotherapy drug, 142
Chemotherapy-induced nausea and vomiting
    (CINV), 142
Chloramphenicol, 127
Chloride secretion activators, for constipation,
    90–91t
Chloroprocaine, 97
Chlorthalidone, for hypertension, 20–22t
Cholinergic agonists, for glaucoma, 146
Cholinergic fibers, 11
Cholinesterase inhibitors, for Alzheimer disease, 105
Chronic pulmonary disorder (COPD),
    pharmacotherapy for, 48f, 49–50
Ciclesonide (Alvesco), 45
Cidofovir, nephrotoxicity, 129
Cilostazol, 36
Cinchonism, 140
Class I antiarrhythmic drugs, 30
Class II antiarrhythmic drugs, 30
Class III antiarrhythmic drugs, 30
Class IV antiarrhythmic drugs, 31
Clearance (CL), 7–8
Clindamycin, 127
  for acne vulgaris, 154
Clinical pharmacology, 1, 2f
Clobetasol propionate, 155t

Clonidine, 13
    for hypertension, 20–22t
Clopidogrel, 37
    for acute coronary syndrome, 25–30
Clotrimazole troches, for thrush, 151
Clozapine, 115
Cluster headaches, drugs for, 104–105
Coal tar shampoo, for psoriasis, 155
Cobicistat, 136–137
Cockcroft-Gault formula, 165
Colchicine, low-dose, for gout, 53
Combined estrogen-progestin oral contraceptives
    (COCs), 65
Combined hormonal contraceptives (CHC), 65
Competitive antagonists, 4
Conjunctivitis, 146–147
Constipation, drugs for, 81, 88f, 90–91t
Corticosteroids, 74
Cough and cold medications, for pediatric patients,
    162–163
COVID-19 virus, 136
COX-2 selective inhibitors, 52
"Coxibs," 52
Crisaborole, for atopic dermatitis, 155
Crohn disease, 81–87
Cromolyn sodium (Opticrom), for allergic
    conjunctivitis, 147
Cushing syndrome, corticosteroids and, 74
Cutaneous candidiasis, pharmacologic treatment
    of, 151
Cyclooxygenase (COX) nonselective nonsteroidal
    antiinflammatory drugs, adverse drug events
    of, 165
Cyclophosphamide, 58
Cyclosporine, 53
    for psoriasis, 155–157
Cytomegalovirus (CMV), 129

D
Dabigatran, 42
Dalfopristin, 127–128
Dantrolene, antidote for MH, 100
Dapagliflozin, for heart failure, 23–24t
Daptomycin, for cell membrane disruptors, 128
Daridorexant, 93–96
Darunavir, 136–137
Dasatinib, 142–143
Deep tendon reflexes, loss, magnesium sulfate
    and, 160
Delirium stage, 97
Denosumab, for osteoporosis, 78
Dependence, 5
Dermatologic pharmacology, 150–158
    allergic contact dermatitis, 154–155
    cutaneous and mucosal candidiasis, 151
    pediculosis, 151–154
    psoriasis, 155–158, 156f
    scabies, 151–154
    skin infections, 150, 152f
    skin infestations, 150, 152f
Desonide, 155t
Dexamethasone, 86t
Dexrazoxane, 142
Dextroamphetamine-amphetamine, 118
Diabetes mellitus, drugs for, 74–75, 74t, 76f
Diaper dermatitis, pharmacologic treatment of, 151
Dicyclomine, 12
Dietary fiber, for constipation, 81

Diflorasone diacetate, 155t
Digoxin, 31
    for heart failure, 23–24t
Dihydroergotamine, for migraines, 104
Diltiazem, 31
    for angina, 17, 25t
    for hypertension, 20–22t
Dimenhydrinate, 86t
Dipeptidyl peptidase 4 (DPP-4) inhibitors, for
    diabetes mellitus, 75
Diphenoxylate, 81, 108
Dipyridamole, 36
Direct factor Xa inhibitors, 37–42
Direct thrombin inhibitors, 42
Direct-acting parasympathomimetic agents, 11
Disease-modifying antirheumatic agents, 58–59, 60f
Disopyramide, 30
DNA/nucleic acid synthesis inhibitors, 128
Dobutamine, 12
Docusate salts, for constipation, 90–91t
Dofetilide (po), 30
Dolasetron, 86t
Donepezil, 11
    for Alzheimer disease, 105
Dopamine D2 receptors blockers, 114–115
Doripenem, 126
Dorzolamide, for glaucoma, 146
Dose response curve, 4, 5f
Dose-dependent cardiovascular depression, 100
Dose-dependent respiratory depression, 97
Dose-limiting toxicity, of opioids, 108
Doxazosin, 13
    for hypertension, 20–22t
Dronabinol, 86t
Drug dosage, for pediatric patients, 162–163
Drug interactions, mechanisms of, 8
Dry eye disease (DED), 146
Dry-powder inhaler (DPI), 44
Dual orexin receptor antagonists (DORAs), 93–96
Dupilumab, 48
    for atopic dermatitis, 155
Dyslipidemia, treatment of, 31–36, 34f

E
Echinocandins, 137, 140
Eclampsia, pharmacotherapy for, 160
Edoxaban, 37–42
Edrophonium, 11
Eicosanoids, 51–52
Elective induction, definition of, 161
Eletriptan, for migraines, 104
Eluxadoline, for inflammatory bowel disease, 87
Emergency contraception (EC), 65, 70
Empagliflozin, for heart failure, 23–24t
Enalapril
    for heart failure, 23–24t
    for hypertension, 20–22t
Enalaprilat, 20–22t
Endocrine drugs, hormones and, 64–79
    for adrenal hormones, 74
    for androgens and male reproductive system,
        70–71, 72f
    for endocrine pancreas and diabetes mellitus,
        74–75, 74t, 76f
    for female hormones, 65–70, 68f
    for osteoporosis, 75–78
    thyroid and antithyroid medications, 64–65, 67f
Endocrine pancreas, 74–75, 76f

Enoxaparin, 37
Enteral route of administration, 6
Enzalutamide, 143
Epidermal growth factor receptors (EGFRs), 143
Epinastine (Elestat), for allergic conjunctivitis, 147
Epinephrine, 10, 97
Eplerenone
    for heart failure, 23–24t
    for hypertension, 20–22t
Eprosartan, for hypertension, 20–22t
Eptifibatide, 37
    for acute coronary syndrome, 25–30
Eptinezumab, for migraines, 104–105
Erectile dysfunction (ED), 71
Ergotamine, for migraines, 104
Ergots, for migraines, 104
Erlotinib, 143
Ertapenem, 126
Erysipelas, pharmacologic treatment of, 151
Erythromycin, topical, for acne vulgaris, 154
Eslicarbazepine, for focal seizures, 101
Estazolam, 93
Ethacrynic acid, for hypertension, 20–22t
Ethambutol, 128–129
Ethosuximide, narrow-spectrum AED, 101
Etomidate, 97
Evinacumab, 36
Excretion, 7–8
Exemestane, 143
Eye diseases, drug therapy for, 146–149
Ezetimibe, for dyslipidemia, 36

F
Facilitated diffusion, 6
Famciclovir, 129
Febuxostat, for gout, 53
Feces, 7
Felodipine, for angina, 25t
Female hormones, 65–70, 68f
Fentanyl, 108
Ferrous sulfate, for iron deficiency anemia, 62
Fibrates, 31–36
Fibrinolytic drugs, 42
    for acute coronary syndrome, 30
Fifth generation ceftaroline, 126
First-generation antidepressants, 114
First-order kinetics, 8
First-pass effect, 6
First-trimester medication abortion, 70
5-Aminosalicylates (5-ASA), for ulcerative colitis,
    81–87
Flecainide, 30
Fluconazole, for vulvovaginitis, 151
Fluid intake, for constipation, 81
Flu-like syndrome, 129
Fluorometholone, for allergic conjunctivitis, 147
Fluoroquinolones, 128
Flurazepam, 93
Fluticasone (ArmonAir, Arnuity, Flovent), 45
Fluticasone propionate, 155t
Folate inhibitors, 128
Folic acid
    deficiency, 62
    for psoriasis, 155–157
Folliculitis, pharmacologic treatment of, 151
Fondaparinux, 37
Formoterol, 12
Fosaprepitant, 86t

Foscarnet, 129
Fosinopril, 20–22t
Fosphenytoin, IV, 101
Fourth-generation cephalosporin cefepime, 126
Fremanezumab subcutaneous, for migraines, 104–105
Frovatriptan, for migraines, 104
Furosemide, for hypertension, 20–22t
Furuncles, pharmacologic treatment of, 151

G

Gabapentin, 101
Galantamine, 11
    for Alzheimer disease, 105
Galcanezumab, subcutaneous, for migraines, 104–105
Ganciclovir, 129
Ganglionic blockers, 11
Gap 0 phase (G$_0$), cell cycle, 143t
Gap 1 phase (G$_1$), cell cycle, 143t
Gap 2 phase (G$_2$), cell cycle, 143t
Gastroesophageal reflux disease (GERD), 80, 83f
Gastrointestinal pharmacology, 80–92
    antiemetic drugs, 81, 85f, 86t
    for constipation, 81, 88f, 90–91t
    for inflammatory bowel disease, 81–87
    for peptic ulcer disease, 80–81
GDM. see Gestational diabetes mellitus
General anesthetics, 97
Generalized absence seizures, 101
Genitourinary syndrome of menopause (GSM), 70
Geriatric pharmacology, 165–166
Gestational diabetes mellitus (GDM), pharmacotherapy for, 159–160
Gestational hypertension, pharmacotherapy for, 160
Glaucoma, 146
GLP-1 receptor agonists, for diabetes mellitus, 75
Glucocorticoids, for inflammatory bowel disease, 87
Glucocorticosteroids, 45, 74
α-Glucosidase inhibitors, for diabetes mellitus, 75
Glutamate, 100
Glycerin suppository, for constipation, 90–91t
Glycopeptide vancomycin, 126–127
Gout, treatment of, 52–53, 57f
Gradual tapering, 93
Granisetron, 86t
Griseofulvin, oral, for skin infections, 150
Guanabenz methyldopa, 13
Guanfacine, 13
Guselkumab, for psoriasis, 158

H

Half-life (T$_{1/2}$), 8
Heart failure, treatment of, 16–17, 23–24t, 26f
Helicobacter pylori, 80–81
Hematopoietic growth factors, anemia and, 62
Heparin, 37
Hepatic steatosis, 136
Hepatitis B, 129
Hepatitis C virus, 136
Hepatobiliary excretion, 7
Hepatotoxicity, 100
Histamine, 51
Histamine 2 receptor antagonists (H2RAs), 80
Histamine-receptor antagonists, 96
HMG coenzyme A reductase inhibitors (statins), 31
Hormonal therapies, 143

Hormones and endocrine drugs, 64–79
    for adrenal hormones, 74
    for androgens and male reproductive system, 70–71, 72f
    for endocrine pancreas and diabetes mellitus, 74–75, 74t, 76f
    for female hormones, 65–70, 68f
    for osteoporosis, 75–78
    thyroid and antithyroid medications, 64–65, 67f
Human leukocyte antigen-B*1502 allele, 100–101
Hydralazine/isosorbide dinitrate, for heart failure, 23–24t
Hydrochlorothiazide, for hypertension, 20–22t
Hydrocortisone valerate, 155t
Hydroxychloroquine (HCQ), for rheumatoid arthritis, 58–59
Hyperprolactinemia, 115
Hyperreactive response, 5
Hypersensitivity, 5
Hypertension, treatment of, 16, 18f, 20–22t
Hypertensive emergencies, 16
Hyperthyroidism, 64
Hyperuricemia, 52
Hyponatremia, 101
Hyporeactive response, 5
Hypothyroidism, 64

I

Ibalizumab, 137
Ibuprofen, for dyslipidemia, 36
Ibutilide, 30
Idarucizumab, 42
Idiosyncrasy, 5
IL inhibitors, 59
IL-17 blockers, 59
Imatinib, 142–143
Imipenem, 126
Immunomodulators
    for asthma, 48
    for inflammatory bowel disease, 87
Immunosuppressants, 53–58
Impetigo, pharmacologic treatment of, 151
Indacaterol, 12
Indapamide, for hypertension, 20–22t
Indirect-acting parasympathomimetic agents, 11
Indomethacin, for preterm labor, 160
Induction, 8
Induction of labor, definition of, 161
Infectious conjunctivitis, 147
Infectious disease, drug therapy for, 121–141
    antibacterial drugs, 121–129, 122f, 124f
    antiparasitic drugs, 140
    antivirals, 129–137, 130f, 132f, 134f
Inflammatory bowel disease, 81–87
    medication for, 87
Inhaled anesthetics, 97
Inhaled glucocorticosteroids (ICS), 45
Inhibition, 8
Insomnia, treatment of, 93–96
Insulin degludec, 74t
Insulin glargine, 74t
Insulin therapy, for gestational diabetes mellitus, 160
Insulins, 74–75, 74t
Integrase strand transfer inhibitors (INSTIs), 137
Interleukin (IL)-17 pathway, inhibitors of, for psoriasis, 158
Intermediate-acting neutral protamine hagedorn (NPH), 74t

International normalized ratio, 37
Intertrigo, pharmacologic treatment of, 151
Intraarticular glucocorticosteroid, for gout, 52–53
Intramuscular penicillin, 126
Inverse agonists, 4
Ipratropium, 12, 45
Irbesartan, for hypertension, 20–22t
Iron deficiency anemia, 62
Isoproterenol, 12
Isosorbide mononitrate, for angina, 17, 25t
Isotretinoin, oral, for acne vulgaris, 154
Isradipine, for hypertension, 20–22t
Itraconazole, oral, for onychomycosis, 150
IV iron, for anemia, 62
Ivabradine, 31
    for heart failure, 23–24t
Ivermectin, 140
    oral, for scabies, 151–154
Ixekizumab, 59

K

Ketamine, 97
Ketotifen fumarate (Ketotifen), for allergic conjunctivitis, 147
Kidney, 7
Kinase inhibitors, 59

L

Labetalol, 12
    for hypertension, 16, 20–22t
Lacosamide, 104
Lactation, pharmacologic considerations during, 159
Lactic acidosis, 127, 136
Lactulose, for constipation, 90–91t
Lamotrigine, 101
Lasmiditan, for migraines, 104
Lefamulin, 128
Leflunomide (LEF), for rheumatoid arthritis, 58–59
Lemborexant, 93–96
Letrozole, 143
Leucovorin, 142
Leukocytes, decrease of, sirolimus and, 53–58
Leukotriene receptor antagonists, for asthma, 45
Levamulin, 127
Levetiracetam, 101
Levobunolol, for glaucoma, 146
Levodopa, for Parkinson disease, 105, 107f
Lidocaine, 97
Linaclotide, for constipation, 90–91t
Linezolid, 127
Lisinopril
    for heart failure, 23–24t
    for hypertension, 20–22t
Lithium
    for bipolar disorder, 115
    narrow therapeutic index, 115
    renal effects of, 115
Liver, 7
Loading dose, 8
Local anesthetic drugs, 96
Lodoxamide tromethamine (Alomide), for allergic conjunctivitis, 147
Lomitapide, for dyslipidemia, 36
Long-acting analog, 74t
Long-acting beta-adrenergic agonists inhaled (LABAs), 45
Long-acting nitrates, for angina, 25t

Loop diuretics
for heart failure, 16–17, 23–24t
for hypertension, 20–22t
Loperamide, 81, 108
Losartan
for heart failure, 23–24t
for hypertension, 20–22t
Loteprednol, for allergic conjunctivitis, 147
Low-dose colchicine, for gout, 53
Low-molecular-weight heparin (LMWH)
for acute coronary syndrome, 30
as anticoagulant, 37
Lubiprostone, for constipation, 90–91t
Lumigan (bimatoprost), 146
Luteinizing hormone-releasing agonists, 143

M

Macrolides, 127
Magnesium salts, for constipation, 90–91t
Magnesium sulfate
for constipation, 90–91t
for preeclampsia, 160
Magnesium toxicity, pharmacotherapy for, 160
Maintenance doses, 8
Male reproductive system, 70–71, 72f
Malignant hyperthermia (MH), 100
Mast cell stabilizers, for allergic conjunctivitis, 147
Meclizine, 86t
Medical pharmacology, introduction to, 1, 2f
Medrysone (HMS), for allergic conjunctivitis, 147
Medullary depression, 97
Meglitinides, for diabetes mellitus, 75
Melatonin-receptor agonists, 96
Memantine, for Alzheimer disease, 108
Menopausal hormone therapy (MHT), 70
Menopause, 70
Mepivacaine, 97
Mepolizumab, 48
Mercaptopurine, 58
Meropenem, 126
Mesalamine, for ulcerative colitis, 81–87
Mesna, 142
Metabolism, 7
Metformin
for diabetes mellitus, 75
for gestational diabetes mellitus, 160
Methimazole, for hyperthyroidism, 64
Methohexital, 97
Methotrexate, 142
for psoriasis, 155–157
for rheumatoid arthritis, 58
Methylcellulose, for constipation, 90–91t
Metipranolol, for glaucoma, 146
Metoclopramide, 86t
Metoprolol, 12
for angina, 25t
for hypertension, 20–22t
Metoprolol succinate, 23–24t
Micafungin, 140
Miconazole mucoadhesive buccal tablets, for thrush, 151
Mifepristone, for abortion, 70
Migraines, drugs for, 104–105
Mild to moderate agonists, 108
Mineralocorticoid receptor antagonists (MRA), for heart failure, 23–24t
Mirtazapine, 114

Misoprostol
for abortion, 70
for induction of labor, 161
Mitosis (M), cell cycle, 143t
Mixed receptor actions, 108
Moexipril, 20–22t
Monoamine oxidase inhibitors, for psychiatric disorders, 114
Monoamine oxidase type B (MAO B) inhibitors, for Parkinson disease, 105
Monosodium urate crystal deposition disease, 52
Montelukast (Singulair), oral, for pediatric patients, 162–163
Morphine, 108
Mucosal candidiasis, pharmacologic treatment of, 151
Multidrug-resistant gram-negative infections, 126
Mupirocin, topical, for pediatric patients, 162–163
Muscarinic agonists, 11
Muscarinic receptor antagonists, 45
Mycophenolate mofetil (MMF), 58
Myocarditis, 115

N

Naloxone, 109
Naltrexone, 109
Naratriptan, for migraines, 104
Natural penicillins, 126
Nebivolol, for hypertension, 20–22t
Nebulizers, 44
Nedocromil, for allergic conjunctivitis, 147
Nefazodone, 114
Negative chronotropic effect, 10
Neostigmine, 11
Nephrotoxicity, tacrolimus and, 53
Netarsudil, for glaucoma, 146
Netupitant, 86t
Neuroleptic malignant syndrome (NMS), 115
Neuromuscular blockers, 100
Neurotoxicity, 97
Nicardipine, for hypertension, 16, 20–22t
Nicotinic acid derivatives (niacin), 36
Nicotinic (N) type receptors, 11
Nifedipine
for hypertension, 20–22t
for preterm labor, 160
Nilotinib, 142–143
Nisoldipine, for hypertension, 20–22t
Nitrate tolerance, 17
Nitrates, for angina, 17
Nitroglycerin
for acute coronary syndrome, 25
for angina, 17, 25t
for hypertension, 16
Non-benzodiazepine receptor agonists, 93
Non-beta-lactam cell wall inhibitors, 126–127
Noncompetitive antagonists, 4
Non-ergot dopamine agonists, for Parkinson disease, 105
Nonnucleoside reverse transcriptase inhibitors (NNRTIs), 136
Non-oral hormonal contraceptives, 65
Nonsteroidal antiinflammatory drugs (NSAIDs), 52, 55f
Nonstructural proteins 3/4A (NS3/4A) protease inhibitors (PIs), 136
Norepinephrine (NE), 10
NS5A inhibitors, 136

NS5B nonnucleoside polymerase inhibitors (NNPIs), 136
NS5B nucleoside polymerase inhibitors (NPIs), 136
Nystatin
swish and swallow, for thrush, 151
topical, for pediatric patients, 162–163

O

Ocular therapeutics, pharmacology of, 146–147, 148f
Olmesartan, for hypertension, 20–22t
Olsalazine, for ulcerative colitis, 81–87
Omalizumab, 48
Ondansetron, 86t
Onychomycosis, pharmacologic treatment of, 150
Open-angle glaucoma include alpha-2 adrenergic agonists, 146
Opioid addiction, 109
Opioid use disorder (OUD), 109
Opioids, 108–109, 111f
Oral naloxegol, for constipation, 81
Oropharyngeal candidiasis, pharmacologic treatment of, 151
Oseltamivir, 129
Osmotic laxatives, for constipation, 81, 90–91t
Ospemifene, 70
Osteoporosis, 75–78
Oxazolidinones, 127
Oxcarbazepine, for focal seizures, 101
Oxybutynin, 12
Oxytocin, synthetic, for induction of labor, 161

P

P2Y12 receptor blockers, for acute coronary syndrome, 25–30
Palonosetron, 86t
Parasympatholytic drugs, 11–12
Parasympathomimetic drugs, 11–12
Parathyroid hormone-related protein (PTHrP) analogs, for osteoporosis, 78
Parenteral penicillin, 126
Parenteral route of administration, 6–7
Parkinson disease, drugs for, 105, 107f
Partial agonist, 4
Pazopanib, 143
PCSK9 inhibitors, 36
Pediatric pharmacology, 162–164, 163f
Pediculosis, pharmacologic treatment of, 151–154
Pegloticase, for gout, 53
Pemirolast (Alamast), for allergic conjunctivitis, 147
Penicillin G, 126
Penicillin V, 126
Peptic ulcer disease, treatment of, 80–81
Peptidoglycan, 126
Perampanel, 101
Peripheral neuropathy, 128–129
Peripherally acting opioid antagonists (PAMORA), 109
Permethrin 5% cream, for scabies, 151–154
Pharmacodynamics, 1, 4–5
Pharmacogenetics, 1
Pharmacogenomics, 1
Pharmacokinetics, 1, 5–6
Pharmacology
defined, 1
dermatologic, 150–158
allergic contact dermatitis, 154–155
cutaneous and mucosal candidiasis, 151
pediculosis, 151–154

Pharmacology (*Continued*)
 psoriasis, 155–158, 156f
 scabies, 151–154
 skin infections, 150, 152f
 geriatric, 165–166
 of ocular therapeutics, 146–147, 148f
 pediatric, 162–164, 163f
 of select conditions during pregnancy, 159–161
  considerations for, 159
  induction of labor, 161
Pharmacotherapeutics, 1
Pharmacotherapy, for pregnancy-associated conditions, 159–161
Phase I metabolic reactions, 7
Phase II metabolic reactions, 7
Phenelzine, for psychiatric disorders, 114
Phenoxybenzamine, 13
Phentolamine, 13
Phenylephrine, 12
Phenytoin, 101
Phosphodiesterase type 5 (PDE5) inhibitors, for erectile dysfunction, 71
Physostigmine, 11
Pilocarpine, 11
 for glaucoma, 146
Pimecrolimus cream, for atopic dermatitis, 155
Pinocytosis, 6
Pioglitazone, for diabetes mellitus, 75
Piperacillin, 126
Pivoxil, 126
Placebo, 5
Placental barrier, 7
Platelets, decrease of, sirolimus and, 53–58
Plecanatide, for constipation, 90–91t
Pleuromutilins, 127, 128
Polyenes, 137
Polyenes nystatin, 137
Polyethylene glycol (PEG)-electrolyte solutions, for constipation, 90–91t
Polypharmacy, in older adults, 165
Positive chronotropic effect, 11
Postattachment inhibitor, 137
Potassium blocking, 30–31
Potassium sparing diuretics, for hypertension, 20–22t
Potency, 4
Potentiation, 8
Pralidoxime, 11
Prasugrel, 37
 for acute coronary syndrome, 25–30
Praziquantel, 140
Prazosin, 13
Prazosin, for hypertension, 20–22t
Prednisolone
 for allergic conjunctivitis, 147
 for pediatric patients, 162–163
Prednisone, oral, for pediatric patients, 162–163
Preeclampsia, pharmacotherapy for, 160
Pregabalin, 101
Preganglionic fibers, 11
Pregnancy, select conditions during, pharmacology of, 159–161
 considerations for, 159
 induction of labor, 161
Pressurized metered-dose inhaler (pMDI), 44
Preterm labor, pharmacotherapy for, 160
Procainamide, 30
Procaine, 97

Prochlorperazine, 86t
Progestin-only contraceptive, 65
Promethazine, 86t
Propafenone, 30
Prophylaxis, 121
Propofol, 97
Propranolol, for hypertension, 20–22t
Prostaglandin analogs, for glaucoma, 146
Protamine sulfate, 37
Protein synthesis inhibitors, 121
Proton-pump inhibitors (PPIs), 80
Prucalopride, for constipation, 90–91t
Psoralen plus ultraviolet A (PUVA), for psoriasis, 155–157
Psoriasis, pharmacologic treatment of, 155–158, 156f
Psychopharmacology, 109–118
 antidepressants, 109–114, 113f
 antipsychotic medications, 114–115, 117f
 anxiolytics, 115
 attention-deficit hyperactivity disorder, 115–118
 medications for bipolar disorder, 115
Psyllium, for constipation, 90–91t
Pulmonary pharmacology, 44–50
 for asthma, 44
 for COPD, 48f, 49–50
Pure antagonists, 108
PUVA. *see* Psoralen plus ultraviolet A
Pyrantel, 140
Pyrazinamide, 128–129
Pyridostigmine, 11

Q

QT prolongation, 115
Quazepam, 93
Quinapril, for hypertension, 20–22t
Quinidine, 30, 140
Quinine, 140
Quinupristin, 127–128

R

Radioiodine, for hyperthyroidism, 64–65
Ramipril
 for heart failure, 23–24t
 for hypertension, 20–22t
Ranolazine, for angina, 17, 25t
Rapid-acting insulin analog, 74t
Rapid-acting insulin glulisine, 74t
Receptors, 4
Rectal (PR) route of administration, 6
Relative infant dose, 159
Remdesivir, 136
Renal insufficiency, 129
Renin-angiotensin system inhibitors (ARNI), for heart failure, 23–24t
Reslizumab, 48
Reteplase, 42
Retinoids, topical, for acne vulgaris, 154
Rheumatoid arthritis (RA), drugs for, 58, 60f
Rifampin, 128–129
Rifaximin, for inflammatory bowel disease, 87
Rimegepant, for migraines, 104–105
Rimexolone (Vexol), for allergic conjunctivitis, 147
Risankizumab, for psoriasis, 158
Rivaroxaban, 37–42
Rivastigmine, 11
 for Alzheimer disease, 105
Rizatriptan, for migraines, 104

Rolapitant, 86t
Romosozumab, for osteoporosis, 78
Ropivacaine, 97
Route of administration, 6–7
Rufinamide, 104

S

Salmeterol, 12
Scabies, pharmacologic treatment of, 151–154
Scopolamine, 12
 transdermal, 86t
Screening tool of older people's prescriptions (STOPP), in geriatric pharmacology, 166
Screening tool to alert to right treatment (START), in geriatric pharmacology, 166
Second-generation antidepressants, 109
Secukinumab, 59
Sedative hypnotics, 93–96, 95f
Seizures disorders, 114
Selective serotonin reuptake inhibitors (SSRIs), 109
Selenium sulfide, shampoo, for tinea versicolor, 150
Semisynthetic penicillins, 126
Serotonin 5-hydroxytryptamine, for constipation, 90–91t
Serotonin syndrome, 114, 127
Serotonin-norepinephrine reuptake inhibitors (SNRI), 109, 118
Sevoflurane, 100
Short-acting beta-adrenergic agonists inhaled (SABAs), 45
Short-acting nitrates, for angina, 25t
Short-acting regular human insulin, 74t
Significant cognitive impairment, 101
Silodosin, 13
Singulair. *see* Montelukast
Sirolimus (Rapamycin), 53–58
Skin abscesses, pharmacologic treatment of, 151
Skin infections, pharmacologic treatment of, 150, 152f
Skin infestations, pharmacologic treatment of, 150, 152f
Sodium channel modulators, 100
Sodium nitroprusside, for hypertension, 16
Sodium-glucose cotransporter 2 (SGLT2) inhibitors, for heart failure, 23–24t
Soft tissue infections, bacterial, pharmacologic treatment of, 151
Soft-mist inhaler (SMI), 44
Solute carriers (SLC), 6
Sorafenib, 143
Sorbitol, for constipation, 90–91t
Sotalol, 30
Sotrovimab, 136
Spinosad 0.9% topical suspension, for scabies, 151–154
Spironolactone
 for acne vulgaris, 154
 for heart failure, 23–24t
 for hypertension, 20–22t
START. *see* Screening tool to alert to right treatment
Steady state, 8
Steroidal compounds, 100
Stimulant laxatives, for constipation, 90–91t
Stiripentol, 104
Stool softeners, for constipation, 90–91t
STOPP. *see* Screening tool of older people's prescriptions
Streptogramins, 127–128

Strong agonists, 108
Subcutaneous methylnaltrexone, for constipation, 81
Subcutaneous sumatriptan, 105
Sublingual (SL) route of administration, 6
Sulfasalazine
   for inflammatory bowel disease, 81–87
   for rheumatoid arthritis, 58–59
   for ulcerative colitis, 81–87
Sulfonamides, 128
Sulfonylureas, for diabetes mellitus, 75
Sumatriptan, 104
   intranasal, 105
Sunitinib, 143
Supratherapeutic doses, 4
Surgical anesthesia, 97
Suvorexant, 93–96
Sympathetic nervous system, 10
Sympathomimetics, 12–13, 14f
Synergism, 8
Synthesis phase (S), cell cycle, 143t
Synthetic fibers polycarbophil, for constipation, 90–91t
Synthetic oxytocin, for induction of labor, 161
Systemic steroids, for asthma, 45

T

Tachyphylaxis, 5
Tacrolimus, 53
   for atopic dermatitis, 155
Tamsulosin, 13
Tardive dyskinesia (TD), 114–115
Tasimelteon, 96
Tazarotene, for psoriasis, 155
Tedizolid, 127
Telmisartan, for hypertension, 20–22t
Temazepam, 93
Tendinopathies, peripheral neuropathy, 128
Tenecteplase, 42
Teratogen, 1
   pregnancy and, 159
Teratology, 1
Terazosin, 13
   for hypertension, 20–22t
Terbinafine, oral, for onychomycosis, 150
Terbutaline, for preterm labor, 160
Teriparatide, 78
Testosterone replacement therapy (TRT), 71
Tetracaine, 97
Tetracyclines, for acne vulgaris, 154
Tetraiodothyronine (T4), 64
Theophylline, 45
Therapeutic index (T.I.), 4–5
Thiazide type diuretics, for hypertension, 16, 20–22t
Thiazolidinediones (TZD), for diabetes mellitus, 75
Thionamides, for hyperthyroidism, 64

Thrombocytopenia, 127
Thrush, pharmacologic treatment of, 151
Thyroid dysfunction, 115
Thyroid medications, 64–65, 67f
Tiagabine, 104
Ticagrelor, 37
   for acute coronary syndrome, 25–30
Ticarcillin, 126
Ticlopidine, 37
Tildrakizumab, for psoriasis, 158
Timolol, for glaucoma, 146
Tinea barbae, pharmacologic treatment of, 150
Tinea capitis, pharmacologic treatment of, 150
Tinea corporis, 150
Tinea cruris, 150
Tinea faciei, 150
Tinea manuum, 150
Tinea pedis, 150
Tinea unguium, pharmacologic treatment of, 150
Tinea versicolor, pharmacologic treatment of, 150
Tinzaparin, 37
Tiotropium, 12
Tirofiban, 37
   for acute coronary syndrome, 25–30
TNF-alpha inhibitors, for psoriasis, 157–158
Tocolytic drugs, for preterm labor, 160
Tofacitinib, 59
Tolerance, 5
Topical carbonic anhydrase inhibitors, for glaucoma, 146
Topical corticosteroid, for atopic dermatitis, 155, 155t
Topical glucocorticoids, for allergic conjunctivitis, 147
Topical ocular medications, for glaucoma, 146
Topical ophthalmic steroids, 147
Topical pediculicides, for pediculosis, 154
Topiramate, broad-spectrum AED, 101
Torsemide, for hypertension, 20–22t
Toxicology, 1
Trandolapril, 20–22t
Tranylcypromine, for psychiatric disorders, 114
Travatan Z (travoprost), 146
Trazodone, 114
Triamcinolone acetonide, 155t
Tricyclic antidepressants (TCAs), 114
Triiodothyronine (T3), 64
Triptans, for migraines, 104
Tumor necrosis factor (TNF) inhibitors, 59
Type I hypersensitivity reactions, 5
Type II hypersensitivity reactions, 5
Type III hypersensitivity reactions, 5
Type IV hypersensitivity reactions, 5
Tyramine, 114
Tyrosine kinase inhibitors (TKIs), 142–143

U

Ulcerative colitis, 81–87
Ultra-long-acting analog, 74t
Unclassified siderophore, 126
Unfractionated heparin (UFH), 37
   for acute coronary syndrome, 30
Uricosuric agents, for gout, 53
US Food and Drug Administration drug development, 4
Ustekinumab, for psoriasis, 158

V

Vaborbactam, 126
Vaginal estrogens, 70
Valaciclovir, 129
Valganciclovir, 129
Valproate, 100
   for bipolar disorder, 115
   broad-spectrum AED, 101
Valproic acid, 100
Valsartan
   for heart failure, 23–24t
   for hypertension, 20–22t
Valved holding chambers (VHCs), 44
Vascular endothelial growth factor (VEGF), 143
Vasoconstrictor, for allergic conjunctivitis, 147
Verapamil, 31, 105
   for angina, 17, 25t
   for hypertension, 20–22t
Vilazodone, 114
Vitamin B12 deficiency, megaloblastic anemia and, 62
Vitamin D analogs, topical, for psoriasis, 155
Vitamin E, for Alzheimer disease, 108
Vitamin K, 37
Vitamin K antagonist (VKA), 37
Volume of distribution (Vd), 7
Vorapaxar, 37
Vortioxetine, 114
Vulvovaginitis, pharmacologic treatment of, 151

W

Warfarin, 37
West nomogram, for body surface area, 163f

X

Xalatan (latanoprost), 146

Z

Zero-order kinetics, 8
Zinc pyrithione, shampoo, for tinea versicolor, 150
Zioptan (tafluprost), 146
Zolmitriptan, 104, 105
Zonisamide, 101